Pharmacology

Pharmacology

Edited by
Phoenix McWilliams

Larsen & Keller
www.larsen-keller.com

Pharmacology
Edited by Phoenix McWilliams
ISBN: 978-1-63549-217-0 (Hardback)

© 2017 Larsen & Keller

⊟ Larsen & Keller

Published by Larsen and Keller Education,
5 Penn Plaza,
19th Floor,
New York, NY 10001, USA

Cataloging-in-Publication Data

Pharmacology / edited by Phoenix McWilliams.
    p. cm.
Includes bibliographical references and index.
ISBN 978-1-63549-217-0
1. Pharmacology. 2. Drugs. I. McWilliams, Phoenix.
RM300 .P43 2017
615.1--dc23

The publisher's policy is to use permanent paper from mills that operate a sustainable forestry policy. Furthermore, the publisher ensures that the text paper and cover boards used have met acceptable environmental accreditation standards.

Printed and bound in the United States of America.

For more information regarding Larsen and Keller Education and its products, please visit the publisher's website www.larsen-keller.com

Table of Contents

Preface

Pharmacology as a field of medicinal sciences and biology is concerned with the production, analysis, synthesis, design, and composition of drugs. Pharmacology is divided into two categories namely, pharmacokinetics and pharmacodynamics. This book is a compilation of chapters that discuss the most vital concepts of this field. It unfolds the innovative aspects of this subject, which will be crucial for the holistic understanding of the field. It will prove to be immensely beneficial to students involved in this area at various levels. For someone with an interest and eye for detail, this textbook covers the most significant topics in of pharmacology.

To facilitate a deeper understanding of the contents of this book a short introduction of every chapter is written below:

Chapter 1- Pharmacology is a branch of medicine that concerns itself with the study of medicinal drugs. Drugs in this subject are defined into certain categories such as man-made, natural or endogenous. The main areas of this subject are pharmacodynamics and pharmacokinetics. This chapter will provide an integrated understanding of pharmacology

Chapter 2- Clinical pharmacology is the study of medicinal drugs; it helps in connecting the gap between medical practice and laboratory science. Clinical pharmacology helps in the promotion of the safety of prescription and to minimize its side-effects. The other branches of pharmacology are neuropharmacology, psychopharmacology, pharmacogenetics, pharmacogenomics, pharmacoepidemiology and toxicology. This section is a compilation of the various branches of pharmacology that form an integral part of the broader subject matter.

Chapter 3- Drug design is the process of finding new medicines. It involves the design of molecules that are complementary in shape and charge. The features elucidated in the chapter are drug discovery, new chemical entity, high-throughput screening, drug development, pre-clinical development, clinical trial etc. This chapter provides a plethora of interdisciplinary topics for a better comprehension on the topic of drugs.

Chapter 4- Pharmaceutical drugs are used to diagnose and cure diseases. Some of the different types of drug classes are antiplatelet drugs, anticoagulants, prescription drugs, anti-diabetic medications and generic drugs. Pharmaceutical drugs are best understood in confluence with the major topics listed in the following section.

Chapter 5- Pharmacokinetics is a branch of pharmacology; it is the study of how an organism is affected by drugs. It includes the effects of dosage and the adverse reactions to drugs. The aspects explained in the section are clearance, biological half-life, bioavailability, adverse drug reaction, ADME, drug metabolism and others. The chapter serves as a source to understand the major categories related to pharmacokinetics and pharmacodynamics.

Chapter 6- Enzyme inhibitor is a molecule that helps in binding enzymes. They are also used in decreasing the activities of enzymes; decreasing the activities of enzymes helps in correcting metabolic imbalances and is also used in pesticides. The features elucidated are dissociation constant, homeostasis, cytochrome P450, alcohol dehydrogenase and epoxide hydrolase. This section is an overview on enzyme inhibitors.

I owe the completion of this book to the never-ending support of my family, who supported me throughout the project.

Editor

Introduction to Pharmacology

Pharmacology is a branch of medicine that concerns itself with the study of medicinal drugs. Drugs in this subject are defined into certain categories such as man-made, natural or endogenous. The main areas of this subject are pharmacodynamics and pharmacokinetics. This chapter will provide an integrated understanding of pharmacology.

Pharmacology

Pharmacology is the branch of medicine and biology concerned with the study of drug action, where a drug can be broadly defined as any man-made, natural, or endogenous (from within body) molecule which exerts a biochemical and/or physiological effect on the cell, tissue, organ, or organism (sometimes the word pharmacon is used as a term to encompass these endogenous and exogenous bioactive species). More specifically, it is the study of the interactions that occur between a living organism and chemicals that affect normal or abnormal biochemical function. If substances have medicinal properties, they are considered pharmaceuticals.

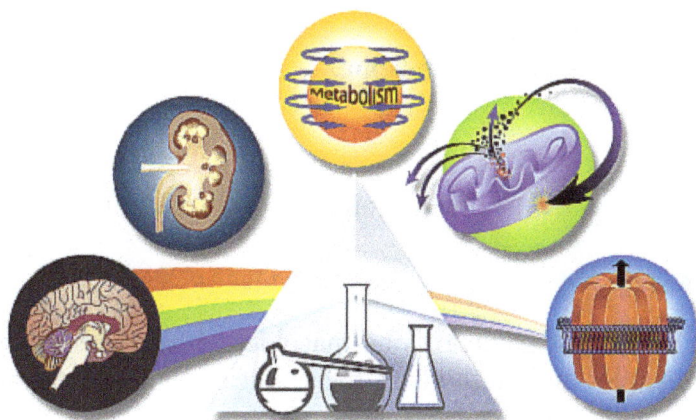

A variety of topics involved with pharmacology, including neuropharmacology, renal pharmacology, human metabolism, intracellular metabolism, and intracellular regulation

The field encompasses drug composition and properties, synthesis and drug design, molecular and cellular mechanisms, organ/systems mechanisms, signal transduction/cellular communication, molecular diagnostics, interactions, toxicology, chemical biology, therapy, and medical applications and antipathogenic capabilities. The two main areas of pharmacology are pharmacodynamics and pharmacokinetics. The former studies the effects of the drug on biological systems, and the latter the effects of biological systems on the drug. In broad terms, pharmacodynamics discusses the chemicals with biological receptors, and pharmacokinetics discusses the absorption, distribution, metabolism, and excretion (ADME) of chemicals from the biological systems. Pharmacology is not synonymous with pharmacy and the two terms are frequently confused. Pharmacology, a biomedical science, deals with the research, discovery, and characterization of chemicals which show biological effects and the elucidation of cellular and organismal function in relation to these chemicals. In contrast, pharmacy, a health services profession, is concerned with application of the principles learned from pharmacology in its clinical settings; whether it be in a dispensing or clinical care role. In either field, the primary contrast between the two are their distinctions between direct-patient care, for pharmacy practice, and the science-oriented research field, driven by pharmacology.

The origins of clinical pharmacology date back to the Middle Ages in Avicenna's *The Canon of Medicine*, Peter of Spain's *Commentary on Isaac*, and John of St Amand's *Commentary on the Antedotary of Nicholas*. Clinical pharmacology owes much of its foundation to the work of William Withering. Pharmacology as a scientific discipline did not further advance until the mid-19th century amid the great biomedical resurgence of that period. Before the second half of the nineteenth century, the remarkable potency and specificity of the actions of drugs such as morphine, quinine and digitalis were explained vaguely and with reference to extraordinary chemical powers and affinities to certain organs or tissues. The first pharmacology department was set up by Rudolf Buchheim in 1847, in recognition of the need to understand how therapeutic drugs and poisons produced their effects.

Early pharmacologists focused on natural substances, mainly plant extracts. Pharmacology developed in the 19th century as a biomedical science that applied the principles of scientific experimentation to therapeutic contexts. Today pharmacologists use genetics, molecular biology, chemistry, and other advanced tools to transform information about molecular mechanisms and targets into therapies directed against disease, defects or pathogens, and create methods for preventative care, diagnostics, and ultimately personalized medicine.

Divisions

The discipline of pharmacology can be divided into many sub disciplines each with a specific focus.

Clinical Pharmacology

Clinical pharmacology is the basic science of pharmacology with an added focus on the application of pharmacological principles and methods in the medical clinic and towards patient care and outcomes.

Neuropharmacology

Neuropharmacology is the study of the effects of medication on central and peripheral nervous system functioning.

Psychopharmacology

Psychopharmacology, also known as behavioral pharmacology, is the study of the effects of medication on the psyche (psychology), observing changed behaviors of the body and mind, and how molecular events are manifest in a measurable behavioral form. This is similar to the closely related ethnopharmacology. Psychopharmacology is an interdisciplinary field which studies behavioral effects of psychoactive drugs. It incorporates approaches and techniques from neuro-pharmacology, animal behavior and behavioral neuroscience, and is interested in the behavioral and neurobiological mechanisms of action of psychoactive drugs. Another goal of behavioral pharmacology is to develop animal behavioral models to screen chemical compounds with therapeutic potentials. People in this field (called behavioral pharmacologists) typically use small animals (e.g. rodents) to study psychotherapeutic drugs such as antipsychotics, antide-pressants and anxiolytics, and drugs of abuse such as nicotine, cocaine, methamphetamine, etc. study of drugs which affect behavior. *Ethopharmacology* is a term which has been in use since the 1960s and derives from the Greek word *"ethos"* meaning character and "pharmacology" the study of drug actions and mechanism.

Cardiovascular Pharmacology

Cardiovascular pharmacology is the study of the effects of drugs on the entire cardiovascular sys-tem, including the heart and blood vessels.

Pharmacogenetics

Pharmacogenetics is clinical testing of genetic variation that gives rise to differing response to drugs.

Pharmacogenomics

Pharmacogenomics is the application of genomic technologies to drug discovery and further char-acterization of older drugs.

Pharmacoepidemiology

Pharmacoepidemiology is the study of the effects of drugs in large numbers of people.

Systems pharmacology

Systems pharmacology is the application of systems biology principles to the field of pharmacol-ogy.

Toxicology

Toxicology is the study of the adverse effects, molecular targets, and characterization of drugs or any chemical substance in excess (including those beneficial in lower doses).

Theoretical Pharmacology

Theoretical pharmacology is a relatively new and rapidly expanding field of research activity in which many of the techniques of computational chemistry, in particular computational quantum chemistry and the method of molecular mechanics, are proving to be of great value. Theoreti-cal pharmacologists aim at rationalizing the relation between the activity of a particular drug, as observed experimentally, and its structural features as derived from computer experiments. They aim to find structure—activity relations. Furthermore, on the basis of the structure of a given organic molecule, the theoretical pharmacologist aims at predicting the biological activity of new drugs that are of the same general type as existing drugs. More ambitiously, it aims to predict entirely new classes of drugs, tailor-made for specific purposes.

Posology

Posology is the study of how medicines are dosed. It also depends upon various factors including age, climate, weight, sex, and time of administration. It is derived from the Greek words posos meaning how much and logos meaning science.

Pharmacognosy

Pharmacognosy is a branch of pharmacology dealing especially with the composition, use, and development of medicinal substances of biological origin and especially medicinal substances obtained from plants.

Environmental Pharmacology

Environmental pharmacology is a new discipline. Focus is being given to understand gene–environment interaction, drug-environment interaction and toxin-environment interaction. There is a close collaboration between environmental science and medicine in addressing these issues, as healthcare itself can be a cause of environmental damage or remediation. Human health and ecology are intimately related. Demand for more pharmaceutical products may place the public at risk through the destruction of species. The entry of chemicals and drugs into the aquatic ecosystem is a more serious concern today. In addition, the production of some illegal drugs pollutes drinking water supply by releasing carcinogens. This field is intimately linked with Public Health fields.

Dental Pharmacology

Dental pharmacology relates to the study of drugs commonly used in the treatment of dental disease.

Scientific Background

The study of chemicals requires intimate knowledge of the biological system affected. With the knowledge of cell biology and biochemistry increasing, the field of pharmacology has also changed substantially. It has become possible, through molecular analysis of receptors, to design chemicals that act on specific cellular signaling or metabolic pathways by affecting sites directly on cell-surface receptors (which modulate and mediate cellular signaling pathways controlling cellular function).

A chemical has, from the pharmacological point-of-view, various properties. Pharmacokinetics describes the effect of the body on the chemical (e.g. half-life and volume of distribution), and pharmacodynamics describes the chemical's effect on the body (desired or toxic).

When describing the pharmacokinetic properties of the chemical that is the active ingredient or active pharmaceutical ingredient (API), pharmacologists are often interested in *L-ADME*:

- Liberation – How is the API disintegrated (for solid oral forms (breaking down into smaller particles)), dispersed, or dissolved from the medication?

- Absorption – How is the API absorbed (through the skin, the intestine, the oral mucosa)?

- Distribution – How does the API spread through the organism?

- Metabolism – Is the API converted chemically inside the body, and into which substances. Are these active (as well)? Could they be toxic?

- Excretion – How is the API excreted (through the bile, urine, breath, skin)?

Medication is said to have a narrow or wide *therapeutic index* or *therapeutic window*. This describes the ratio of desired effect to toxic effect. A compound with a narrow therapeutic index (close to one) exerts its desired effect at a dose close to its toxic dose. A compound with a wide therapeutic index (greater than five) exerts its desired effect at a dose substantially below its toxic dose. Those with a narrow margin are more difficult to dose and administer, and may require therapeutic drug monitoring (examples are warfarin, some antiepileptics, aminoglycoside antibiotics). Most anti-cancer drugs have a narrow therapeutic margin: toxic side-effects are almost always encountered at doses used to kill tumors.

Medicine Development and Safety Testing

Development of medication is a vital concern to medicine, but also has strong economical and political implications. To protect the consumer and prevent abuse, many governments regulate the manufacture, sale, and administration of medication. In the United States, the main body that regulates pharmaceuticals is the Food and Drug Administration and they enforce standards set by the United States Pharmacopoeia. In the European Union, the main body that regulates pharmaceuticals is the EMA and they enforce standards set by the European Pharmacopoeia.

The metabolic stability and the reactivity of a library of candidate drug compounds have to be assessed for drug metabolism and toxicological studies. Many methods have been proposed for quantitative predictions in drug metabolism; one example of a recent computational method is SPORCalc. If the chemical structure of a medicinal compound is altered slightly, this could slightly or dramatically alter the medicinal properties of the compound depending on the level of alteration as it relates to the structural composition of the substrate or receptor site on which it exerts its medicinal effect, a concept referred to as the structural activity relationship (SAR). This means that when a useful activity has been identified, chemists will make many similar compounds called analogues, in an attempt to maximize the desired medicinal effect(s) of the compound. This development phase can take anywhere from a few years to a decade or more and is very expensive.

These new analogues need to be developed. It needs to be determined how safe the medicine is for human consumption, its stability in the human body and the best form for delivery to the desired organ system, like tablet or aerosol. After extensive testing, which can take up to 6 years, the new medicine is ready for marketing and selling.

As a result of the long time required to develop analogues and test a new medicine and the fact that of every 5000 potential new medicines typically only one will ever reach the open market, this is an expensive way of doing things, often costing over 1 billion dollars. To recoup this outlay pharmaceutical companies may do a number of things:

- Carefully research the demand for their potential new product before spending an outlay of company funds.

- Obtain a patent on the new medicine preventing other companies from producing that medicine for a certain allocation of time.

Drug Legislation and Safety

In the United States, the Food and Drug Administration (FDA) is responsible for creating guidelines for the approval and use of drugs. The FDA requires that all approved drugs fulfill two requirements:

1. The drug must be found to be effective against the disease for which it is seeking approval (where 'effective' means only that the drug performed better than placebo or competitors in at least two trials).

2. The drug must meet safety criteria by being subject to animal and controlled human testing.

Gaining FDA approval usually takes several years to attain. Testing done on animals must be extensive and must include several species to help in the evaluation of both the effectiveness and toxicity of the drug. The dosage of any drug approved for use is intended to fall within a range in which the drug produces a therapeutic effect or desired outcome.

The safety and effectiveness of prescription drugs in the U.S. is regulated by the federal Prescription Drug Marketing Act of 1987.

The Medicines and Healthcare products Regulatory Agency (MHRA) has a similar role in the UK.

Education

Students of pharmacology are trained as biomedical scientists, studying the effects of drugs on living organisms. This can lead to new drug discoveries, as well as a better understanding of the way in which the human body works.

Students of pharmacology must have detailed working knowledge of aspects in physiology, pathology and chemistry. During a typical degree they will cover areas such as (but not limited to) biochemistry, cell biology, basic physiology, genetics & the Central Dogma, medical microbiology, neuroscience, and depending on the department's interests, bio-organic chemistry and/or chemical biology.

Modern Pharmacology is highly interdisciplinary. Graduate programs accept students from most biological and chemical backgrounds. With the increasing drive towards biophysical and computational research to describe systems, pharmacologists may even consider themselves mainly physical scientists. In many instances, Analytical Chemistry is closely related to the studies and needs of pharmacological research. Therefore, many institutions will include pharmacology under a Chemistry or Biochemistry Department, especially if a separate Pharmacology Dept. does not exist. What makes an institutional department independent of another, or exist in the first place, is usually an artifact of historical times.

Whereas a pharmacy student will eventually work in a pharmacy dispensing medications, a pharmacologist will typically work within a laboratory setting. Careers for a pharmacologist include academic positions (medical and non-medical), governmental positions, private industrial positions, science writing, scientific patents and law, consultation, biotech and pharmaceutical employment, the alcohol industry, food industry, forensics/law enforcement, public health, and environmental/ecological sciences.

Pharmacy

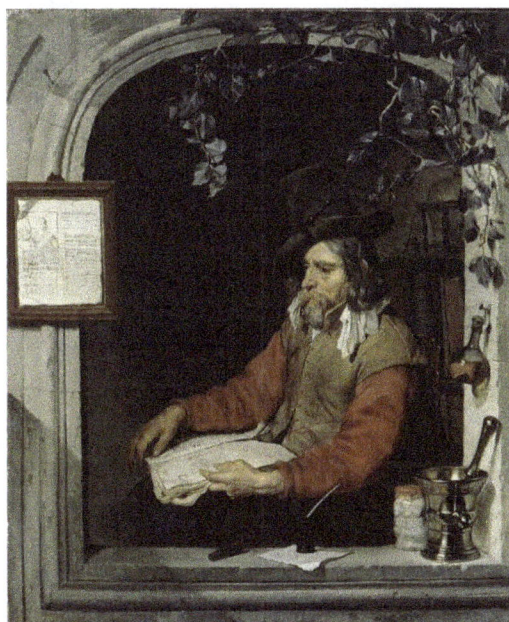

The Apothecary or The Chemist by Gabriël Metsu (c. 1651–67)

Pharmacy is the science and technique of preparing and dispensing drugs. It is a health profession that links health sciences with chemical sciences and aims to ensure the safe and effective use of pharmaceutical drugs.

The scope of pharmacy practice includes more traditional roles such as compounding and dispensing medications, and it also includes more modern services related to health care, including clinical services, reviewing medications for safety and efficacy, and providing drug information. Pharmacists, therefore, are the experts on drug therapy and are the primary health professionals who optimize use of medication for the benefit of the patients.

An establishment in which pharmacy (in the first sense) is practiced is called a pharmacy (this term is more common in the United States) or a chemist's (which is more common in Great Britain). In the United States and Canada, drugstores commonly sell medicines, as well as miscellaneous items such as confectionery, cosmetics, office supplies, toys, hair care products and magazines and occasionally refreshments and groceries.

The word *pharmacy* is derived from its root word *pharma*, which had first been used sometime in the 15th–17th centuries. However, the original Greek roots from *pharmakos* imply sorcery or even poison. In addition to pharma responsibilities, the pharma offered general medical advice and a range of services that are now performed solely by other specialist practitioners, such as surgery and midwifery. The pharma (as it was referred to) often operated through a retail shop which, in addition to ingredients for medicines, sold tobacco and patent medicines. Often the place that did this was called an apothecary and several languages have this as the dominant term, though their practices are more akin to a modern pharmacy, in English the term apothecary would today be seen as outdated or only appropriate if herbal remedies were on offer to a large extent. The pharmas also used many other herbs not listed.

In its investigation of herbal and chemical ingredients, the work of the pharma may be regarded as a precursor of the modern sciences of chemistry and pharmacology, prior to the formulation of the scientific method.

Disciplines

The field of pharmacy can generally be divided into three primary disciplines:

- Pharmaceutics
- Medicinal Chemistry and Pharmacognosy
- Pharmacy Practice

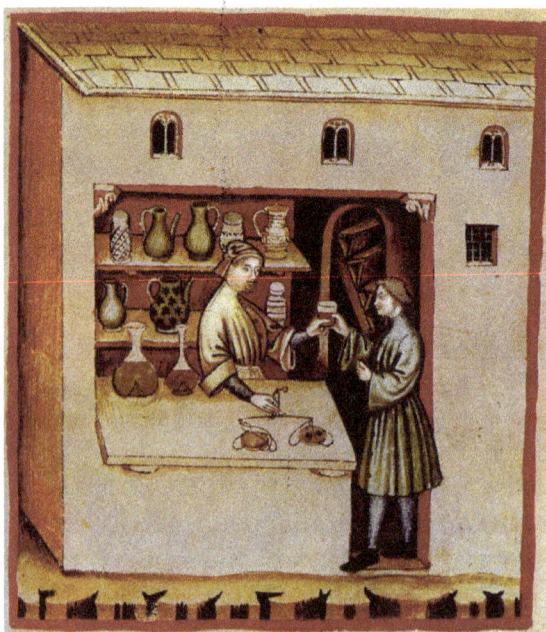

Pharmacy, tacuinum sanitatis casanatensis (14th century)

The boundaries between these disciplines and with other sciences, such as biochemistry, are not always clear-cut. Often, collaborative teams from various disciplines (pharmacists and other scientists) work together toward the introduction of new therapeutics and methods for patient care. However, pharmacy is not a basic or biomedical science in its typical form. Medicinal chemistry is also a distinct branch of synthetic chemistry combining pharmacology, organic chemistry, and chemical biology.

Pharmacology is sometimes considered as the 4th discipline of pharmacy. Although pharmacology is essential to the study of pharmacy, it is not specific to pharmacy. Both disciplines are distinct.Those who wish to practice both pharmacy (patient oriented) and pharmacology (a biomedical science requiring the scientific method) receive separate training and degrees unique to either discipline.

Pharmacoinformatics is considered another new discipline, for systematic drug discovery and development with efficiency and safety.

Professionals

The World Health Organization estimates that there are at least 2.6 million pharmacists and other pharmaceutical personnel worldwide.

Pharmacists

Pharmacists are healthcare professionals with specialised education and training who perform various roles to ensure optimal health outcomes for their patients through the quality use of medicines. Pharmacists may also be small-business proprietors, owning the pharmacy in which they practice. Since pharmacists know about the mode of action of a particular drug, and its metabolism and physiological effects on the human body in great detail, they play an important role in optimisation of a drug treatment for an individual.

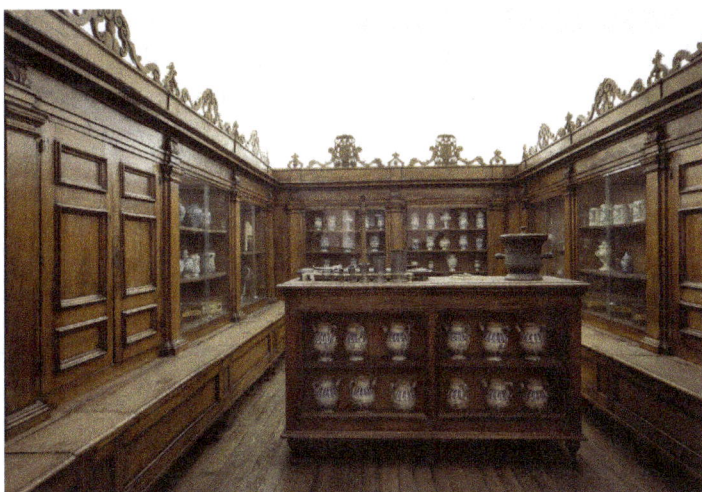

Convent pharmacy exhibited at the Museo nazionale della scienza e della tecnologia Leonardo da Vinci of Milan.

Pharmacists are represented internationally by the International Pharmaceutical Federation (FIP). They are represented at the national level by professional organisations such as the Royal Pharmaceutical Society in the UK, the Pharmaceutical Society of Australia (PSA), the Canadian Pharmacists Association (CPhA),the Pakistan Pharmacists Association (PPA), and the American Pharmacists Association (APhA).

In some cases, the representative body is also the registering body, which is responsible for the regulation and ethics of the profession.

In the United States, specializations in pharmacy practice recognized by the Board of Pharmacy Specialties include: cardiovascular, infectious disease, oncology, pharmacotherapy, nuclear, nutrition, and psychiatry. The Commission for Certification in Geriatric Pharmacy certifies pharmacists in geriatric pharmacy practice. The American Board of Applied Toxicology certifies pharmacists and other medical professionals in applied toxicology.

Pharmacy Technicians

Pharmacy technicians support the work of pharmacists and other health professionals by performing a variety of pharmacy related functions, including dispensing prescription drugs and other medical devices to patients and instructing on their use. They may also perform administrative duties in pharmaceutical practice, such as reviewing prescription requests with medics's offices and insurance companies to ensure correct medications are provided and payment is received.

A Pharmacy Technician in the UK is considered a health care professional and often does not work under the direct supervision of a pharmacist (if employed in a hospital pharmacy) but instead is supervised and managed by other senior pharmacy technicians. In the UK the role of a PhT has grown and responsibility has been passed on to them to manage the pharmacy department and specialised areas in pharmacy practice allowing pharmacists the time to specialise in their expert field as medication consultants spending more time working with patients and in research. A pharmacy technician once qualified has to register as a professional on the General Pharmaceutical Council (GPhC) register. The GPhC is the governing body for pharmacy health care professionals and this is who regulates the practice of pharmacists and pharmacy technicians.

In the US, pharmacy technicians perform their duties under supervision of pharmacists. Although they may perform, under supervision, most dispensing, compounding and other tasks, they are not generally allowed to perform the role of counseling patients on the proper use of their medications.

History

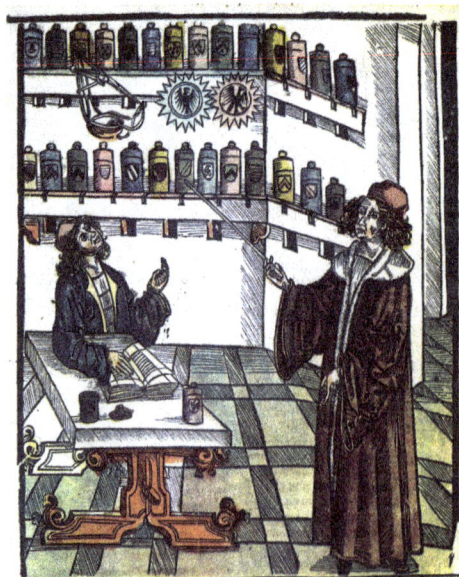

Physician and Pharmacist, illustration from *Medicinarius* (1505) by Hieronymus Brunschwig.

The earliest known compilation of medicinal substances was the *Sushruta Samhita*, an Indian Ayurvedic treatise attributed to Sushruta in the 6th century BC. However, the earliest text as preserved dates to the 3rd or 4th century AD.

Many Sumerian (late 6th millennium BC – early 2nd millennium BC) cuneiform clay tablets record prescriptions for medicine.

Ancient Egyptian pharmacological knowledge was recorded in various papyri such as the *Ebers Papyrus* of 1550 BC, and the *Edwin Smith Papyrus* of the 16th century BC.

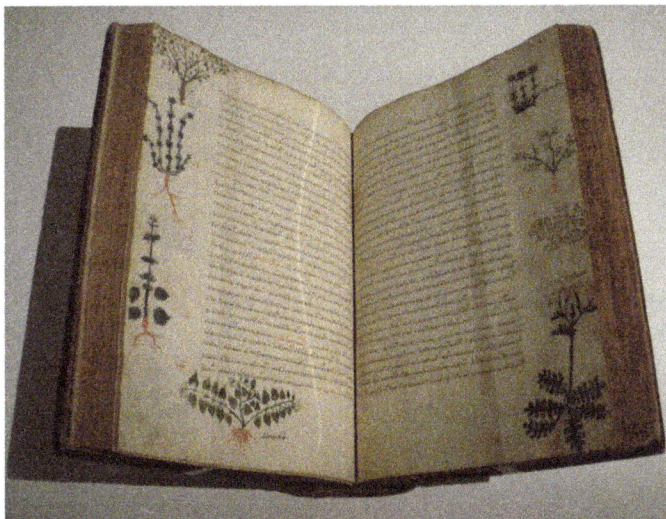

Dioscorides, *De Materia Medica*, Byzantium, 15th century

In Ancient Greece, Diocles of Carystus (4th century BC) was one of several men studying the medicinal properties of plants. He wrote several treatises on the topic. The Latin translation *De Materia Medica* (*Concerning medical substances*) was used a basis for many medieval texts, and was built upon by many middle eastern scientists during the Islamic Golden Age. The title coined the term *materia medica*.

The earliest known Chinese manual on materia medica is the *Shennong Bencao Jing* (*The Divine Farmer's Herb-Root Classic*), dating back to the 1st century AD. It was compiled during the Han dynasty and was attributed to the mythical Shennong. Earlier literature included lists of prescriptions for specific ailments, exemplified by a manuscript "Recipes for 52 Ailments", found in the Mawangdui, sealed in 168 BC. Further details on Chinese pharmacy can be found in the Pharmacy in China article.

In Japan, at the end of the Asuka period (538–710) and the early Nara period (710–794), the men who fulfilled roles similar to those of modern pharmacists were highly respected. The place of pharmacists in society was expressly defined in the Taihō Code (701) and re-stated in the Yōrō Code (718). Ranked positions in the pre-Heian Imperial court were established; and this organizational structure remained largely intact until the Meiji Restoration (1868). In this highly stable hierarchy, the pharmacists—and even pharmacist assistants—were assigned status superior to all others in health-related fields such as physicians and acupuncturists. In the Imperial household, the pharmacist was even ranked above the two personal physicians of the Emperor.

There is a stone sign for a pharmacy with a tripod, a mortar, and a pestle opposite one for a doctor in the Arcadian Way in Ephesus near Kusadasi in Turkey. The current Ephesus dates back to 400 BC and was the site of the Temple of Artemis, one of the seven wonders of the world.

In Baghdad the first pharmacies, or drug stores, were established in 754, under the Abbasid Caliphate during the Islamic Golden Age. By the 9th century, these pharmacies were state-regulated.

The advances made in the Middle East in botany and chemistry led medicine in medieval Islam substantially to develop pharmacology. Muhammad ibn Zakarīya Rāzi (Rhazes) (865–915), for instance, acted to promote the medical uses of chemical compounds. Abu al-Qasim al-Zahrawi (Abulcasis) (936–1013) pioneered the preparation of medicines by sublimation and distillation. His *Liber servitoris* is of particular interest, as it provides the reader with recipes and explains how to prepare the `simples' from which were compounded the complex drugs then generally used. Sabur Ibn Sahl (d 869), was, however, the first physician to initiate pharmacopoedia, describing a large variety of drugs and remedies for ailments. Al-Biruni (973–1050) wrote one of the most valuable Islamic works on pharmacology, entitled *Kitab al-Saydalah* (*The Book of Drugs*), in which he detailed the properties of drugs and outlined the role of pharmacy and the functions and duties of the pharmacist. Avicenna, too, described no less than 700 preparations, their properties, modes of action, and their indications. He devoted in fact a whole volume to simple drugs in *The Canon of Medicine*. Of great impact were also the works by al-Maridini of Baghdad and Cairo, and Ibn al-Wafid (1008–1074), both of which were printed in Latin more than fifty times, appearing as *De Medicinis universalibus et particularibus* by 'Mesue' the younger, and the *Medicamentis simplicibus* by 'Abenguefit'. Peter of Abano (1250–1316) translated and added a supplement to the work of al-Maridini under the title *De Veneris*. Al-Muwaffaq's contributions in the field are also pioneering. Living in the 10th century, he wrote *The foundations of the true properties of Remedies*, amongst others describing arsenious oxide, and being acquainted with silicic acid. He made clear distinction between sodium carbonate and potassium carbonate, and drew attention to the poisonous nature of copper compounds, especially copper vitriol, and also lead compounds. He also describes the distillation of sea-water for drinking.

In Europe pharmacy-like shops began to appear during the 12th century. In 1240 emperor Frederic II issued a decree by which the physician's and the apothecary's professions were separated. The first pharmacy in Europe (still working) was opened in 1241 in Trier, Germany.

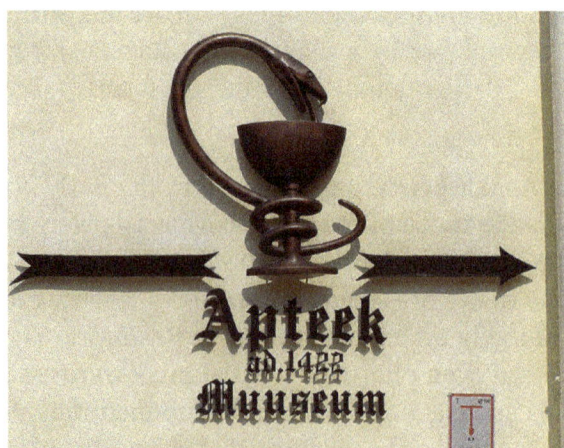

Sign of the Town Hall Pharmacy in Tallinn, operating continuously from at least 1422

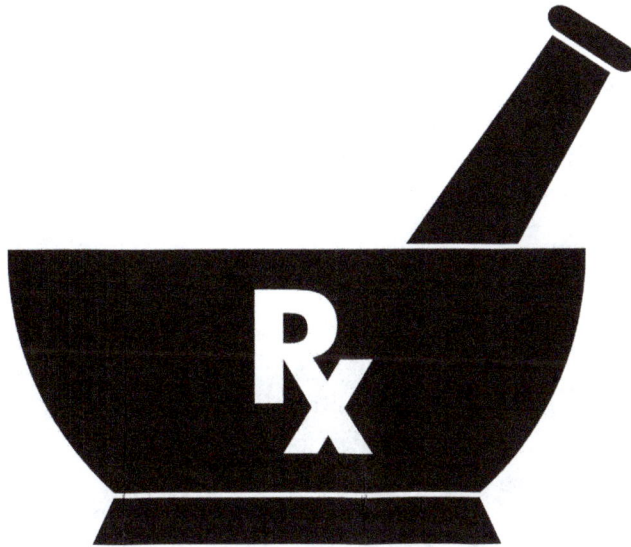

The mortar and pestle, one of the internationally recognized symbols to represent the pharmacy profession

In Europe there are old pharmacies still operating in Dubrovnik, Croatia, located inside the Franciscan monastery, opened in 1317; and in the Town Hall Square of Tallinn, Estonia, dating from at least 1422. The oldest is claimed to have been set up in 1221 in the Church of Santa Maria Novella in Florence, Italy, which now houses a perfume museum. The medieval Esteve Pharmacy, located in Llívia, a Catalan enclave close to Puigcerdà, also now a museum, dates back to the 15th century, keeping albarellos from the 16th and 17th centuries, old prescription books and antique drugs.

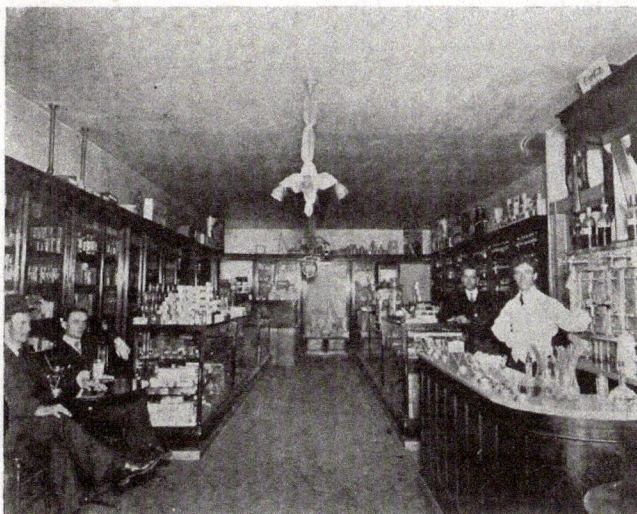

Interior of A. E. Lathrop's Drug Store—Simsbury, Conn.

Typical American drug store with a soda fountain, about 1905

Types of Pharmacy Practice Areas

Pharmacists practice in a variety of areas including community pharmacies, hospitals, clinics, extended care facilities, psychiatric hospitals, and regulatory agencies. Pharmacists can specialize in various areas of practice including but not limited to: hematology/oncology, infectious diseases, ambulatory care, nutrition support, drug information, critical care, pediatrics, etc.

Community Pharmacy

A pharmacy (commonly the chemist in Australia, New Zealand and the UK; or drugstore in North America; retail pharmacy in industry terminology; or Apothecary, historically) is the place where most pharmacists practice the profession of pharmacy. It is the community pharmacy where the dichotomy of the profession exists—health professionals who are also retailers.

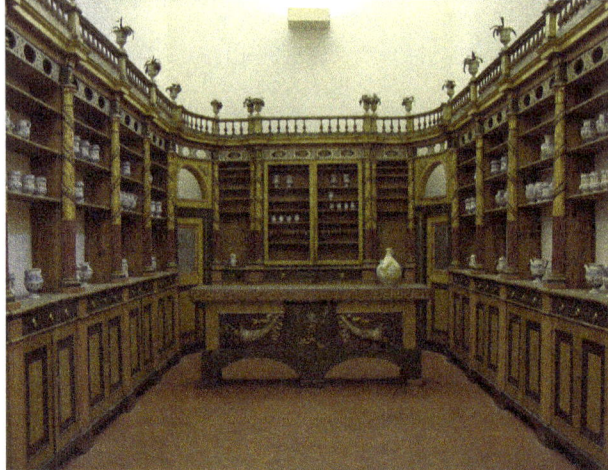
19th-century Italian pharmacy

Community pharmacies usually consist of a retail storefront with a dispensary where medications are stored and dispensed. According to Sharif Kaf al-Ghazal, the opening of the first drugstores are recorded by Muslim pharmacists in Baghdad in 754.

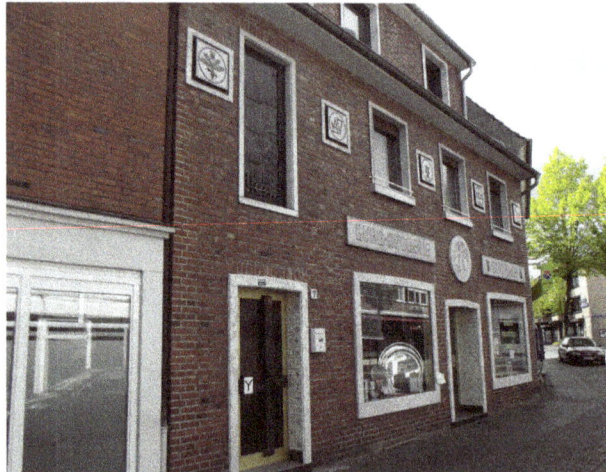
Classic symbols at the wall of a former German pharmacy

In most countries, the dispensary is subject to pharmacy legislation; with requirements for storage conditions, compulsory texts, equipment, etc., specified in legislation. Where it was once the case that pharmacists stayed within the dispensary compounding/dispensing medications, there has been an increasing trend towards the use of trained pharmacy technicians while the pharmacist spends more time communicating with patients. Pharmacy technicians are now more dependent upon automation to assist them in their new role dealing with patients' prescriptions and patient safety issues.

Pharmacies are typically required to have a pharmacist on-duty at all times when open. It is also often a requirement that the owner of a pharmacy must be a registered pharmacist, although this is not the case in all jurisdictions, such that many retailers (including supermarkets and mass merchandisers) now include a pharmacy as a department of their store.

Likewise, many pharmacies are now rather grocery store-like in their design. In addition to medicines and prescriptions, many now sell a diverse arrangement of additional items such as cosmetics, shampoo, office supplies, confections, snack foods, durable medical equipment, greeting cards, and provide photo processing services.

Hospital Pharmacy

Pharmacies within hospitals differ considerably from community pharmacies. Some pharmacists in hospital pharmacies may have more complex clinical medication management issues whereas pharmacists in community pharmacies often have more complex business and customer relations issues.

Because of the complexity of medications including specific indications, effectiveness of treatment regimens, safety of medications (i.e., drug interactions) and patient compliance issues (in the hospital and at home) many pharmacists practicing in hospitals gain more education and training after pharmacy school through a pharmacy practice residency and sometimes followed by another residency in a specific area. Those pharmacists are often referred to as clinical pharmacists and they often specialize in various disciplines of pharmacy. For example, there are pharmacists who specialize in hematology/oncology, HIV/AIDS, infectious disease, critical care, emergency medicine, toxicology, nuclear pharmacy, pain management, psychiatry, anti-coagulation clinics, herbal medicine, neurology/epilepsy management, pediatrics, neonatal pharmacists and more.

Hospital pharmacies can often be found within the premises of the hospital. Hospital pharmacies usually stock a larger range of medications, including more specialized medications, than would be feasible in the community setting. Most hospital medications are unit-dose, or a single dose of medicine. Hospital pharmacists and trained pharmacy technicians compound sterile products for patients including total parenteral nutrition (TPN), and other medications given intravenously. This is a complex process that requires adequate training of personnel, quality assurance of products, and adequate facilities. Several hospital pharmacies have decided to outsource high risk preparations and some other compounding functions to companies who specialize in compounding. The high cost of medications and drug-related technology, combined with the potential impact of medications and pharmacy services on patient-care outcomes and patient safety, make it imperative that hospital pharmacies perform at the highest level possible.

Clinical Pharmacy

Pharmacists provide direct patient care services that optimizes the use of medication and promotes health, wellness, and disease prevention. Clinical pharmacists care for patients in all health care settings, but the clinical pharmacy movement initially began inside hospitals and clinics. Clinical pharmacists often collaborate with physicians and other healthcare professionals to improve pharmaceutical care. Clinical pharmacists are now an integral part of the interdisciplinary approach to patient care. They often participate in patient care rounds for drug product selection.

The clinical pharmacist's role involves creating a comprehensive drug therapy plan for patient-specific problems, identifying goals of therapy, and reviewing all prescribed medications prior to dispensing and administration to the patient. The review process often involves an evaluation of the appropriateness of the drug therapy (e.g., drug choice, dose, route, frequency, and duration of therapy) and its efficacy. The pharmacist must also monitor for potential drug interactions, adverse drug reactions, and assess patient drug allergies while designing and initiating a drug therapy plan.

Ambulatory Care Pharmacy

Since the emergence of modern clinical pharmacy, ambulatory care pharmacy practice has emerged as a unique pharmacy practice setting. Ambulatory care pharmacy is based primarily on pharmacotherapy services that a pharmacist provides in a clinic. Pharmacists in this setting often do not dispense drugs, but rather see patients in office visits to manage chronic disease states.

In the U.S. federal health care system (including the VA, the Indian Health Service, and NIH) ambulatory care pharmacists are given full independent prescribing authority. In some states such North Carolina and New Mexico these pharmacist clinicians are given collaborative prescriptive and diagnostic authority. In 2011 the board of Pharmaceutical Specialties approved ambulatory care pharmacy practice as a separate board certification. The official designation for pharmacists who pass the ambulatory care pharmacy specialty certification exam will be Board Certified Ambulatory Care Pharmacist and these pharmacists will carry the initials BCACP.

Compounding Pharmacy

Compounding is the practice of preparing drugs in new forms. For example, if a drug manufacturer only provides a drug as a tablet, a compounding pharmacist might make a medicated lollipop that contains the drug. Patients who have difficulty swallowing the tablet may prefer to suck the medicated lollipop instead.

Another form of compounding is by mixing different strengths (g,mg,mcg) of capsules or tablets to yield the desired amount of medication indicated by the physician, physician assistant, Nurse Practitioner, or clinical pharmacist practitioner. This form of compounding is found at community or hospital pharmacies or in-home administration therapy.

Compounding pharmacies specialize in compounding, although many also dispense the same non-compounded drugs that patients can obtain from community pharmacies.

Consultant Pharmacy

Consultant pharmacy practice focuses more on medication regimen review (i.e. "cognitive services") than on actual dispensing of drugs. Consultant pharmacists most typically work in nursing homes, but are increasingly branching into other institutions and non-institutional settings. Traditionally consultant pharmacists were usually independent business owners, though in the United States many now work for several large pharmacy management companies (primarily Omnicare, Kindred Healthcare and PharMerica). This trend may be gradually reversing as consultant pharmacists begin to work directly with patients, primarily because many elderly people are now taking numerous medications but continue to live outside of institutional settings. Some community pharmacies employ consultant pharmacists and/or provide consulting services.

The main principle of consultant pharmacy is developed by Hepler and Strand in 1990.

Internet Pharmacy

Since about the year 2000, a growing number of Internet pharmacies have been established worldwide. Many of these pharmacies are similar to community pharmacies, and in fact, many of them are actually operated by brick-and-mortar community pharmacies that serve consumers online and those that walk in their door. The primary difference is the method by which the medications are requested and received. Some customers consider this to be more convenient and private method rather than traveling to a community drugstore where another customer might overhear about the drugs that they take. Internet pharmacies (also known as online pharmacies) are also recommended to some patients by their physicians if they are homebound.

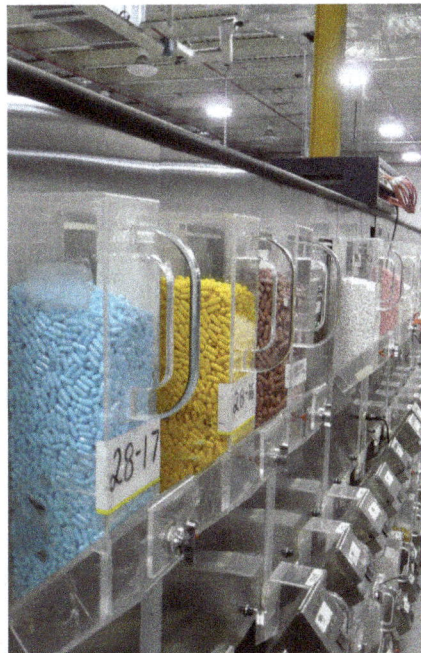

Canisters of pills from a mail order pharmacy.

While most Internet pharmacies sell prescription drugs and require a valid prescription, some Internet pharmacies sell prescription drugs without requiring a prescription. Many customers order drugs from such pharmacies to avoid the "inconvenience" of visiting a doctor or to obtain medications which their doctors were unwilling to prescribe. However, this practice has been criticized as potentially dangerous, especially by those who feel that only doctors can reliably assess contraindications, risk/benefit ratios, and an individual's overall suitability for use of a medication. There also have been reports of such pharmacies dispensing substandard products.

Of particular concern with Internet pharmacies is the ease with which people, youth in particular, can obtain controlled substances (e.g., Vicodin, generically known as hydrocodone) via the Internet without a prescription issued by a doctor/practitioner who has an established doctor-patient relationship. There are many instances where a practitioner issues a prescription, brokered by an Internet server, for a controlled substance to a "patient" s/he has never met. In the United States, in order for a prescription for a controlled substance to be valid, it must be issued for a legitimate medical purpose by a licensed practitioner acting in the course of legitimate doctor-patient relationship. The filling pharmacy has a corresponding responsibility to ensure that the prescription is valid. Often, individual state laws outline what defines a valid patient-doctor relationship.

Canada is home to dozens of licensed Internet pharmacies, many of which sell their lower-cost prescription drugs to U.S. consumers, who pay one of the world's highest drug prices. In recent years, many consumers in the US and in other countries with high drug costs, have turned to licensed Internet pharmacies in India, Israel and the UK, which often have even lower prices than in Canada.

In the United States, there has been a push to legalize importation of medications from Canada and other countries, in order to reduce consumer costs. While in most cases importation of prescription medications violates Food and Drug Administration (FDA) regulations and federal laws, enforcement is generally targeted at international drug suppliers, rather than consumers. There is no known case of any U.S. citizens buying Canadian drugs for personal use with a prescription, who has ever been charged by authorities.

Veterinary Pharmacy

Veterinary pharmacies, sometimes called *animal pharmacies*, may fall in the category of hospital pharmacy, retail pharmacy or mail-order pharmacy. Veterinary pharmacies stock different varieties and different strengths of medications to fulfill the pharmaceutical needs of animals. Because the needs of animals, as well as the regulations on veterinary medicine, are often very different from those related to people, veterinary pharmacy is often kept separate from regular pharmacies.

Nuclear Pharmacy

Nuclear pharmacy focuses on preparing radioactive materials for diagnostic tests and for treating certain diseases. Nuclear pharmacists undergo additional training specific to handling radioactive materials, and unlike in community and hospital pharmacies, nuclear pharmacists typically do not interact directly with patients.

Military Pharmacy

Military pharmacy is an entirely different working environment due to the fact that technicians perform most duties that in a civilian sector would be illegal. State laws of Technician patient counseling and medication checking by a pharmacist do not apply.

Pharmacy Informatics

Pharmacy informatics is the combination of pharmacy practice science and applied information science. Pharmacy informaticists work in many practice areas of pharmacy, however, they may also work in information technology departments or for healthcare information technology vendor companies. As a practice area and specialist domain, pharmacy informatics is growing quickly to meet the needs of major national and international patient information projects and health system interoperability goals. Pharmacists in this area are trained to participate in medication management system development, deployment and optimization.

Specialty Pharmacy

Specialty pharmacies supply high cost injectable, oral, infused, or inhaled medications that are used for chronic and complex disease states such as cancer, hepatitis, and rheumatoid arthritis. Unlike a traditional community pharmacy where prescriptions for any common medication can be brought in and filled, specialty pharmacies carry novel medications that need to be properly stored, administered, carefully monitored, and clinically managed. In addition to supplying these drugs, specialty pharmacies also provide lab monitoring, adherence counseling, and assist patients with cost-containment strategies needed to obtain their expensive specialty drugs. It is currently the fastest growing sector of the pharmaceutical industry with 19 of 28 newly FDA approved medications in 2013 being specialty drugs.

Due to the demand for clinicians who can properly manage these specific patient populations, the Specialty Pharmacy Certification Board has developed a new certification exam to certify specialty pharmacists. Along with the 100 question computerized multiple-choice exam, pharmacists must also complete 3,000 hours of specialty pharmacy practice within the past three years as well as 30 hours of specialty pharmacist continuing education within the past two years.

Issues in Pharmacy

Separation of Prescribing from Dispensing

In most jurisdictions (such as the United States), pharmacists are regulated separately from physicians. These jurisdictions also usually specify that *only* pharmacists may supply scheduled pharmaceuticals to the public, and that pharmacists cannot form business partnerships with physicians or give them "kickback" payments. However, the American Medical Association (AMA) Code of Ethics provides that physicians may dispense drugs within their office practices as long as there is no patient exploitation and patients have the right to a written prescription that can be filled elsewhere. 7 to 10 percent of American physicians practices reportedly dispense drugs on their own.

In some rural areas in the United Kingdom, there are dispensing physicians who are allowed to both prescribe and dispense prescription-only medicines to their patients from within their practices. The law requires that the GP practice be located in a designated rural area and that there is also a specified, minimum distance (currently 1.6 kilometres) between a patient's home and the nearest retail pharmacy. This law also exists in Austria for general physicians if the nearest pharmacy is more than 4 kilometers away, or where none is registered in the city.

In other jurisdictions (particularly in Asian countries such as China, Malaysia, and Singapore), doctors are allowed to dispense drugs themselves and the practice of pharmacy is sometimes integrated with that of the physician, particularly in traditional Chinese medicine.

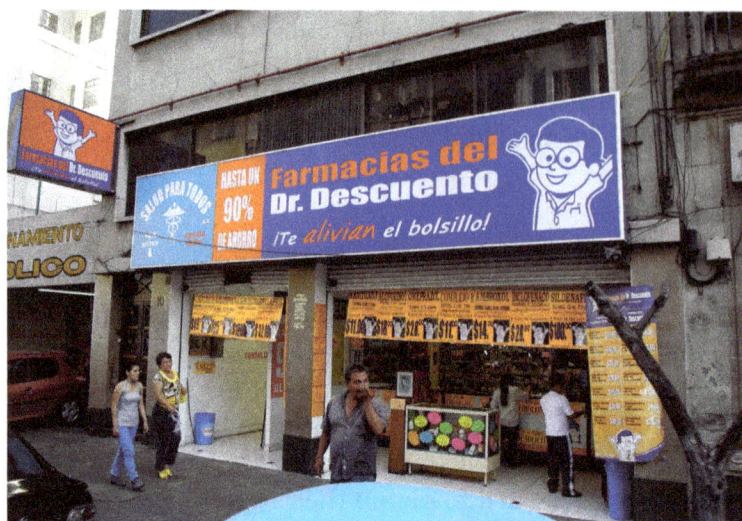

One of a chain of pharmacies in Mexico City, Mexico, named "Doctor Discount," March 2010.

In Canada it is common for a medical clinic and a pharmacy to be located together and for the ownership in both enterprises to be common, but licensed separately.

The reason for the majority rule is the high risk of a conflict of interest and/or the avoidance of absolute powers. Otherwise, the physician has a financial self-interest in "diagnosing" as many conditions as possible, and in exaggerating their seriousness, because he or she can then sell more medications to the patient. Such self-interest directly conflicts with the patient's interest in obtaining cost-effective medication and avoiding the unnecessary use of medication that may have side-effects. This system reflects much similarity to the checks and balances system of the U.S. and many other governments.

A campaign for separation has begun in many countries and has already been successful (as in Korea). As many of the remaining nations move towards separation, resistance and lobbying from dispensing doctors who have pecuniary interests may prove a major stumbling block (e.g. in Malaysia).

The Future of Pharmacy

In the coming decades, pharmacists are expected to become more integral within the health care system. Rather than simply dispensing medication, pharmacists are increasingly expected to be compensated for their patient care skills. In particular, Medication Therapy Management (MTM) includes the clinical services that pharmacists can provide for their patients. Such services include the thorough analysis of all medication (prescription, non-prescription, and herbals) currently being taken by an individual. The result is a reconciliation of medication and patient education resulting in increased patient health outcomes and decreased costs to the health care system.

This shift has already commenced in some countries; for instance, pharmacists in Australia receive remuneration from the Australian Government for conducting comprehensive Home Medicines Reviews. In Canada, pharmacists in certain provinces have limited prescribing rights (as in Alberta and British Columbia) or are remunerated by their provincial government for expanded services such as medications reviews (Medschecks in Ontario). In the United Kingdom, pharmacists who undertake additional training are obtaining prescribing rights and this is because of pharmacy education. They are also being paid for by the government for medicine use reviews. In Scotland the pharmacist can write prescriptions for Scottish registered patients of their regular medications, for the majority of drugs, except for controlled drugs, when the patient is unable to see their doctor, as could happen if they are away from home or the doctor is unavailable. In the United States, pharmaceutical care or clinical pharmacy has had an evolving influence on the practice of pharmacy. Moreover, the Doctor of Pharmacy (Pharm. D.) degree is now required before entering practice and some pharmacists now complete one or two years of residency or fellowship training following graduation. In addition, consultant pharmacists, who traditionally operated primarily in nursing homes are now expanding into direct consultation with patients, under the banner of "senior care pharmacy."

In addition to patient care, pharmacies will be a focal point for medical adherence initiatives. There is enough evidence to show that integrated pharmacy based initiatives significantly impact adherence for chronic patients. For example, a study published in NIH shows "pharmacy based interventions improved patients' medication adherence rates by 2.1 percent and increased physicians' initiation rates by 38 percent, compared to the control group".

References

- Newton, David; Alasdair Thorpe; Chris Otter (2004). Revise A2 Chemistry. Heinemann Educational Publishers. p. 1. ISBN 0-435-58347-6.

- Edward Kremers, Glenn Sonnedecker (1986). "Kremers and Urdang's History of pharmacy". Amer. Inst. History of Pharmacy. p.17. ISBN 0931292174

2

Branches of Pharmacology

Clinical pharmacology is the study of medicinal drugs; it helps in connecting the gap between medical practice and laboratory science. Clinical pharmacology helps in the promotion of the safety of prescription and to minimize its side-effects. The other branches of pharmacology are neuropharmacology, psychopharmacology, pharmacogenetics, pharmacogenomics, pharmacoepidemiology and toxicology. This section is a compilation of the various branches of pharmacology that form an integral part of the broader subject matter.

Clinical Pharmacology

Clinical pharmacology is the science of drugs and their clinical use. It is underpinned by the basic science of pharmacology, with added focus on the application of pharmacological principles and quantitative methods in the real world. It has a broad scope, from the discovery of new target molecules, to the effects of drug usage in whole populations.

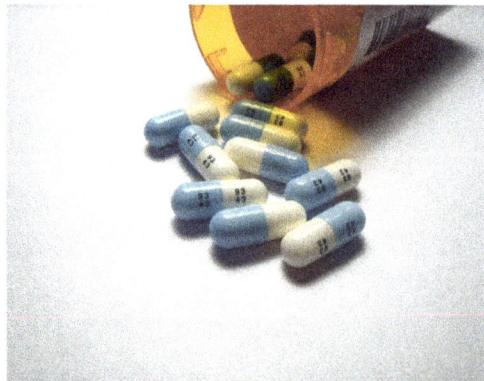

Clinical pharmacology connects the gap between medical practice and laboratory science. The main objective is to promote the safety of prescription, maximise the drug effects and minimise the side effects. It is important that there be association with pharmacists skilled in areas of drug information, medication safety and other aspects of pharmacy practice related to clinical pharmacology. In fact, in countries such as USA, Netherlands and France, pharmacists train to become clinical pharmacologists. Therefore, clinical pharmacology is not specific to medicine.

Clinical pharmacologists usually have a rigorous medical and scientific training which enables them to evaluate evidence and produce new data through well designed studies. Clinical pharmacologists must have access to enough outpatients for clinical care, teaching and education, and research as well be supervised by medical specialists. Their responsibilities to patients include, but are not limited to analyzing adverse drug effects, therapeutics, and toxicology including reproductive toxicology, cardiovascular risks, perioperative drug management and psychopharmacology.

In addition, the application of genetic, biochemical, or virotherapeutical techniques has led to a clear appreciation of the mechanisms involved in drug action.

Branches

- Pharmacodynamics - finding out what drugs do to the body and how. This includes not just the cellular and molecular aspects, but also more relevant clinical measurements. For example, not just the biology of salbutamol, a beta2-adrenergic receptor agonist, but the peak flow rate of both healthy volunteers and real patients.

- Pharmacokinetics - what happens to the drug while in the body. This involves the body systems for handling the drug, usually divided into the following classification:

    o Absorption

    o Distribution

    o Metabolism

    o Excretion.

- Rational Prescribing - using the right medication, at the right dose, using the right route and frequency of administration for the patient, and stopping the drug appropriately.

- Adverse Drug Effects

- Toxicology

- Drug interactions

- Drug development - usually culminating in some form of clinical trial.

Neuropharmacology

Neuropharmacology is the study of how drugs affect cellular function in the nervous system, and the neural mechanisms through which they influence behavior. There are two main branches of neuropharmacology: behavioral and molecular. Behavioral neuropharmacology focuses on the study of how drugs affect human behavior (neuropsychopharmacology), including the study of how drug dependence and addiction affect the human brain. Molecular neuropharmacology involves the study of neurons and their neurochemical interactions, with the overall goal of developing drugs that have beneficial effects on neurological function. Both of these fields are closely connected, since both are concerned with the interactions of neurotransmitters, neuropeptides, neurohormones, neuromodulators, enzymes, second messengers, co-transporters, ion channels, and receptor proteins in the central and peripheral nervous systems. Studying these interactions, researchers are developing drugs to treat many different neurological disorders, including pain, neurodegenerative diseases such as Parkinson's disease and Alzheimer's disease, psychological disorders, addiction, and many others.

History

Neuropharmacology did not appear in the scientific field until, in the early part of the 20th century, scientists were able to figure out a basic understanding of the nervous system and how nerves communicate between one another. Before this discovery, there were drugs that had been found that demonstrated some type of influence on the nervous system. In the 1930s, French scientists began working with a compound called phenothiazine in the hope of synthesizing a drug that would be able to combat malaria. Though this drug showed very little hope in the use against malaria-infected individuals, it was found to have sedative effects along with what appeared to be beneficial effects toward patients with Parkinson's disease. This black box method, wherein an investigator would administer a drug and examine the response without knowing how to relate drug action to patient response, was the main approach to this field, until, in the late 1940s and early 1950s, scientists were able to identify specific neurotransmitters, such as norepinephrine (involved in the constriction of blood vessels and the increase in heart rate and blood pressure), dopamine (the chemical whose shortage is involved in Parkinson's disease), and serotonin (soon to be recognized as deeply connected to depression). In the 1950s, scientists also became better able to measure levels of specific neurochemicals in the body and thus correlate these levels with behavior. The invention of the voltage clamp in 1949 allowed for the study of ion channels and the nerve action potential. These two major historical events in neuropharmacology allowed scientists not only to study how information is transferred from one neuron to another but also to study how a neuron processes this information within itself.

Overview

Neuropharmacology is a very broad region of science that encompasses many aspects of the nervous system from single neuron manipulation to entire areas of the brain, spinal cord, and peripheral nerves. To better understand the basis behind drug development, one must first understand how neurons communicate with one another. This article will focus on both behavioral and molecular neuropharmacology; the major receptors, ion channels, and neurotransmitters manipulated through drug action and how people with a neurological disorder benefit from this drug action.

Neurochemical Interactions

To understand the potential advances in medicine that neuropharmacology can bring, it is important to understand how human behavior and thought processes are transferred from neuron to neuron and how medications can alter the chemical foundations of these processes.

Neurons are known as excitable cells because on its surface membrane there are an abundance of proteins known as ion-channels that allow small charged particles to pass in and out of the cell. The structure of the neuron allows chemical information to be received by its dendrites, propagated through the perikaryon (cell body) and down its axon, and eventually passing on to other neurons through its axon terminal.

These voltage-gated ion channels allow for rapid depolarization throughout the cell. This depolarization, if it reaches a certain threshold, will cause an action potential. Once the action potential reaches the axon terminal, it will cause an influx of calcium ions into the cell. The calcium ions will then cause vesicles, small packets filled with neurotransmitters, to bind to the cell membrane and release its contents into the synapse. This cell is known as the pre-synaptic neuron, and the cell that interacts with the neurotransmitters released is known as the post-synaptic neuron. Once the neurotransmitter is released into the synapse, it can either bind to receptors on the post-synaptic cell, the pre-synaptic cell can re-uptake it and save it for later transmission, or it can be broken down by enzymes in the synapse specific to that certain neurotransmitter. These three different actions are major areas where drug action can affect communication between neurons.

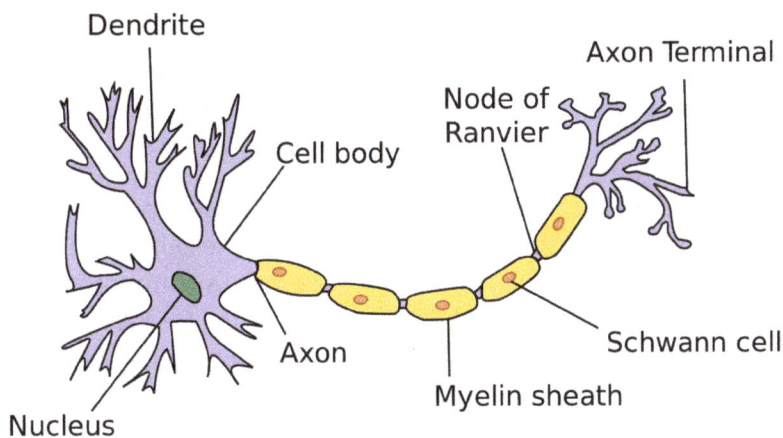

Labeling of different parts of a neuron

There are two types of receptors that neurotransmitters interact with on a post-synaptic neuron. The first types of receptors are ligand-gated ion channels or LGICs. LGIC receptors are the fastest types of transduction from chemical signal to electrical signal. Once the neurotransmitter binds to the receptor, it will cause a conformational change that will allow ions to directly flow into the cell. The second types are known as G-protein-coupled receptors or GPCRs. These are much slower than LGICs due to an increase in the amount of biochemical reactions that must take place intracellularly. Once the neurotransmitter binds to the GPCR protein, it causes a cascade of intracellular interactions that can lead to many different types of changes in cellular biochemistry, physiology, and gene expression. Neurotransmitter/receptor interactions in the field of neuropharmacology are extremely important because many drugs that are developed today have to do with disrupting this binding process.

Molecular Neuropharmacology

Molecular neuropharmacology involves the study of neurons and their neurochemical interactions, and receptors on neurons, with the goal of developing new drugs that will treat neurological disorders such as pain, neurodegenerative diseases, and psychological disorders (also known in this case as neuropsychopharmacology). There are a few technical words that must be defined when relating neurotransmission to receptor action:

1. Agonist — a molecule that binds to a receptor protein and activates that receptor

2. Competitive antagonist — a molecule that binds to the same site on the receptor protein as the agonist, preventing activation of the receptor

3. Non-competitive antagonist — a molecule that binds to a receptor protein on a different site than that of the agonist, but causes a conformational change in the protein that does not allow activation.

The following neurotransmitter/receptor interactions can be affected by synthetic compounds that act as one of the three above. Sodium/potassium ion channels can also be manipulated throughout a neuron to induce inhibitory effects of action potentials.

GABA

The GABA neurotransmitter mediates the fast synaptic inhibition in the central nervous system. When GABA is released from its pre-synaptic cell, it will bind to a receptor (most likely the $GABA_A$ receptor) that causes the post-synaptic cell to hyperpolarize (stay below its action potential threshold). This will counteract the effect of any excitatory manipulation from other neurotransmitter/receptor interactions.

This $GABA_A$ receptor contains many binding sites that allow conformational changes and are the primary target for drug development. The most common of these binding sites, benzodiazepine, allows for both agonist and antagonist effects on the receptor. A common drug, diazepam, acts as an allosteric enhancer at this binding site. Another receptor for GABA, known as $GABA_B$, can be enhanced by a molecule called baclofen. This molecule acts as an agonist, therefore activating the receptor, and is known to help control and decrease spastic movement.

Dopamine

The dopamine neurotransmitter mediates synaptic transmission by binding to five specific GPCRs. These five receptor proteins are separated into two classes due to whether the response elicits an excitatory or inhibitory response on the post-synaptic cell. There are many types of drugs, legal and illegal, that effect dopamine and its interactions in the brain. With Parkinson's disease, a disease that decreases the amount of dopamine in the brain, the dopamine precursor Levodopa is given to the patient due to the fact that dopamine cannot cross the blood–brain barrier and L-dopa can. Some dopamine agonists are also given to Parkinson's patients that have a disorder known as restless leg syndrome or RLS. Some examples of these are ropinirole and pramipexole.

Psychological disorders like that of attention deficit hyperactivity disorder (ADHD) can be treated with drugs like methylphenidate (also known as Ritalin), which block the re-uptake of dopamine by the pre-synaptic cell, thereby providing an increase of dopamine left in the synaptic gap. This increase in synaptic dopamine will increase binding to receptors of the post-synaptic cell. This same mechanism is also used by other illegal and more potent stimulant drugs such as cocaine.

Serotonin

The serotonin neurotransmitter has the ability to mediate synaptic transmission through either GPCR's or LGIC receptors. Depending on what part of the brain region serotonin is being acted upon, will depend on whether the output is either increasing or decreasing post-synaptic responses. The most popular and widely used drugs in the regulation of serotonin during depression are known as SSRI's or selective serotonin reuptake inhibitors. These drugs inhibit the transport of serotonin back into the pre-synaptic neuron, leaving more serotonin in the synaptic gap to be used.

Before the discovery of SSRIs, there were also very many drugs that inhibited the enzyme that breaks down serotonin. MAOIs or monoamine oxidase inhibitors increased the amount of serotonin in the pre-synaptic cell, but had many side-effects including intense migraines and high blood pressure. This was eventually linked to the drug's interacting with a common chemical known as tyramine found in many types of food.

Ion Channels

Ion channels located on the surface membrane of the neuron allows for an influx of sodium ions and outward movement of potassium ions during an action potential. Selectively blocking these ion channels will decrease the likelihood of an action potential to occur. The drug riluzole is a neuroprotective drug that blocks sodium ion channels. Since these channels cannot activate, there is no action potential, and the neuron does not perform any transduction of chemical signals into electrical signals and the signal does not move on. This drug is used as an anesthetic as well as a sedative.

Behavioral Neuropharmacology

One form of behavioral neuropharmacology focuses on the study of drug dependence and how drug addiction affects the human mind. Most research has shown that the major part of the brain that reinforces addiction through neurochemical reward is the nucleus accumbens. The image to the right shows how dopamine is projected into this area. Chronic alcohol abuse can cause dependence and addiction. How this addiction occurs is described below.

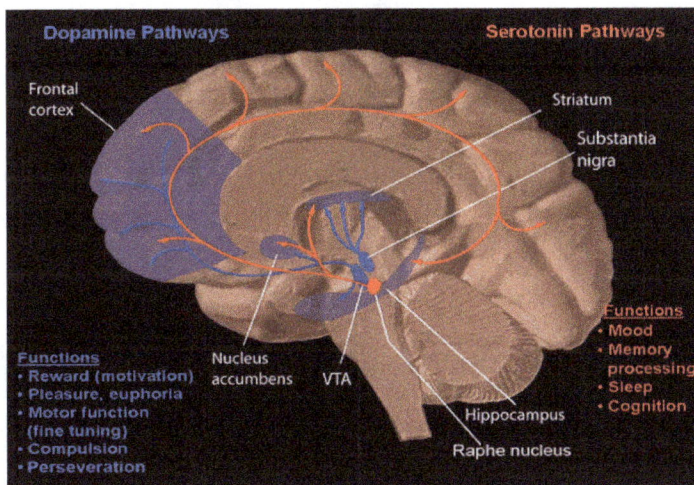

Dopamine and serotonin pathway

Ethanol

Alcohol's rewarding and reinforcing (i.e., addictive) properties are mediated through its effects on dopamine neurons in the mesolimbic reward pathway, which connects the ventral tegmental area to the nucleus accumbens (NAcc). One of alcohol's primary effects is the allosteric inhibition of NMDA receptors and facilitation of $GABA_A$ receptors (e.g., enhanced $GABA_A$ receptor-mediated chloride flux through allosteric regulation of the receptor). At high doses, ethanol inhibits most ligand gated ion channels and voltage gated ion channels in neurons as well. Alcohol inhibits sodium-potassium pumps in the cerebellum and this is likely how it impairs cerebellar computation and body co-ordination.

With acute alcohol consumption, dopamine is released in the synapses of the mesolimbic pathway, in turn heightening activation of postsynaptic D1 receptors. The activation of these receptors triggers postsynaptic internal signaling events through protein kinase A which ultimately phosphorylate cAMP response element binding protein (CREB), inducing CREB-mediated changes in gene expression.

With chronic alcohol intake, consumption of ethanol similarly induces CREB phosphorylation through the D1 receptor pathway, but it also alters NMDA receptor function through phosphorylation mechanisms; an adaptive downregulation of the D1 receptor pathway and CREB function occurs as well. Chronic consumption is also associated with an effect on CREB phosphorylation and function via postsynaptic NMDA receptor signaling cascades through a MAPK/ERK pathway and CAMK-mediated pathway. These modifications to CREB function in the mesolimbic pathway induce expression (i.e., increase gene expression) of ΔFosB in the NAcc, where ΔFosB is the "master control protein" that, when overexpressed in the NAcc, is necessary and sufficient for the development and maintenance of an addictive state (i.e., its overexpression in the nucleus accumbens produces and then directly modulates compulsive alcohol consumption).

Research

Parkinson's Disease

Parkinson's disease is a neurodegenerative disease described by the selective loss of dopaminergic neurons located in the substantia nigra. Today, the most commonly used drug to combat this disease is levodopa or L-DOPA. This precursor to dopamine can penetrate through the blood–brain barrier, whereas the neurotransmitter dopamine cannot. There has been extensive research to determine whether L-dopa is a better treatment for Parkinson's disease rather than other dopamine agonists. Some believe that the long-term use of L-dopa will compromise neuroprotection and, thus, eventually lead to dopaminergic cell death. Though there has been no proof, in-vivo or in-vitro, some still believe that the better long-term use of dopamine agonists be better for the patient.

Alzheimer's Disease

While there are a variety of hypotheses that have been proposed for the cause of Alzheimer's disease, the knowledge of this disease is far from complete to explain, making it difficult to develop methods for treatment. In the brain of Alzheimer's patients, both neuronal nicotinic acetylcholine (nACh) receptors and NMDA receptors are known to be down-regulated. Thus, four anticholinesterases have been developed and approved by the U.S. Food and Drug Administration (FDA) for the treatment in the U.S.A. However, these are not ideal drugs, considering their side-effects and limited effectiveness. One promising drug, nefiracetam, is being developed for the treatment of Alzheimer's and other patients with dementia, and has unique actions in potentiating the activity of both nACh receptors and NMDA receptors.

Future

With an increase in technology and our understanding of the nervous system, the development of drugs will continue to rise with an increase in drug sensitivity and specificity. Structure-activity relationship or SARs is a major area of research within neuropharmacology that tries to modify the effect or the potency (i.e., activity) of bioactive chemical compounds by modifying their chemical structure.

Psychopharmacology

Psychopharmacology is the scientific study of the effects drugs have on mood, sensation, thinking, and behavior. It is distinguished from neuropsychopharmacology, which emphasizes the correlation between drug-induced changes in the functioning of cells in the nervous system and changes in consciousness and behavior.

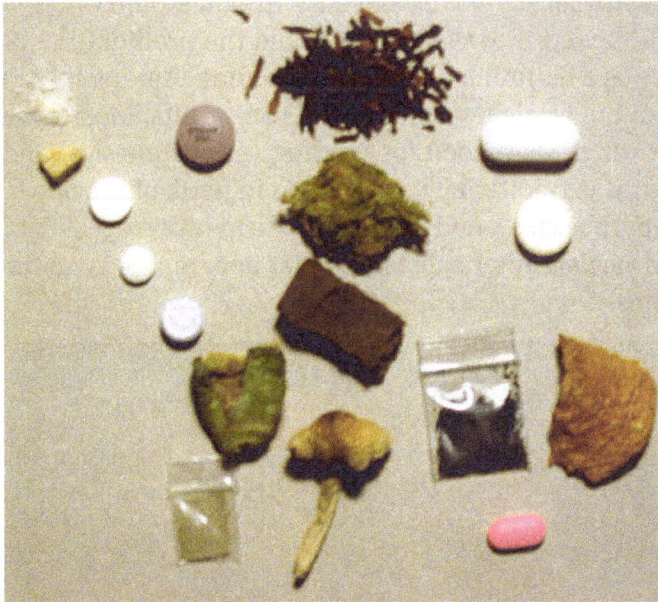

An arrangement of psychoactive drugs

The field of psychopharmacology studies a wide range of substances with various types of psychoactive properties, focusing primarily on the chemical interactions with the brain.

Psychoactive drugs interact with particular target sites or receptors found in the nervous system to induce widespread changes in physiological or psychological functions. The specific interaction between drugs and their receptors is referred to as "drug action", and the widespread changes in physiological or psychological function is referred to as "drug effect". These drugs may originate from natural sources such as plants and animals, or from artificial sources such as chemical synthesis in the laboratory.

Historical Overview

Early Psychopharmacology

Not often mentioned or included in the field of psychopharmacology today, are psychoactive substances not identified as useful in modern mental health settings or references. These substances are naturally occurring, but nonetheless psychoactive, and are compounds identified through the work of ethnobotanists and ethnomycologists (and others who study the native use of naturally occurring psychoactive drugs). However, although these substances have been used throughout history by various cultures, and have a profound effect on mentality and brain function, they have not always attained the degree of scrutinous evaluation that lab-made compounds have. Nevertheless, some, such as psilocybin and mescaline, have provided a basis of study for the compounds that are used and examined in the field today. Hunter-gatherer societies tended to favor psychedelics, dissociatives and deliriants, and today their use can still be observed in many surviving tribal cultures. The exact drug used depends on what the particular ecosystem a given tribe lives in can support, and are typically found growing wild. Such drugs include various psychedelic mushrooms containing psilocybin, muscimol, and muscarine (to name a few), and cacti containing mescaline and other chemicals, along with myriad other psychoactive-chemical-containing plants. These societies generally attach spiritual significance to such drug use, and often incorporate it into their religious practices. With the dawn of the Neolithic and the proliferation of agriculture, new psychoactives came into use as a natural by-product of farming. Among them were opium, cannabis, and alcohol derived from the fermentation of cereals and fruits. Most societies began developing herblores, lists of herbs which were good for treating various physical and mental ailments. For example, St. John's Wort was traditionally prescribed in parts of Europe for depression (in addition to use as a general-purpose tea), and Chinese medicine developed elaborate lists of herbs and preparations. These and various other substances that have an effect on the brain are still used as remedies in many cultures.

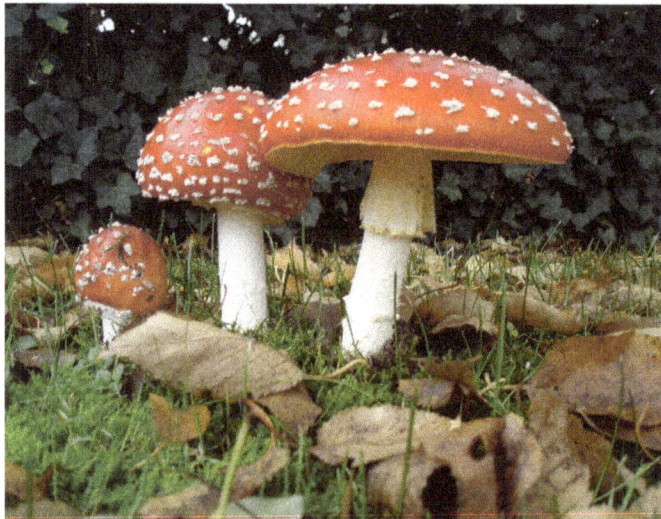

The common muscimol-bearing mushroom *Amanita muscaria*, also known as the "Fly Agaric"

Modern Psychopharmacology

The dawn of contemporary psychopharmacology marked the beginning of the use of psychiatric drugs to treat psychological illnesses. It brought with it the use of opiates and barbiturates for the management of acute behavioral issues in patients. In the early stages, psychopharmacology was primarily used for sedation. Then with the 1950s came the establishment of chlorpromazine for psychoses, lithium carbonate for mania, and then in rapid succession, the development of tricyclic antidepressants, monoamine oxidase inhibitors, benzodiazepines, among other antipsychotics and antidepressants. A defining feature of this era includes an evolution of research methods, with the establishment of placebo-controlled, double blind studies, and the development of methods for analyzing blood levels with respect to clinical outcome and increased sophistication in clinical trials. The early 1960s revealed a revolutionary model by Julius Axelrod describing nerve signals and synaptic transmission, which was followed by a drastic increase of biochemical brain research into the effects of psychotropic agents on brain chemistry. After the 1960s, the field of psychiatry shifted to incorporate the indications for and efficacy of pharmacological treatments, and began to focus on the use and toxicities of these medications. The 1970s and 1980s were further marked by a better understanding of the synaptic aspects of the action mechanisms of drugs. However, the model has its critics, too – notably Joanna Moncrieff and the Critical Psychiatry Network.

Chemical signaling

Neurotransmitters

Psychoactive drugs exert their sensory and behavioral effects almost entirely by acting on neurotransmitters and by modifying one or more aspects of synaptic transmission. Neurotransmitters can be viewed as chemicals through which neurons primarily communicate; psychoactive drugs affect the mind by altering this communication. Drugs may act by 1) serving as a precursor for the neurotransmitter; 2) inhibiting neurotransmitter synthesis; 3) preventing storage of neurotransmitter in the presynaptic vesicle; 4) stimulating or inhibiting neurotransmitter release; 5) stimulating or blocking post-synaptic receptors; 6) stimulating autoreceptors, inhibiting neurotransmitter release; 7) blocking autoreceptors, increasing neurotransmitter release; 8) inhibiting neurotransmission breakdown; or 9) blocking neurotransmitter reuptake by the presynaptic neuron.

Hormones

The other central method through which drugs act is by affecting communications between cells through hormones. Neurotransmitters can usually only travel a microscopic distance before reaching their target at the other side of the synaptic cleft, while hormones can travel long distances before reaching target cells anywhere in the body. Thus, the endocrine system is a critical focus of psychopharmacology because 1) drugs can alter the secretion of many hormones; 2) hormones may alter the behavioral responses to drugs; 3) hormones themselves sometimes have psychoactive properties; and 4) the secretion of some hormones, especially those dependent on the pituitary gland, is controlled by neurotransmitter systems in the brain.

Psychopharmacological Substances

Alcohol

Alcohol is a depressant, the effects of which may vary according to dosage amount, frequency, and chronicity. As a member of the sedative-hypnotic class, at the lowest doses, the individual feels relaxed and less anxious. In quiet settings, the user may feel drowsy, but in settings with increased sensory stimulation, individuals may feel uninhibited and more confident. High doses of alcohol rapidly consumed may produce amnesia for the events that occur during intoxication. Other effects include reduced coordination, which leads to slurred speech, impaired fine-motor skills, and delayed reaction time. The effects of alcohol on the body's neurochemistry are more difficult to examine than some other drugs. This is because the chemical nature of the substance makes it easy to penetrate into the brain, and it also influences the phospholipid bilayer of neurons. This allows alcohol to have a widespread impact on many normal cell functions and modifies the actions of several neurotransmitter systems. Alcohol inhibits glutamate (a major excitatory neurotransmitter in the nervous system) neurotransmission by reducing the effectiveness at the NMDA receptor, which is related to memory loss associated with intoxication. It also modulates the function of GABA, a major inhibitory amino acid neurotransmitter. The reinforcing qualities of alcohol leading to repeated use – and thus also the mechanisms of withdrawal from chronic alcohol use – are partially due to the substance's action on the dopamine system. This is also due to alcohol's effect on the opioid systems, or endorphins, that have opiate-like effects, such as modulating pain, mood, feeding, reinforcement, and response to stress.

Antidepressants

Antidepressants reduce symptoms of mood disorders primarily through the regulation of norepinephrine and serotonin (particularly the 5-HT receptors). After chronic use, neurons adapt to the change in biochemistry, resulting in a change in pre- and postsynaptic receptor density and second messenger function.

Monoamine oxidase inhibitors (MAOIs) are the oldest class of antidepressants. They inhibit monoamine oxidase, the enzyme that metabolizes the monoamine neurotransmitters in the presynaptic terminals that are not contained in protective synaptic vesicles. The inhibition of the enzyme increases the amount of neurotransmitter available for release. It increases norepinephrine, dopamine, and 5-HT and thus increases the action of the transmitters at their receptors. MAOIs have been somewhat disfavored because of their reputation for more serious side effects.

Tricyclic antidepressants (TCAs) work through binding to the presynaptic transporter proteins and blocking the reuptake of norepinephrine or 5-HT into the presynaptic terminal, prolonging the duration of transmitter action at the synapse.

Selective serotonin reuptake inhibitors (SSRIs) selectively block the reuptake of serotonin (5-HT) through their inhibiting effects on the sodium/potassium ATP-dependent serotonin transporter in presynaptic neurons. This increases the availability of 5-HT in the synaptic cleft. The main parameters to consider in choosing an antidepressant are side effects and safety. Most SSRIs are available generically and are relatively inexpensive. Older antidepressants, such as the TCAs and MAOIs usually require more visits and monitoring, and this may offset the low expense of the drugs. The SSRIs are relatively safe in overdose and better tolerated than the TCAs and MAOIs for most patients.

Antipsychotics

All antipsychotic substances, except clozapine, are relatively potent postsynaptic dopamine receptor blockers (dopamine antagonists). All of the effective antipsychotics, except clozapine, act on the nigrostriatal system. For an antipsychotic to be effective, it generally requires a dopamine antagonism of 60%-80% of dopamine D_2 receptors.

First generation (typical) antipsychotics: Traditional neuroleptics modify several neurotransmitter systems, but their clinical effectiveness is most likely due to their ability to antagonize dopamine transmission by competitively blocking the receptors or by inhibiting dopamine release. The most serious and troublesome side effects of these classical antipsychotics are movement disorders that resemble the symptoms of Parkinson's disease, because the neuroleptics antagonize dopamine receptors broadly, also reducing the normal dopamine-mediated inhibition of cholinergic cells in the striatum.

Second-generation (atypical) antipsychotics: The concept of "atypicality" is from the finding that the second generation antipsychotics (SGAs) had a greater serotonin/dopamine ratio than did earlier drugs, and might be associated with improved efficacy (particularly for the negative symptoms of psychosis) and reduced extrapyramidal side effects. Some of the efficacy of atypical antipsychotics may be due to 5-HT$_2$ antagonism or the blockade of other dopamine receptors. Agents that purely block 5-HT$_2$ or dopamine receptors other than D$_2$ have often failed as effective antipsychotics.

Benzodiazepines

Benzodiazepines are often used to reduce anxiety symptoms, muscle tension, seizure disorders, insomnia, symptoms of alcohol withdrawal, and panic attack symptoms. Their action is primarily on specific benzodiazepine sites on the GABA$_A$ receptor. This receptor complex is thought to mediate the anxiolytic, sedative, and anticonvulsant actions of the benzodiazepines. Use of benzodiazepines carries the risk of tolerance (necessitating increased dosage), dependence, and abuse. Taking these drugs for a long period of time can lead to withdrawal symptoms upon abrupt discontinuation.

Hallucinogens

Hallucinogens cause perceptual and cognitive distortions without delirium. The state of intoxication is often called a "trip". Onset is the first stage after an individual ingests (LSD, psilocybin, or mescaline) or smokes (dimethyltryptamine) the substance. This stage may consist of visual effects, with an intensification of colors and the appearance of geometric patterns that can be seen with one's eyes closed. This is followed by a plateau phase, where the subjective sense of time begins to slow and the visual effects increase in intensity. The user may experience synesthesia, a crossing-over of sensations (for example, one may "see" sounds and "hear" colors). In addition to the sensory-perceptual effects, hallucinogenic substances may induce feelings of depersonalization, emotional shifts to a euphoric or anxious/fearful state, and a disruption of logical thought. Hallucinogens are classified chemically as either indoleamines (specifically tryptamines), sharing a common structure with serotonin, or as phenethylamines, which share a common structure with norepinephrine. Both classes of these drugs are agonists at the 5-HT$_2$ receptors; this is thought to be the central component of their hallucinogenic properties. Activation of 5-HT$_{2A}$ may be particularly important for hallucinogenic activity. However, repeated exposure to hallucinogens leads to rapid tolerance, likely through down-regulation of these receptors in specific target cells.

Hypnotics

Hypnotics are often used to treat the symptoms of insomnia, or other sleep disorders. Benzodiazepines are still among the most widely prescribed sedative-hypnotics in the United States today. Certain non-benzodiazepine drugs are used as hypnotics as well. Although they lack the chemical structure of the benzodiazepines, their sedative effect is similarly through action on the GABAA receptor. They also have a reputation of being less addictive than benzodiazepines. Melatonin, a naturally-occurring hormone, is often used over the counter (OTC) to treat insomnia and jet lag. This hormone appears to be excreted by the pineal gland early during the sleep cycle and may contribute to human circadian rhythms. Because OTC melatonin supplements are not subject to careful and consistent manufacturing, more specific melatonin agonists are sometimes preferred. They are used for their action on melatonin receptors in the suprachiasmatic nucleus, responsible for sleep-wake cycles. Many barbiturates have or had an FDA-approved indication for use as sed-ative-hypnotics, but have become less widely used because of their limited safety margin in over-dose, their potential for dependence, and the degree of central nervous system depression they induce. The amino-acid L-tryptophan is also available OTC, and seems to be free of dependence or abuse liability. However, it is not as powerful as the traditional hypnotics. Because of the possible role of serotonin in sleep patterns, a new generation of 5-HT$_2$ antagonists are in current develop-ment as hypnotics.

Cannabis and the Cannabinoids

Cannabis consumption produces a dose-dependent state of intoxication in humans. There is com-monly increased blood flow to the skin, which leads to sensations of warmth or flushing, and heart rate is also increased. It also frequently induces increased hunger. Iversen (2000) categorized the subjective and behavioral effects often associated with cannabis into three stages. The first is the "buzz," a brief period of initial responding, where the main effects are lightheadedness or slight dizziness, in addition to possible tingling sensations in the extremities or other parts of the body. The "high" is characterized by feelings of euphoria and exhilaration characterized by mild psychedelia, as well as a sense of disinhibition. If the individual has taken a sufficiently large dose of cannabis, the level of intoxication progresses to the stage of being "stoned," and the user may feel calm, relaxed, and possibly in a dreamlike state. Sensory reactions may include the feeling of floating, enhanced visual and auditory perception, visual illusions, or the perception of the slowing of time passage, which are somewhat psychedelic in nature.

There exist two primary CNS cannabinoid receptors, on which marijuana and the cannabinoids act. Both the CB1 receptor and CB2 receptor are found in the brain. The CB2 receptor is also found in the immune system. CB$_1$ is expressed at high densities in the basal ganglia, cerebellum, hippo-campus, and cerebral cortex. Receptor activation can inhibit cAMP formation, inhibit voltage-sen-sitive calcium ion channels, and activate potassium ion channels. Many CB$_1$ receptors are located on axon terminals, where they act to inhibit the release of various neurotransmitters. In combina-tion, these drug actions work to alter various functions of the central nervous system including the motor system, memory, and various cognitive processes.

Opiates

The opiate drugs, which include drugs like heroin, morphine, and oxycodone, belong to the class of narcotic analgesics, which reduce pain without producing unconsciousness, but do produce a sense of relaxation and sleep, and at high doses, may result in coma and death. The ability of opiates (both endogenous and exogenous) to relieve pain depends on a complex set of neuronal pathways at the spinal cord level, as well as various locations above the spinal cord. Small endor-phin neurons in the spinal cord act on receptors to decrease the conduction of pain signals from the spinal cord to higher brain centers. Descending neurons originating in the periaqueductal gray give rise to two pathways that further block pain signals in the spinal cord. The pathways begin in the locus coeruleus (noradrenaline) and the nucleus of raphe (serotonin). Similar to other abused substances, opiate drugs increase dopamine release in the nucleus accumbens. Opiates are more likely to produce physical dependence than any other class of psychoactive drugs, and can lead to painful withdrawal symptoms if discontinued abruptly after regular use.

Stimulants

Cocaine is one of the more common stimulants, and is a complex drug that interacts with various neurotransmitter systems. It commonly cause heightened alertness, increased confidence, feelings of exhilaration, reduced fatigue, and a generalized sense of well-being. The effects of cocaine are similar to those of the amphetamines, though cocaine tends to have a shorter duration of effect. In high doses and/or with prolonged use, cocaine can result in a number of negative effects as well, including irritability, anxiety, exhaustion, total insomnia, and even psychotic symptomatology. Most of the behavioral and physiological actions of cocaine can be explained by its ability to block the reuptake of the two catecholamines, dopamine and norepinephrine, as well as serotonin. Cocaine binds to transporters that normally clear these transmitters from the synaptic cleft, inhibiting their function. This leads to increased levels of neurotransmitter in the cleft and transmission at the synapses. Based on in-vitro studies using rat brain tissue, cocaine binds most strongly to the serotonin transporter, followed by the dopamine transporter, and then the norepinephrine transporter.

Amphetamines tend to cause the same behavioral and subjective effects of cocaine. Various forms of amphetamine are commonly used to treat the symptoms of attention deficit hyperactivity disorder (ADHD) and narcolepsy, or are used recreationally. Amphetamine and methamphetamine are indirect agonists of the catecholaminergic systems. They block catecholamine reuptake, in addition to releasing catecholamines from nerve terminals. There is evidence that dopamine receptors play a central role in the behavioral responses of animals to cocaine, amphetamines, and other psychostimulant drugs. One action causes the dopamine molecules to be released from inside the vesicles into the cytoplasm of the nerve terminal, which are then transported outside by the mesolimbic dopamine pathway to the nucleus accumbens. This plays a key role in the rewarding and reinforcing effects of cocaine and amphetamine in animals, and is the primary mechanism for amphetamine dependence.

Psychopharmacological Research

In psychopharmacology, researchers are interested in any substance that crosses the blood–brain barrier and thus has an effect on behavior, mood or cognition. Drugs are researched for their physiochemical properties, physical side effects, and psychological side effects. Researchers in psychopharmacology study a variety of different psychoactive substances that include alcohol, cannabinoids, club drugs, psychedelics, opiates, nicotine, caffeine, psychomotor stimulants, inhalants, and anabolic-androgenic steroids. They also study drugs used in the treatment of affective and anxiety disorders, as well as schizophrenia.

Clinical studies are often very specific, typically beginning with animal testing, and ending with human testing. In the human testing phase, there is often a group of subjects, one group is given a placebo, and the other is administered a carefully measured therapeutic dose of the drug in question. After all of the testing is completed, the drug is proposed to the concerned regulatory authority (e.g. the U.S. FDA), and is either commercially introduced to the public via prescription, or deemed safe enough for over the counter sale.

Though particular drugs are prescribed for specific symptoms or syndromes, they are usually not specific to the treatment of any single mental disorder. Because of their ability to modify the behavior of even the most disturbed patients, the antipsychotic, antianxiety, and antidepressant agents have greatly affected the management of the hospitalized mentally ill, enabling hospital staff to devote more of their attention to therapeutic efforts and enabling many patients to lead relatively normal lives outside of the hospital.

A somewhat controversial application of psychopharmacology is "cosmetic psychiatry": persons who do not meet criteria for any psychiatric disorder are nevertheless prescribed psychotropic medication. The antidepressant bupropion is then prescribed to increase perceived energy levels and assertiveness while diminishing the need for sleep. The antihypertensive compound propranolol is sometimes chosen to eliminate the discomfort of day-to-day anxiety. Fluoxetine in nondepressed people can produce a feeling of generalized well-being. Pramipexole, a treatment for restless leg syndrome, can dramatically increase libido in women. These and other off-label lifestyle applications of medications are not uncommon. Although occasionally reported in the medical literature no guidelines for such usage have been developed. There is also a potential for the misuse of prescription psychoactive drugs by elderly persons, who may have multiple drug prescriptions.

Pharmacogenetics

Pharmacogenetics is the study of inherited genetic differences in drug metabolic pathways which can affect individual responses to drugs, both in terms of therapeutic effect as well as adverse effects. The term *pharmacogenetics* is often used interchangeably with the term *pharmacogenomics* which also investigates the role of acquired and inherited genetic differences in relation to drug response and drug behavior through a systematic examination of genes, gene products, and inter- and intra-individual variation in gene expression and function.

In oncology, *pharmacogenetics* historically is the study of germline mutations (e.g., single-nucleotide polymorphisms affecting genes coding for liver enzymes responsible for drug deposition and pharmacokinetics), whereas *pharmacogenomics* refers to somatic mutations in tumoral DNA leading to alteration in drug response (e.g., KRAS mutations in patients treated with anti-Her1 biologics).

Predicting Drug-drug Interactions

Much of current clinical interest is at the level of pharmacogenetics, involving variation in genes involved in drug metabolism with a particular emphasis on improving drug safety. The wider use of pharmacogenetic testing is viewed by many as an outstanding opportunity to improve prescribing safety and efficacy. Driving this trend are the 106,000 deaths and 2.2 Million serious events caused by adverse drug reactions in the US each year. As such ADRs are responsible for 5-7% of hospital admissions in the US and Europe, lead to the withdrawal of 4% of new medicines, and cost society an amount equal to the costs of drug treatment.

Comparisons of the list of drugs most commonly implicated in adverse drug reactions with the list of metabolizing enzymes with known polymorphisms found that drugs commonly involved in adverse drug reactions were also those that were metabolized by enzymes with known polymorphisms.

Scientists and doctors are using this new technology for a variety of things, one being improving the efficacy of drugs. In psychology, we can predict quite accurately which anti-depressant a patient will best respond to by simply looking into their genetic code. This is a huge step from the previous practice of adjusting and experimenting with different medications to get the best response. Antidepressants also have a large percentage of unresponsive patients and poor prediction rate of ADRs (adverse drug reactions). In depressed patients, 30% are not helped by antidepressants. In psychopharmacological therapy, a patient must be on a drug for 2 weeks before the effects can be fully examined and evaluated. For a patient in that 30%, this could mean months of trying medications to find an antidote to their pain. Any assistance in predicting a patient's drug reaction to psychopharmacological therapy should be taken advantage of. Pharmacogenetics is a very useful and important tool in predicting which drugs will be effective in various patients. The drug Plavix blocks platelet reception and is the second best selling prescription drug in the world, however, it is known to warrant different responses among patients. GWAS studies have linked the gene CYP2C19 to those who cannot normally metabolize Plavix. Plavix is given to patients after receiving a stent in the coronary artery to prevent clotting.

Stent clots almost always result in heart attack or sudden death, fortunately it only occurs in 1 or 2% of the population. That 1 or 2% are those with the CYP2C19 SNP. This finding has been applied in at least two hospitals, Scripps and Vanderbilt University, where patients who are candidates for heart stents are screened for the CYP2C19 variants.

Another newfound use of pharmacogenetics involves the use of Vitamin E. The Technion Israel Institute of Technology observed that vitamin E can be used to in certain genotypes to lower the risk of cardiovascular disease in patients with diabetes, but in the same patients with another genotype, vitamin E can raise the risk of cardiovascular disease. A study was carried out, showing vitamin E is able to increase the function of HDL in those with the genotype haptoglobin 2-2 who suffer from diabetes. HDL is a lipoprotein that removes cholesterol from the blood and is associated with a reduced risk of atherosclerosis and heart disease. However, if you have the misfortune to possess the genotype haptoglobin 2-1, the study shows that this same treatment can drastically decrease your HDL function and cause cardiovascular disease.

Pharmacogenetics is a rising concern in clinical oncology, because the therapeutic window of most anticancer drugs is narrow and patients with impaired ability to detoxify drugs will undergo life-threatening toxicities. In particular, genetic deregulations affecting genes coding for DPD, UGT1A1, TPMT, CDA and CYP2D6 are now considered as critical issues for patients treated with 5-FU/capecitabine, irinotecan, mercaptopurine/azathioprine, gemcitabine/capecitabine/AraC and tamoxifen, respectively. The decision to use pharmacogenetic techniques is influenced by the relative costs of genotyping technologies and the cost of providing a treatment to a patient with an incompatible genotype. When available, phenotype-based approaches proved their usefulness while being cost-effective.

In the search for informative correlates of psychotropic drug response, pharmacogenetics has several advantages:

- The genotype of an individual is essentially invariable and remains unaffected by the treatment itself.

- Molecular biology techniques provide an accurate assessment of the genotype of an individual.

- There has been a dramatic increase in the amount of genomic information that is available. This information provides the necessary data for comprehensive studies of individual genes and broad investigation of genome-wide variation.

- The ease of accessibility to genotype information through peripheral blood or saliva sampling and advances in molecular techniques has increased the feasibility of DNA collection and genotyping in large-scale clinical trials.

History

The first observations of genetic variation in drug response date from the 1950s, involving the muscle relaxant suxamethonium chloride, and drugs metabolized by N-acetyltransferase. One in 3500 Caucasians has less efficient variant of the enzyme (butyrylcholinesterase) that metabolizes suxamethonium chloride. As a consequence, the drug's effect is prolonged, with slower recovery from surgical paralysis. Variation in the N-acetyltransferase gene divides people into "slow acetylators" and "fast acetylators", with very different half-lives and blood concentrations of such important drugs as isoniazid (antituberculosis) and procainamide (antiarrhythmic). As part of the inborn system for clearing the body of xenobiotics, the cytochrome P450 oxidases (CYPs) are heavily involved in drug metabolism, and genetic variations in CYPs affect large populations. One member of the CYP superfamily, CYP2D6, now has over 75 known allelic variations, some of which lead to no activity, and some to enhanced activity. An estimated 29% of people in parts of East Africa may have multiple copies of the gene, and will therefore not be adequately treated with standard doses of drugs such as the painkiller codeine (which is activated by the enzyme). The first study using Genome-wide association studies (GWAS) linked age-related macular degeneration (AMD) with a SNP located on chromosome 1 that increased one's risk of AMD. AMD is the most common cause of blindness, affecting more than seven million Americans. Until this study in 2005, we only knew about the inflammation of the retinal tissue causing AMD, not the genes responsible.

Thiopurines and TPMT (Thiopurine Methyl Transferase)

One of the earliest tests for a genetic variation resulting in a clinically important consequence was on the enzyme thiopurine methyltransferase (TPMT). TPMT metabolizes 6-mercaptopurine and azathioprine, two thiopurine drugs used in a range of indications, from childhood leukemia to autoimmune diseases. In people with a deficiency in TPMT activity, thiopurine metabolism must proceed by other pathways, one of which leads to the active thiopurine metabolite that is toxic to the bone marrow at high concentrations. Deficiency of TPMT affects a small proportion of people, though seriously. One in 300 people have two variant alleles and lack TPMT activity; these people need only 6-10% of the standard dose of the drug, and, if treated with the full dose, are at risk of severe bone marrow suppression. For them, genotype predicts clinical outcome, a prerequisite for an effective pharmacogenetic test. In 85-90% of affected people, this deficiency results from one of three common variant alleles. Around 10% of people are heterozygous – they carry one variant allele – and produce a reduced quantity of functional enzyme. Overall, they are at greater risk of adverse effects, although as individuals their genotype is not necessarily predictive of their clinical outcome, which makes the interpretation of a clinical test difficult. Recent research suggests that patients who are heterozygous may have a better response to treatment, which raises whether people who have two wild-type alleles could tolerate a higher therapeutic dose. The US Food and Drug Administration (FDA) have recently deliberated the inclusion of a recommendation for testing for TPMT deficiency to the prescribing information for 6-mercaptopurine and azathioprine. The information previously carried the warning that inherited deficiency of the enzyme could increase the risk of severe bone marrow suppression. It now carries the recommendation that people who develop bone marrow suppression while receiving 6-mercaptopurine or azathioprine be tested for TPMT deficiency.

Hepatitis C

A polymorphism near a human interferon gene is predictive of the effectiveness of an artificial interferon treatment for Hepatitis C. For genotype 1 hepatitis C treated with Pegylated interferon-alpha-2a or Pegylated interferon-alpha-2b (brand names Pegasys or PEG-Intron) combined with ribavirin, it has been shown that genetic polymorphisms near the human IL28B gene, encoding interferon lambda 3, are associated with significant differences in response to the treatment. Genotype 1 hepatitis C patients carrying certain genetic variant alleles near the IL28B gene are more probable to achieve sustained virological response after the treatment than others, and demonstrated that the same genetic variants are also associated with the natural clearance of the genotype 1 hepatitis C virus.

Integrating into the Health Care System

Despite the many successes, most drugs are not tested using GWAS. However, it is estimated that over 25% of common medication have some type of genetic information that could be used in the medical field. If the use of personalized medicine is widely adopted and used, it will make medical trials more efficient. This will lower the costs that come about due to adverse drug side effects and prescription of drugs that have been proven ineffective in certain genotypes. It is very costly when a clinical trial is put to a stop by licensing authorities because of the small population who experiences adverse drug reactions. With the new push for pharmacogenetics, it is possible to develop and license a drug specifically intended for those who are the small population genetically at risk for adverse side effects.

The ability to test and analyze an individual's DNA to determine if the body can break down certain drugs through the biochemical pathways has application in all fields of medicine. Pharmacogenetics gives those in the health care industry a potential solution to help prevent the significant amount of deaths that occur each year due to drug reactions and side effects. The companies or laboratories that perform this testing can do so acrossed all categories or drugs whether it be for high blood pressure, gastrointestinal, urological, psychotropic or anti-anxiety drugs. Results can be presented showing which drugs the body is capable of breaking down normally versus the drugs the body cannot break down normally. This test only needs to be done once and can provide valuable information such as a summary of an individual's genetic polymorphisms, which could help in a situation such as being a patient in the emergency room.

Technological Advances

As the cost per genetic test decreases, the development of personalized drug therapies will increase. Technology now allows for genetic analysis of hundreds of target genes involved in medication metabolism and response in less than 24 hours for under $1,000. This a huge step towards bringing pharmacogenetic technology into everyday medical decisions. Likewise, companies like deCODE genetics, Navigenics and 23andMe offer genome scans. The companies use the same genotyping chips that are used in GWAS studies and provide customers with a write-up of individual risk for various traits and diseases and testing for 500,000 known SNPs. Costs range from $995 to $2500 and include updates with new data from studies as they become available. The more expensive packages even included a telephone session with a genetics counselor to discuss the results.

Ethics

Pharmacogenetics has become a controversial issue in the area of bioethics. It's a new topic to the medical field, as well as the public. This new technique will have a huge impact on society, influencing the treatment of both common and rare diseases. As a new topic in the medical field the ethics behind it are still not clear. However, ethical issues and their possible solutions are already being addressed.

There are three main ethical issues that have risen from pharmacogenetics. First, would there be a type equity at both drug development and the accessibility to tests. The concern of accessibility to the test is whether it is going to be available directly to patients via the internet, or over the counter. The second concern regards the confidentiality of storage and usage of genetic information. Thirdly, would patients have the control over being tested.

One concern that has risen is the ethical decision health providers must take with respect to educating the patient of the risks and benefits of medicine developed by this new technology. Pharmacogenetics is a new process that may increase the benefits of medicine while decreasing the risk. However clinicians have been unsuccessful in educating patients regarding the concept of benefits over risk. The Nuffield Council reported that patients and health professionals have adequate information about pharmacogenetics tests and medicine. Health care providers will also encounter an ethical decision in deciding to tell their patients that only certain individuals will benefit from the new medicine due to their genetic make-up. Another ethical concern is that patients who have not taken the test be able to have access to this type of medicine. If access is given by the doctor the medicine could negatively impact the patient's health. The ethical issues behind pharmacogenetics tests, as well as medicine, are still a concern and policies will need to be implemented in the future.

Pharmacogenomics

Pharmacogenomics is the study of the role of the genome in drug response. Its name (*pharmaco-* + *genomics*) reflects its combining of pharmacology and genomics. Pharmacogenomics can be defined as the technology that analyzes how the genetic makeup of an individual affects his/her response to drugs. It deals with the influence of acquired and inherited genetic variation on drug response in patients by correlating gene expression or single-nucleotide polymorphisms with pharmacokinetics and pharmacodynamics (drug absorption, distribution, metabolism, and elimination), as well as drug receptor target effects. The term *pharmacogenomics* is often used interchangeably with *pharmacogenetics*. Although both terms relate to drug response based on genetic influences, pharmacogenetics focuses on single drug-gene interactions, while pharmacogenomics encompasses a more genome-wide association approach, incorporating genomics and epigenetics while dealing with the effects of multiple genes on drug response.

Pharmacogenomics aims to develop rational means to optimize drug therapy, with respect to the patients' genotype, to ensure maximum efficacy with minimal adverse effects. Through the utilization of pharmacogenomics, it is hoped that pharmaceutical drug treatments can deviate from what is dubbed as the "one-dose-fits-all" approach. It attempts to eliminate the trial-and-error method of prescribing, allowing physicians to take into consideration their patient's genes, the functionality of these genes, and how this may affect the efficacy of the patient's current or future treatments (and where applicable, provide an explanation for the failure of past treatments). Such approaches promise the advent of precision medicine and even personalized medicine, in which drugs and drug combinations are optimized for narrow subsets of patients or even for each individual's unique genetic makeup. Whether used to explain a patient's response or lack thereof to a treatment, or act as a predictive tool, it hopes to achieve better treatment outcomes, greater efficacy, minimization of the occurrence of drug toxicities and adverse drug reactions (ADRs). For patients who have lack of therapeutic response to a treatment, alternative therapies can be prescribed that would best suit their requirements. In order to provide pharmacogenomic recommendations for a given drug, two possible types of input can be used: genotyping or exome or whole genome sequencing. Sequencing provides many more data points, including detection of mutations that prematurely terminate the synthesized protein (early stop codon).

History

Pharmacogenomics was first recognized by Pythagoras around 510 BC when he made a connection between the dangers of fava bean ingestion with hemolytic anemia and oxidative stress. Interestingly, this identification was later validated and attributed to deficiency of G6PD in the 1950s and called favism. Although the first official publication dates back to 1961, circa 1950s marked the unofficial beginnings of this science. Reports of prolonged paralysis and fatal reactions linked to genetic variants in patients who lacked butyryl-cholinesterase ('pseudocholinesterase') following administration of succinylcholine injection during anesthesia were first reported in 1956. The term pharmacogenetic was first coined in 1959 by Friedrich Vogel of Heidelberg, Germany (although some papers suggest it was 1957). In the late 1960s, twin studies supported the inference of genetic involvement in drug metabolism, with identical twins sharing remarkable similarities to drug response compared to fraternity twins. The term pharmacogenomics first began appearing around the 1990s.

The first FDA approval of a pharmacogenetic test was in 2005 (for alleles in CYP2D6 and CYP2C19).

Drug-metabolizing Enzymes

There are several known genes which are largely responsible for variances in drug metabolism and response. The focus of this article will remain on the genes that are more widely accepted and utilized clinically for brevity.

- Cytochrome P450s
- VKORC1

- TPMT

Cytochrome P450

The most prevalent drug-metabolizing enzymes (DME) are the Cytochrome P450 (CYP) enzymes. The term Cytochrome P450 was coined by Omura and Sato in 1962 to describe the membrane-bound, heme-containing protein characterized by 450 nm spectral peak when complexed with carbon monoxide. The human CYP family consists of 57 genes, with 18 families and 44 subfamilies. CYP proteins are conveniently arranged into these families and subfamilies on the basis of similarities identified between the amino acid sequences. Enzymes that share 35-40% identity are assigned to the same family by an Arabic numeral, and those that share 55-70% make up a particular subfamily with a designated letter. For example, CYP2D6 refers to family 2, subfamily D, and gene number 6.

From a clinical perspective, the most commonly tested CYPs include: CYP2D6, CYP2C19, CYP2C9, CYP3A4 and CYP3A5. These genes account for the metabolism of approximately 80-90% of currently available prescription drugs. The table below provides a summary for some of the medications that take these pathways.

Drug Metabolism of Major CYPs		
Enzyme	**Fraction of drug metabolism (%)**	**Example Drugs**
CYP2C9	10	Tolbutamide, ibuprofen, mefenamic acid, tetrahydrocannabinol, losartan, diclofenac
CYP2C19	5	S-mephenytoin, amitriptyline, diazepam, omeprazole, proguanil, hexobarbital, propranolol, imipramine
CYP2D6	20-30	Debrisoquine, metoprolol, sparteine, propranolol, encainide, codeine, dextromethorphan, clozapine, desipramine, haloperidol, amitriptyline, imipramine
CYP3A4	40-45	Erythromycin, ethinyl estradiol, nifedipine, triazolam, cyclosporine, amitriptyline, imipramine
CYP3A5	<1	Erythromycin, ethinyl estradiol, nifedipine, triazolam, cyclosporine, amitriptyline, aldosterone

CYP2D6

Also known as debrisoquine hydroxylase (named after the drug that led to its discovery), CYP2D6 is the most well-known and extensively studied CYP gene. It is a gene of great interest also due to its highly polymorphic nature, and involvement in a high number of medication metabolisms (both as a major and minor pathway). More than 100 CYP2D6 genetic variants have been identified.

CYP2C19

Discovered in the early 1980s, CYP2C19 is the second most extensively studied and well understood gene in pharmacogenomics. Over 28 genetic variants have been identified for CYP2C19, of which affects the metabolism of several classes of drugs, such as antidepressants and proton pump inhibitors.

CYP2C9

CYP2C9 constitutes the majority of the CYP2C subfamily, representing approximately 20% of the liver content. It is involved in the metabolism of approximately 10% of all drugs, which include medications with narrow therapeutic windows such as warfarin and tolbutamide. There are approximately 57 genetic variants associated with CYP2C9.

CYP3A4 and CYP3A5

The CYP3A family is the most abundantly found in the liver, with CYP3A4 accounting for 29% of the liver content. These enzymes also cover between 40-50% of the current prescription drugs, with the CYP3A4 accounting for 40-45% of these medications. CYP3A5 has over 11 genetic variants identified at the time of this publication.

VKORC1

The vitamin K epoxide reductase complex subunit 1 (VKORC1) is responsible for the pharmacodynamics of warfarin. VKORC1 along with CYP2C9 are useful for identifying the risk of bleeding during warfarin administration. Warfarin works by inhibiting VKOR, which is encoded by the VKORC1 gene. Individuals with polymorphism in this have an affected response to warfarin treatment.

TPMT

Thiopurine methyltransferase (TPMT) catalyzes the S-methylation of thiopurines, thereby regulating the balance between cytotoxic thioguanine nucleotide and inactive metabolites in hematopoietic cells. TPMT is highly involved in 6-MP metabolism and TMPT activity and TPMT genotype is known to affect the risk of toxicity. Excessive levels of 6-MP can cause myelosuppression and myelotoxicity.

Codeine, clopidogrel, tamoxifen, and warfarin a few examples of medications that follow the above metabolic pathways.

Predictive Prescribing

Patient genotypes are usually categorized into the following predicted phenotypes:

- Ultra-Rapid Metabolizer: Patients with substantially increased metabolic activity.

- Extensive Metabolizer: Normal metabolic activity;

- Intermediate Metabolizer: Patients with reduced metabolic activity; and

- Poor Metabolizer: Patients with little to no functional metabolic activity.

The two extremes of this spectrum are the Poor Metabolizers and Ultra-Rapid Metabolizers. Efficacy of a medication is not only based on the above metabolic statuses, but also the type of drug consumed. Drugs can be classified into two main groups: active drugs and prodrugs. Active drugs refer to drugs that are inactivated during metabolism, and prodrugs are inactive until they are metabolized.

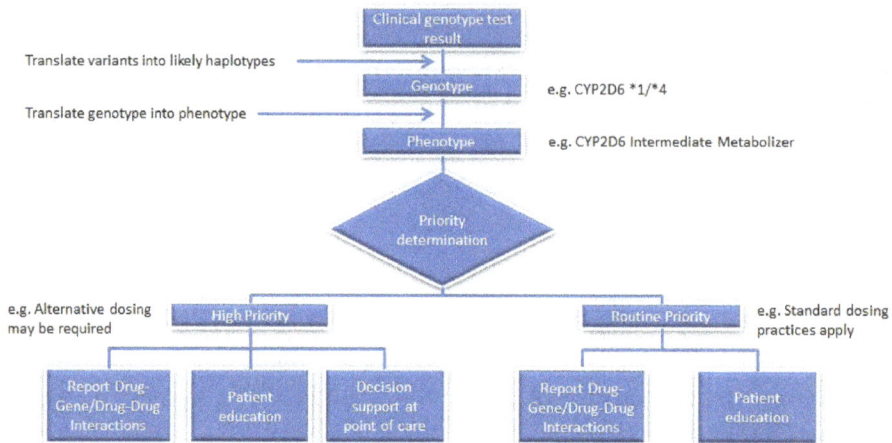

An overall process of how pharmacogenomics functions in a clinical practice. From the raw genotype results, this is then translated to the physical trait, the phenotype. Based on these observations, optimal dosing is evaluated.

For example, we have two patients who are taking codeine for pain relief. Codeine is a prodrug, so it requires conversion from its inactive form to its active form. The active form of codeine is morphine, which provides the therapeutic effect of pain relief. If person A receives one *1 allele each from mother and father to code for the CYP2D6 gene, then that person is considered to have an extensive metabolizer (EM) phenotype, as allele *1 is considered to have a normal-function (this would be represented as CYP2D6 *1/*1). If person B on the other hand had received one *1 allele from the mother and a *4 allele from the father, that individual would be an Intermediate Metabolizer (IM) (the genotype would be CYP2D6 *1/*4). Although both individuals are taking the same dose of codeine, person B could potentially lack the therapeutic benefits of codeine due to the decreased conversion rate of codeine to its active counterpart morphine.

Each phenotype is based upon the allelic variation within the individual genotype. However, several genetic events can influence a same phenotypic trait, and establishing genotype-to-phenotype relationships can thus be far from consensual with many enzymatic patterns. For instance, the influence of the CYP2D6*1/*4 allelic variant on the clinical outcome in patients treated with Tamoxifen remains debated today. In oncology, genes coding for DPD, UGT1A1, TPMT, CDA involved in the pharmacokinetics of 5-FU/capecitabine, irinotecan, 6-mercaptopurine and gemcitabine/cytarabine, respectively, have all been described as being highly polymorphic. A strong body of evidence suggests that patients affected by these genetic polymorphisms will experience severe/lethal toxicities upon drug intake, and that pre-therapeutic screening does help to reduce the risk of treatment-related toxicities through adaptive dosing strategies.

Applications

The list below provides a few more commonly known applications of pharmacogenomics:

- Improve drug safety, and reduce ADRs;

- Tailor treatments to meet patients' unique genetic pre-disposition, identifying optimal dosing;

- Improve drug discovery targeted to human disease; and

- Improve proof of principle for efficacy trials.

Pharmacogenomics may be applied to several areas of medicine, including Pain Management, Cardiology, Oncology, and Psychiatry. A place may also exist in Forensic Pathology, in which pharmacogenomics can be used to determine the cause of death in drug-related deaths where no findings emerge using autopsy.

In cancer treatment, pharmacogenomics tests are used to identify which patients are most likely to respond to certain cancer drugs. In behavioral health, pharmacogenomic tests provide tools for physicians and care givers to better manage medication selection and side effect amelioration. Pharmacogenomics is also known as companion diagnostics, meaning tests being bundled with drugs. Examples include KRAS test with cetuximab and EGFR test with gefitinib. Beside efficacy, germline pharmacogenetics can help to identify patients likely to undergo severe toxicities when given cytotoxics showing impaired detoxification in relation with genetic polymorphism, such as canonical 5-FU.

In cardiovascular disorders, the main concern is response to drugs including warfarin, clopidogrel, beta blockers, and statins.

Example Case Studies

Case A – Antipsychotic adverse reaction

Patient A suffers from schizophrenia. Their treatment included a combination of ziprasidone, olanzapine, trazodone and benzotropine. The patient experienced dizziness and sedation, so they were tapered off ziprasidone and olanzapine, and transition to quetiapine. Trazodone was discontinued. The patient then experienced excessive sweating, tachycardia and neck pain, gained considerable weight and had hallucinations. Five months later, quetiapine was tapered and discontinued, with ziprasidone re-introduction into their treatment due to the excessive weight gain. Although the patient lost the excessive weight they gained, they then developed muscle stiffness, cogwheeling, tremor and night sweats. When benztropine was added they experienced blurry vision. After an additional five months, the patient was switched from ziprasidone to aripiprazole. Over the course of 8 months, patient A gradually experienced more weight gain, sedation, developed difficulty with their gait, stiffness, cogwheel and dyskinetic ocular movements. A pharmacogenomics test later proved the patient had a CYP2D6 *1/*41, with has a predicted phenotype of IM and CYP2C19 *1/*2 with predicted phenotype of IM as well.

Case B – Pain Management

Patient B is a woman who gave birth by caesarian section. Her physician prescribed codeine for post-caesarian pain. She took the standard prescribed dose, however experienced nausea and dizziness while she was taking codeine. She also noticed that her breastfed infant was lethargic and feeding poorly. When the patient mentioned these symptoms to her physician, they recommended that she discontinue codeine use. Within a few days, both the patient and her infant's symptoms were no longer present. It is assumed that if the patient underwent a pharmacogenomic test, it would have revealed she may have had a duplication of the gene CYP2D6 placing her in the Ultra-rapid metabolizer (UM) category, explaining her ADRs to codeine use.

Case C – FDA Warning on Codeine Overdose for Infants

On February 20, 2013, the FDA released a statement addressing a serious concern regarding the connection between children who are known as CYP2D6 UM and fatal reactions to codeine following tonsillectomy and/or adenoidectomy (surgery to remove the tonsils and/or adenoids). They released their strongest Boxed Warning to elucidate the dangers of CYP2D6 UMs consuming codeine. Codeine is converted to morphine by CYP2D6, and those who have UM phenotypes are at danger of producing large amounts of morphine due to the increased function of the gene. The morphine can elevate to life-threatening or fatal amounts, as became evident with the death of three children in August 2012.

Polypharmacy

A potential role pharmacogenomics may play would be to reduce the occurrence of polypharmacy. It is theorized that with tailored drug treatments, patients will not have the need to take several medications that are intended to treat the same condition. In doing so, they could potentially minimize the occurrence of ADRs, have improved treatment outcomes, and can save costs by avoiding purchasing extraneous medications. An example of this can be found in Psychiatry, where patients tend to be receiving more medications than even age-matched non-psychiatric patients. This has been associated with an increased risk of inappropriate prescribing.

The need for pharmacogenomics tailored drug therapies may be most evident in a survey conducted by the Slone Epidemiology Center at Boston University from February 1998 to April 2007. The study elucidated that an average of 82% of adults in the United States are taking at least one medication (prescription or nonprescription drug, vitamin/mineral, herbal/natural supplement), and 29% are taking five or more. The study suggested that those aged 65 years or older continue to be the biggest consumers of medications, with 17-19 % in this age group taking at least ten medications in a given week. Polypharmacy has also shown to have increased since 2000 from 23% to 29%.

Drug Labeling

The U.S. Food and Drug Administration (FDA) appears to be very invested in the science of pharmacogenomics as is demonstrated through the 120 and more FDA-approved drugs that include pharmacogenomic biomarkers in their labels. On May 22, 2005, the FDA issued its first *Guidance for Industry: Pharmacogenomic Data Submissions*, which clarified the type of pharmacogenomic data required to be submitted to the FDA and when. Experts recognized the importance of the FDA's acknowledgement that pharmacogenomics experiments will not bring negative regulatory consequences. The FDA had released its latest guide *Clinical Pharmacogenomics (PGx): Premarket Evaluation in Early-Phase Clinical Studies and Recommendations for Labeling* in January, 2013. The guide is intended to address the use of genomic information during drug development and regulatory review processes.

Challenges

Although there appears to be a general acceptance of the basic tenet of pharmacogenomics amongst physicians and healthcare professionals, several challenges exist that slow the uptake, implementation, and standardization of pharmacogenomics. Some of the concerns raised by physicians include:

- Limitation on how to apply the test into clinical practices and treatment;

- A general feeling of lack of availability of the test;

- The understanding and interpretation of evidence-based research; and

- Ethical, legal and social issues.

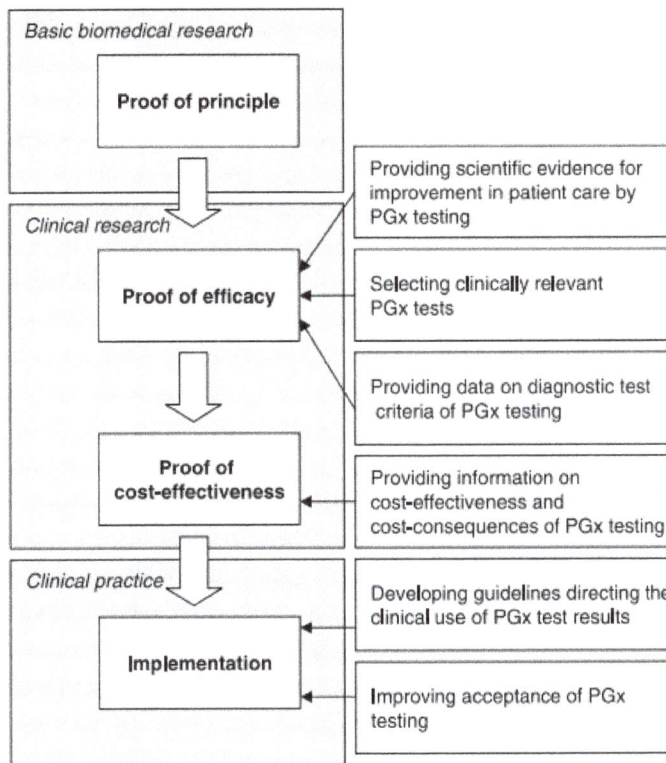

Consecutive phases and associated challenges in Pharmacogenomics.

Issues surrounding the availability of the test include:

- *The lack of availability of scientific data*: Although there are considerable number of DME involved in the metabolic pathways of drugs, only a fraction have sufficient scientific data to validate their use within a clinical setting; and

- *Demonstrating the cost-effectiveness of pharmacogenomics*: Publications for the pharmacoeconomics of pharmacogenomics are scarce, therefore sufficient evidence does not at this time exist to validate the cost-effectiveness and cost-consequences of the test.

Although other factors contribute to the slow progression of pharmacogenomics (such as developing guidelines for clinical use), the above factors appear to be the most prevalent.

Controversies

Some alleles that vary in frequency between specific populations have been shown to be associated with differential responses to specific drugs. The beta blocker atenolol is an anti-hypertensive medication that is shown to more significantly lower the blood pressure of Caucasian patients than

African American patients in the United States. This observation suggests that Caucasian and African American populations have different alleles governing oleic acid biochemistry, which react differentially with atenolol. Similarly, hypersensitivity to the antiretroviral drug abacavir is strongly associated with a single-nucleotide polymorphism that varies in frequency between populations.

The FDA approval of the drug BiDil (isosorbide dinitrate/hydralazine) with a label specifying African-Americans with congestive heart failure, produced a storm of controversy over race-based medicine and fears of genetic stereotyping, even though the label for BiDil did not specify any genetic variants but was based on racial self-identification.

Future

Computational advances in pharmacogenomics has proven to be a blessing in research. As a simple example, for nearly a decade the ability to store more information on a hard drive has enabled us to investigate a human genome sequence cheaper and in more detail with regards to the effects/risks/safety concerns of drugs and other such substances. Such computational advances are expected to continue in the future. The aim is to use the genome sequence data to effectively make decisions in order to minimise the negative impacts on, say, a patient or the health industry in general. A large amount of research in the biomedical sciences regarding Pharmacogenomics as of late stems from combinatorial chemistry, genomic mining, omic technologies and high throughput screening. In order for the field to grow, rich knowledge enterprises and business must work more closely together and adopt simulation strategies. Consequently, more importance must be placed on the role of computational biology with regards to safety and risk assessments. Here, we can find the growing need and importance of being able to manage large, complex data sets, being able to extract information by integrating disparate data so that developments can be made in improving human health.

Pharmacoepidemiology

Pharmacoepidemiology is the study of the uses and effects of drugs in well defined populations.

To accomplish this study, pharmacoepidemiology borrows from both pharmacology and epidemiology. Thus, pharmacoepidemiology is the bridge between both pharmacology and epidemiology. Pharmacology is the study of the effect of drugs and clinical pharmacology is the study of effect of drugs on clinical humans. Part of the task of clinical pharmacology is to provide a risk benefit assessment by effects of drugs in patients:

- doing the studies needed to provide an estimate of the probability of beneficial effects on populations,

- or assessing the probability of adverse effects on populations.

Other parameters relating to drug use may benefit epidemiological methodology. Pharmacoepidemiology then can also be defined as the transparent application of epidemiological methods through pharmacological treatment of conditions to better understand the conditions to be treated.

Epidemiology is the study of the distribution and determinants of diseases and other health states in populations. Epidemiological studies can be divided into two main types:

1. Descriptive epidemiology describes disease and/or exposure and may consist of calculating rates, e.g., incidence and prevalence. Such descriptive studies do not at this time use health control groups and can only generate hypotheses,but not test them. Studies of drug use would generally fall under descriptive studies.

2. Analytic epidemiology includes two types of studies: observational studies, such as case-control and cohort studies, and experimental studies which include clinical trials or randomized clinical trials. The analytic studies compare an exposed group with a control group and usually designed as hypothesis testing by studies.

Pharmacoepidemiology benefits from the methodology developed in general epidemiology and may further develop them for applications of methodology unique to needs of pharmacoepidemiology. There are also some areas that are altogether unique to pharmacoepidemiology, e.g., pharmacovigilance. Pharmacovigilance is a type of continual monitoring of unwanted effects and other safety-related aspects of drugs that are already placed in current growing integrating markets. In practice, pharmacovigilance refers almost exclusively to spontaneous reporting systems which allow health care professionals and others to report adverse drug reactions to the central agency. The central agency combines reports from many sources to produce a more informative profile for drug products than could be done based on reports from fewer health care professionals.

Toxicology

Toxicology is a branch of biology, chemistry, and medicine (more specifically pharmacology) concerned with the study of the adverse effects of chemicals on living organisms. It also studies the harmful effects of chemical, biological and physical agents in biological systems that establishes the extent of damage in living organisms. The relationship between dose and its effects on the exposed organism is of high significance in toxicology. Factors that influence chemical toxicity include the dosage (and whether it is acute or chronic); the route of exposure, the species, age, sex and environment.

History

Dioscorides, a Greek physician in the court of the Roman emperor Nero, made the first attempt to classify plants according to their toxic and therapeutic effect. Ibn Wahshiyya wrote the *Book on Poisons* in the 9th or 10th century. This was followed up in 1360 by Khagendra Mani Darpana.

Mathieu Orfila is considered the modern father of toxicology, having given the subject its first formal treatment in 1813 in his *Traité des poisons*, also called *Toxicologie générale*.

In 1850, Jean Stas became the first person to successfully isolate plant poisons from human tissue. This allowed him to identify the use of nicotine as a poison in the famous Bocarmé murder case, providing the evidence needed to convict the Belgian Count Hippolyte Visart de Bocarmé of killing his brother-in-law.

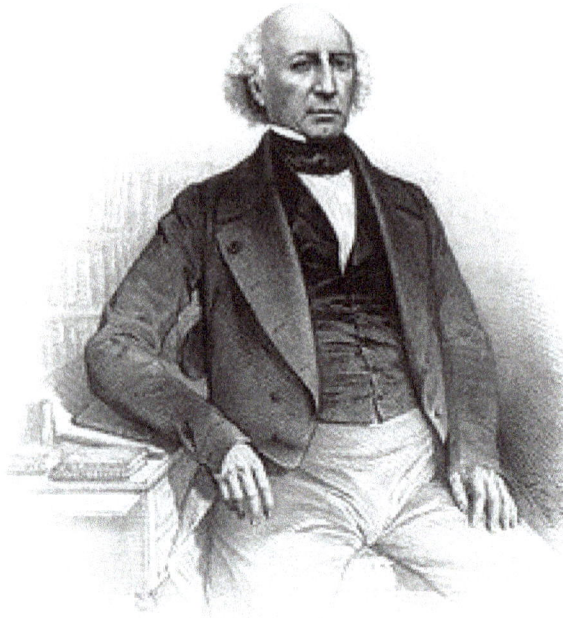

Lithograph of Mathieu Orfila

Theophrastus Phillipus Auroleus Bombastus von Hohenheim (1493–1541) (also referred to as Paracelsus, from his belief that his studies were above or beyond the work of Celsus – a Roman physician from the first century) is also considered «the father» of toxicology. He is credited with the classic toxicology maxim, "*Alle Dinge sind Gift und nichts ist ohne Gift; allein die Dosis macht, dass ein Ding kein Gift ist.*" which translates as, "All things are poisonous and nothing is without poison; only the dose makes a thing not poisonous." This is often condensed to: "The dose makes the poison" or in Latin "Sola dosis facit venenum".

Basic Toxicology

The goal of toxicity assessment is to identify adverse effects of a substance. Adverse effects depend on two main factors: i) routes of exposure (oral, inhalation, or dermal) and ii) dose (duration and concentration of exposure). To explore dose, substances are tested in both acute and chronic models. Generally, different sets of experiments are conducted to determine whether a substance causes cancer and to examine other forms of toxicity.

Factors that influence chemical toxicity:

- Dosage
  - Both large single exposures (acute) and continuous small exposures (chronic) are studied.
- Route of exposure
  - Ingestion, inhalation or skin absorption
- Other factors
  - Species

- Age
- Sex
- Health
- Environment
- Individual characteristics

Testing Methods

Toxicity experiments may be conducted *in vivo* (using the whole animal) or *in vitro* (testing on isolated cells or tissues), or *in silico* (in a computer simulation).

Non-human Animals

The classic experimental tool of toxicology is testing on non-human animals. As of 2014, such animal testing provides information that is not available by other means about how substances function in a living organism.

Alternative Testing Methods

While testing in animal models remains as a method of estimating human effects, there are both ethical and technical concerns with animal testing.

Since the late 1950s, the field of toxicology has sought to reduce or eliminate animal testing under the rubric of "Three Rs" - reduce the number of experiments with animals to the minimum necessary; refine experiments to cause less suffering, and replace *in vivo* experiments with other types, or use more simple forms of life when possible.

Computer modeling is an example of alternative testing methods; using computer models of chemicals and proteins, structure-activity relationships can be determined, and chemical structures that are likely to bind to, and interfere with, proteins with essential functions, can be identified. This work requires expert knowledge in molecular modeling and statistics together with expert judgment in chemistry, biology and toxicology.

In 2007 the National Academy of Sciences published a report called "Toxicity Testing in the 21st Century: A Vision and a Strategy" which opened with a statement: "Change often involves a pivotal event that builds on previous history and opens the door to a new era. Pivotal events in science include the discovery of penicillin, the elucidation of the DNA double helix, and the development of computers. ...Toxicity testing is approaching such a scientific pivot point. It is poised to take advantage of the revolutions in biology and biotechnology. Advances in toxicogenomics, bioinformatics, systems biology, epigenetics, and computational toxicology could transform toxicity testing from a system based on whole-animal testing to one founded primarily on in vitro methods that evaluate changes in biologic processes using cells, cell lines, or cellular components, preferably of human origin." As of 2010 that vision was still unrealized. As of 2014 that vision was still unrealized.

In some cases shifts away from animal studies has been mandated by law or regulation; the European Union (EU) prohibited use of animal testing for cosmetics in 2013.

Dose Response Complexities

Most chemicals display a classic dose response curve – at a low dose (below a threshold), no effect is observed. Some show a phenomenon known as sufficient challenge – a small exposure produces animals that "grow more rapidly, have better general appearance and coat quality, have fewer tumors, and live longer than the control animals". A few chemicals have no well-defined safe level of exposure. These are treated with special care. Some chemicals are subject to bioaccumulation as they are stored in rather than being excreted from the body; these also receive special consideration.

Computational Toxicology

Computational toxicology is a discipline that develops mathematical and computer-based models to better understand and predict adverse health effects caused by chemicals, such as environmental pollutants and pharmaceuticals. Within the *Toxicology in the 21st Century* project, the best predictive models were identified to be Deep Neural Networks, Random Forest, and Support Vector Machines, which can reach the performance of in vitro experiments.

Toxicology as a Profession

A toxicologist is a scientist or medical personnel who specializes in the study of symptoms, mechanisms, treatments and detection of venoms and toxins; especially the poisoning of people. To work as a toxicologist one should obtain a degree in toxicology or a related degree like biology, chemistry or biochemistry. Toxicologists perform many different duties including research in the academic, nonprofit and industrial fields, product safety evaluation, consulting, public service and legal regulation.

Requirements

To work as a toxicologist one should obtain a degree in toxicology or a related degree like biology, chemistry or biochemistry. Bachelor's degree programs in toxicology cover the chemical makeup of toxins and their effects on biochemistry, physiology and ecology. After introductory life science courses are complete, students typically enroll in labs and apply toxicology principles to research and other studies. Advanced students delve into specific sectors, like the pharmaceutical industry or law enforcement, which apply methods of toxicology in their work. The Society of Toxicology (SOT) recommends that undergraduates in postsecondary schools that don't offer a bachelor's degree in toxicology consider attaining a degree in biology or chemistry. Additionally, the SOT advises aspiring toxicologists to take statistics and mathematics courses, as well as gain laboratory experience through lab courses, student research projects and internships.

Duties

Toxicologists perform many more duties including research in the academic, nonprofit and industrial fields, product safety evaluation, consulting, public service and legal regulation. In order to research and assess the effects of chemicals, toxicologists perform carefully designed studies and experiments. These experiments help identify the specific amount of a chemical that may cause harm and potential risks of being near or using products that contain certain chemicals. Research projects may range from assessing the effects of toxic pollutants on the environment to evaluating how the human immune system responds to chemical compounds within pharmaceutical drugs. While the basic duties of toxicologists are to determine the effects of chemicals on organisms and their surroundings, specific job duties may vary based on industry and employment. For example, forensic toxicologists may look for toxic substances in a crime scene, whereas aquatic toxicologists may analyze the toxicity level of wastewater.

Compensation

The salary for jobs in toxicology is dependent on several factors, including level of schooling, specialization, experience. The U.S. Bureau of Labor Statistics (BLS) notes that jobs for biological scientists, which generally include toxicologists, were expected to increase by 21% between 2008 and 2018. The BLS notes that this increase could be due to research and development growth in biotechnology, as well as budget increases for basic and medical research in biological science.

References

- Meyer, J.S.; Quenzer, L.F. (2005). Psychopharmacology: Drugs, The Brain, and Behavior. Sunderland, MA: Sinauer Associates. ISBN 0-87893-534-7.

- Schatzberg, A.F. (2010). Manual of Clinical Psychopharmacology. Washington, DC: American Psychiatric Publishing Inc. ISBN 978-1-58562-377-8.

- The Creative Destruction of Medicine: How the Digital Revolution Will Create Better Health Care. New York: Basic Books. 2012. ISBN 0-465-02550-1.

- Cohen, Nadine (November 2008). Pharmacogenomics and Personalized Medicine (Methods in Pharmacology and Toxicology). Totowa, NJ: Humana Press. p. 6. ISBN 978-1934115046.

- Ritsner, Michael (2013). Polypharmacy in Psychiatry Practice, Volume I. Multiple Medication Strategies. Dordrecht: Springer Science and Business Media. ISBN 978-94-007-5804-9.

- Barh, Debmalya; Dhawan, Dipali; Ganguly, Nirmal Kumar (2013). Omics for Personalized Medicine. India: Springer Media. doi:10.1007/978-81-322-1184-6. ISBN 978-81-322-1183-9.

- Stram, Daniel (2014). Design, Analysis, and Interpretation of Genome-Wide Association Scans. Los Angeles: Springer Science and Business Media. doi:10.1007/978-1-4614-9443-0_8. ISBN 978-1-4614-9442-3.

- Ottoboni, M. Alice (1991). The dose makes the poison : a plain-language guide to toxicology (2nd ed.). New York, N.Y: Van Nostrand Reinhold. ISBN 0-442-00660-8.

- Leeuwen van.C.J.; Vermeire T.G. (2007). Risk assessment of chemicals: An introduction. New York: Springer. pp. 451–479. ISBN 978-1-4020-6102-8.

3

Drug: Design, Discovery and Development

Drug design is the process of finding new medicines. It involves the design of molecules that are complementary in shape and charge. The features elucidated in the chapter are drug discovery, new chemical entity, high-throughput screening, drug development, pre-clinical development, clinical trial etc. This chapter provides a plethora of interdisciplinary topics for a better comprehension on the topic of drugs.

Drug Design

Drug design, often referred to as rational drug design or simply rational design, is the inventive process of finding new medications based on the knowledge of a biological target. The drug is most commonly an organic small molecule that activates or inhibits the function of a biomolecule such as a protein, which in turn results in a therapeutic benefit to the patient. In the most basic sense, drug design involves the design of molecules that are complementary in shape and charge to the biomolecular target with which they interact and therefore will bind to it. Drug design frequently but not necessarily relies on computer modeling techniques. This type of modeling is sometimes referred to as computer-aided drug design. Finally, drug design that relies on the knowledge of the three-dimensional structure of the biomolecular target is known as structure-based drug design. In addition to small molecules, biopharmaceuticals and especially therapeutic antibodies are an increasingly important class of drugs and computational methods for improving the affinity, selectivity, and stability of these protein-based therapeutics have also been developed.

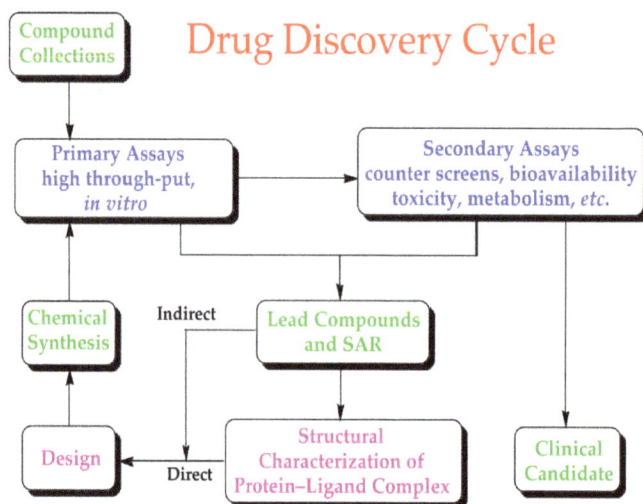

Drug Discovery Cycle

Compound Collections → Primary Assays high through-put, *in vitro* → Secondary Assays counter screens, bioavailability toxicity, metabolism, *etc.*

Chemical Synthesis — Indirect — Lead Compounds and SAR

Design ← Direct — Structural Characterization of Protein–Ligand Complex → Clinical Candidate

The phrase "drug design" is to some extent a misnomer. A more accurate term is ligand design (i.e., design of a molecule that will bind tightly to its target). Although design techniques for prediction of binding affinity are reasonably successful, there are many other properties, such as bioavailability, metabolic half-life, side effects, etc., that first must be optimized before a ligand can become a safe and efficacious drug. These other characteristics are often difficult to predict with rational design techniques. Nevertheless, due to high attrition rates, especially during clinical phases of drug development, more attention is being focused early in the drug design process on selecting candidate drugs whose physicochemical properties are predicted to result in fewer complications during development and hence more likely to lead to an approved, marketed drug. Furthermore, in vitro experiments complemented with computation methods are increasingly used in early drug discovery to select compounds with more favorable ADME (absorption, distribution, metabolism, and excretion) and toxicological profiles.

Drug Targets

A biomolecular target (most commonly a protein or nucleic acid) is a key molecule involved in a particular metabolic or signaling pathway that is associated with a specific disease condition or pathology or to the infectivity or survival of a microbial pathogen. Potential drug targets are not necessarily disease causing but must by definition be disease modifying. In some cases, small molecules will be designed to enhance or inhibit the target function in the specific disease modifying pathway. Small molecules (for example receptor agonists, antagonists, inverse agonists, or modulators; enzyme activators or inhibitors; or ion channel openers or blockers) will be designed that are complementary to the binding site of target. Small molecules (drugs) can be designed so as not to affect any other important "off-target" molecules (often referred to as antitargets) since drug interactions with off-target molecules may lead to undesirable side effects. Due to similarities in binding sites, closely related targets identified through sequence homology have the highest chance of cross reactivity and hence highest side effect potential.

Most commonly, drugs are organic small molecules produced through chemical synthesis, but biopolymer-based drugs (also known as biopharmaceuticals) produced through biological processes are becoming increasingly more common. In addition, mRNA-based gene silencing technologies may have therapeutic applications.

Rational Drug Discovery

In contrast to traditional methods of drug discovery (known as forward pharmacology), which rely on trial-and-error testing of chemical substances on cultured cells or animals, and matching the apparent effects to treatments, rational drug design (also called reverse pharmacology) begins with a hypothesis that modulation of a specific biological target may have therapeutic value. In order for a biomolecule to be selected as a drug target, two essential pieces of information are required. The first is evidence that modulation of the target will be disease modifying. This knowledge may come from, for example, disease linkage studies that show an association between mutations in the biological target and certain disease states. The second is that the target is "druggable". This means that it is capable of binding to a small molecule and that its activity can be modulated by the small molecule.

Once a suitable target has been identified, the target is normally cloned and produced and purified. The purified protein is then used to establish a screening assay. In addition, the three-dimensional structure of the target may be determined.

The search for small molecules that bind to the target is begun by screening libraries of potential drug compounds. This may be done by using the screening assay (a "wet screen"). In addition, if the structure of the target is available, a virtual screen may be performed of candidate drugs. Ideally the candidate drug compounds should be "drug-like", that is they should possess properties that are predicted to lead to oral bioavailability, adequate chemical and metabolic stability, and minimal toxic effects. Several methods are available to estimate druglikeness such as Lipinski's Rule of Five and a range of scoring methods such as lipophilic efficiency. Several methods for predicting drug metabolism have also been proposed in the scientific literature.

Due to the large number of drug properties that must be simultaneously optimized during the design process, multi-objective optimization techniques are sometimes employed. Finally because of the limitations in the current methods for prediction of activity, drug design is still very much reliant on serendipity and bounded rationality.

Computer-aided Drug Design

The most fundamental goal in drug design is to predict whether a given molecule will bind to a target and if so how strongly. Molecular mechanics or molecular dynamics is most often used to estimate the strength of the intermolecular interaction between the small molecule and its biological target. These methods are also used to predict the conformation of the small molecule and to model conformational changes in the target that may occur when the small molecule binds to it. Semi-empirical, ab initio quantum chemistry methods, or density functional theory are often used to provide optimized parameters for the molecular mechanics calculations and also provide an estimate of the electronic properties (electrostatic potential, polarizability, etc.) of the drug candidate that will influence binding affinity.

Molecular mechanics methods may also be used to provide semi-quantitative prediction of the binding affinity. Also, knowledge-based scoring function may be used to provide binding affinity estimates. These methods use linear regression, machine learning, neural nets or other statistical techniques to derive predictive binding affinity equations by fitting experimental affinities to computationally derived interaction energies between the small molecule and the target.

Ideally, the computational method will be able to predict affinity before a compound is synthesized and hence in theory only one compound needs to be synthesized, saving enormous time and cost. The reality is that present computational methods are imperfect and provide, at best, only qualitatively accurate estimates of affinity. In practice it still takes several iterations of design, synthesis, and testing before an optimal drug is discovered. Computational methods have accelerated discovery by reducing the number of iterations required and have often provided novel structures.

Drug design with the help of computers may be used at any of the following stages of drug discovery:

1. hit identification using virtual screening (structure- or ligand-based design)

2. hit-to-lead optimization of affinity and selectivity (structure-based design, QSAR, etc.)

3. lead optimization of other pharmaceutical properties while maintaining affinity

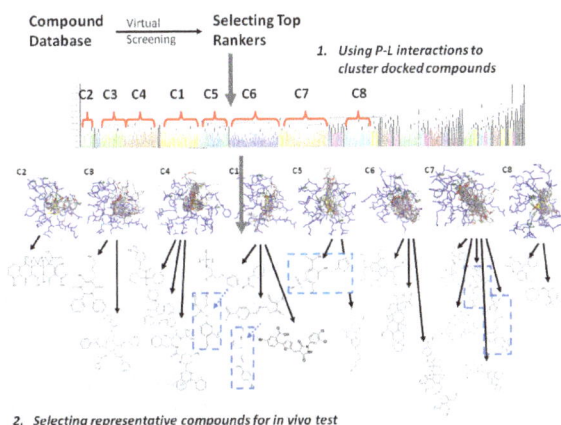

Flowchart of a Usual Clustering Analysis for Structure-Based Drug Design

In order to overcome the insufficient prediction of binding affinity calculated by recent scoring functions, the protein-ligand interaction and compound 3D structure information are used for analysis. For structure-based drug design, several post-screening analyses focusing on protein-ligand interaction have been developed for improving enrichment and effectively mining potential candidates:

- Consensus scoring

    o Selecting candidates by voting of multiple scoring functions

    o May lose the relationship between protein-ligand structural information and scoring criterion

- Cluster analysis

    o Represent and cluster candidates according to protein-ligand 3D information

    o Needs meaningful representation of protein-ligand interactions.

Types

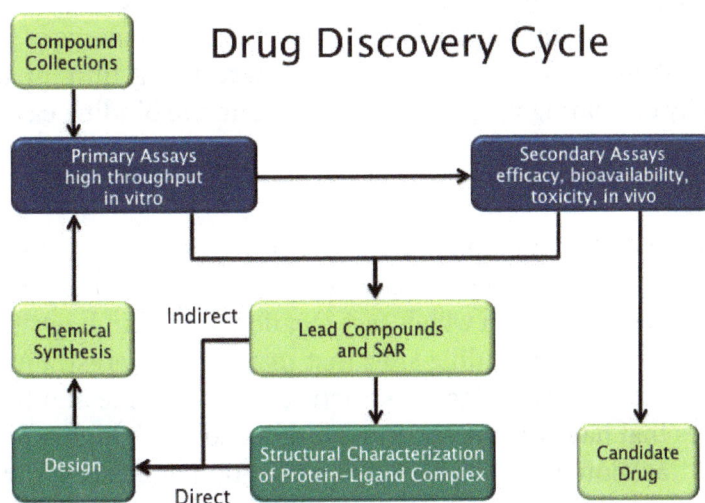

Drug discovery cycle highlighting both ligand-based (indirect) and structure-based (direct) drug design strategies.

There are two major types of drug design. The first is referred to as ligand-based drug design and the second, structure-based drug design.

Ligand-based

Ligand-based drug design (or indirect drug design) relies on knowledge of other molecules that bind to the biological target of interest. These other molecules may be used to derive a pharmacophore model that defines the minimum necessary structural characteristics a molecule must possess in order to bind to the target. In other words, a model of the biological target may be built based on the knowledge of what binds to it, and this model in turn may be used to design new molecular entities that interact with the target. Alternatively, a quantitative structure-activity relationship (QSAR), in which a correlation between calculated properties of molecules and their experimentally determined biological activity, may be derived. These QSAR relationships in turn may be used to predict the activity of new analogs.

Structure-based

Structure-based drug design (or direct drug design) relies on knowledge of the three dimensional structure of the biological target obtained through methods such as x-ray crystallography or NMR spectroscopy. If an experimental structure of a target is not available, it may be possible to create a homology model of the target based on the experimental structure of a related protein. Using the structure of the biological target, candidate drugs that are predicted to bind with high affinity and selectivity to the target may be designed using interactive graphics and the intuition of a medicinal chemist. Alternatively various automated computational procedures may be used to suggest new drug candidates.

Current methods for structure-based drug design can be divided roughly into three main categories. The first method is identification of new ligands for a given receptor by searching large databases of 3D structures of small molecules to find those fitting the binding pocket of the receptor using fast approximate docking programs. This method is known as virtual screening. A second category is de novo design of new ligands. In this method, ligand molecules are built up within the constraints of the binding pocket by assembling small pieces in a stepwise manner. These pieces can be either individual atoms or molecular fragments. The key advantage of such a method is that novel structures, not contained in any database, can be suggested. A third method is the optimization of known ligands by evaluating proposed analogs within the binding cavity.

Binding Site Identification

Binding site identification is the first step in structure based design. If the structure of the target or a sufficiently similar homolog is determined in the presence of a bound ligand, then the ligand should be observable in the structure in which case location of the binding site is trivial. However, there may be unoccupied allosteric binding sites that may be of interest. Furthermore, it may be that only apoprotein (protein without ligand) structures are available and the reliable identification of unoccupied sites that have the potential to bind ligands with high affinity is non-trivial. In brief, binding site identification usually relies on identification of concave surfaces on the protein that can accommodate drug sized molecules that also possess appropriate "hot spots" (hydrophobic surfaces, hydrogen bonding sites, etc.) that drive ligand binding.

Scoring Functions

Structure-based drug design attempts to use the structure of proteins as a basis for designing new ligands by applying the principles of molecular recognition. Selective high affinity binding to the target is generally desirable since it leads to more efficacious drugs with fewer side effects. Thus, one of the most important principles for designing or obtaining potential new ligands is to predict the binding affinity of a certain ligand to its target (and known antitargets) and use the predicted affinity as a criterion for selection.

One early general-purposed empirical scoring function to describe the binding energy of ligands to receptors was developed by Böhm. This empirical scoring function took the form:

$$\Delta G_{bind} = \Delta G_0 + \Delta G_{hb}\Sigma_{h-bonds} + \Delta G_{ionic}\Sigma_{ionic-int} + \Delta G_{lipophilic}|A| + \Delta G_{rot}NROT$$

where:

- ΔG_0 – empirically derived offset that in part corresponds to the overall loss of translational and rotational entropy of the ligand upon binding.

- ΔG_{hb} – contribution from hydrogen bonding

- ΔG_{ionic} – contribution from ionic interactions

- ΔG_{lip} – contribution from lipophilic interactions where $|A_{lipo}|$ is surface area of lipophilic contact between the ligand and receptor

- ΔG_{rot} – entropy penalty due to freezing a rotatable in the ligand bond upon binding

A more general thermodynamic "master" equation is as follows:

$$\Delta G_{bind} = -RT \ln K_d$$

$$K_d = \frac{[Ligand][Receptor]}{[Complex]}$$

$$\Delta G_{bind} = \Delta G_{desolvation} + \Delta G_{motion} + \Delta G_{configuration} + \Delta G_{interaction}$$

where:

- desolvation – enthalpic penalty for removing the ligand from solvent

- motion – entropic penalty for reducing the degrees of freedom when a ligand binds to its receptor

- configuration – conformational strain energy required to put the ligand in its "active" conformation

- interaction – enthalpic gain for "resolvating" the ligand with its receptor

The basic idea is that the overall binding free energy can be decomposed into independent components that are known to be important for the binding process. Each component reflects a certain kind of free energy alteration during the binding process between a ligand and its target receptor.

The Master Equation is the linear combination of these components. According to Gibbs free energy equation, the relation between dissociation equilibrium constant, K_d, and the components of free energy was built.

Various computational methods are used to estimate each of the components of the master equation. For example, the change in polar surface area upon ligand binding can be used to estimate the desolvation energy. The number of rotatable bonds frozen upon ligand binding is proportional to the motion term. The configurational or strain energy can be estimated using molecular mechanics calculations. Finally the interaction energy can be estimated using methods such as the change in non polar surface, statistically derived potentials of mean force, the number of hydrogen bonds formed, etc. In practice, the components of the master equation are fit to experimental data using multiple linear regression. This can be done with a diverse training set including many types of ligands and receptors to produce a less accurate but more general "global" model or a more restricted set of ligands and receptors to produce a more accurate but less general "local" model.

Examples

A particular example of rational drug design involves the use of three-dimensional information about biomolecules obtained from such techniques as X-ray crystallography and NMR spectroscopy. Computer-aided drug design in particular becomes much more tractable when there is a high-resolution structure of a target protein bound to a potent ligand. This approach to drug discovery is sometimes referred to as structure-based drug design. The first unequivocal example of the application of structure-based drug design leading to an approved drug is the carbonic anhydrase inhibitor dorzolamide, which was approved in 1995.

Another important case study in rational drug design is imatinib, a tyrosine kinase inhibitor designed specifically for the *bcr-abl* fusion protein that is characteristic for Philadelphia chromosome-positive leukemias (chronic myelogenous leukemia and occasionally acute lymphocytic leukemia). Imatinib is substantially different from previous drugs for cancer, as most agents of chemotherapy simply target rapidly dividing cells, not differentiating between cancer cells and other tissues.

Additional examples include:

- Many of the atypical antipsychotics
- Cimetidine, the prototypical H_2-receptor antagonist from which the later members of the class were developed
- Selective COX-2 inhibitor NSAIDs
- Enfuvirtide, a peptide HIV entry inhibitor
- Nonbenzodiazepines like zolpidem and zopiclone
- Raltegravir, an HIV integrase inhibitor
- SSRIs (selective serotonin reuptake inhibitors), a class of antidepressants
- Zanamivir, an antiviral drug

Case Studies

- 5-HT3 antagonists
- Acetylcholine receptor agonists
- Angiotensin receptor antagonists
- Bcr-Abl tyrosine-kinase inhibitors
- Cannabinoid receptor antagonists
- CCR5 receptor antagonists
- Cyclooxygenase 2 inhibitors
- Dipeptidyl peptidase-4 inhibitors
- HIV protease inhibitors
- NK1 receptor antagonists
- Non-nucleoside reverse transcriptase inhibitors
- Nucleoside and nucleotide reverse transcriptase inhibitors
- PDE5 inhibitors
- Proton pump inibitors
- Renin inhibitors
- Triptans
- TRPV1 antagonists
- c-Met inhibitors

Criticism

It has been argued that the highly rigid and focused nature of rational drug design suppresses serendipity in drug discovery. Because many of the most significant medical discoveries have been inadvertent, the recent focus on rational drug design may limit the progress of drug discovery. Furthermore, the rational design of a drug may be limited by a crude or incomplete understanding of the underlying molecular processes of the disease it is intended to treat.

Drug Discovery

In the fields of medicine, biotechnology and pharmacology, drug discovery is the process by which new candidate medications are discovered. Historically, drugs were discovered through identifying the active ingredient from traditional remedies or by serendipitous discovery. Later chemical libraries of synthetic small molecules, natural products or extracts were screened in intact cells or whole organisms to identify substances that have a desirable therapeutic effect in a process known as classical pharmacology. Since sequencing of the human genome which allowed rapid cloning and synthesis of large quantities of purified proteins, it has become common practice to use high throughput screening of large compounds libraries against isolated biological targets which are hypothesized to be disease modifying in a process known as reverse pharmacology. Hits from these screens are then tested in cells and then in animals for efficacy.

Modern drug discovery involves the identification of screening hits, medicinal chemistry and optimization of those hits to increase the affinity, selectivity (to reduce the potential of side effects), efficacy/potency, metabolic stability (to increase the half-life), and oral bioavailability. Once a compound that fulfills all of these requirements has been identified, it will begin the process of drug development prior to clinical trials. One or more of these steps may, but not necessarily, involve computer-aided drug design. Modern drug discovery is thus usually a capital-intensive process that involves large investments by pharmaceutical industry corporations as well as national governments (who provide grants and loan guarantees). Despite advances in technology and understanding of biological systems, drug discovery is still a lengthy, "expensive, difficult, and inefficient process" with low rate of new therapeutic discovery. In 2010, the research and development cost of each new molecular entity (NME) was approximately US$1.8 billion. Drug discovery is done by pharmaceutical companies, with research assistance from universities. The "final product" of drug discovery is a patent on the potential drug. The drug requires very expensive Phase I, II and III clinical trials, and most of them fail. Small companies have a critical role, often then selling the rights to larger companies that have the resources to run the clinical trials.

Discovering drugs that may be a commercial success, or a public health success, involves a complex interaction between investors, industry, academia, patent laws, regulatory exclusivity, marketing and the need to balance secrecy with communication. Meanwhile, for disorders whose rarity means that no large commercial success or public health effect can be expected, the orphan drug funding process ensures that people who experience those disorders can have some hope of pharmacotherapeutic advances.

Historical Background

The idea that the effect of a drug in the human body is mediated by specific interactions of the drug molecule with biological macromolecules, (proteins or nucleic acids in most cases) led scientists to the conclusion that individual chemicals are required for the biological activity of the drug. This made for the beginning of the modern era in pharmacology, as pure chemicals, instead of crude extracts, became the standard drugs. Examples of drug compounds isolated from crude preparations are morphine, the active agent in opium, and digoxin, a heart stimulant originating from Digitalis lanata. Organic chemistry also led to the synthesis of many of the natural products isolated from biological sources.

Historically substances, whether crude extracts or purified chemicals were screened for biological activity without knowledge of the biological target. Only after an active substance was identified was an effort made to identify the target. This approach is known as classical pharmacology, forward pharmacology, or phenotypic drug discovery.

Later, small molecules were synthesized to specifically target a known physiological/pathological pathway, rather than adopt the mass screening of banks of stored compounds. This led to great success, such as the work of Gertrude Elion and George H. Hitchings on purine metabolism, the work of James Black on beta blockers and cimetidine, and the discovery of statins by Akira Endo. Another champion of the approach of developing chemical analogues of known active substances was Sir David Jack at Allen and Hanbury's, later Glaxo, who pioneered the first inhaled selective beta2-adrenergic agonist for asthma, the first inhaled steroid for asthma, ranitidine as a successor to cimetidine, and supported the development of the triptans.

Gertrude Elion, working mostly with a group of fewer than 50 people on purine analogues, contributed to the discovery of the first anti-viral; the first immunosuppressant (azathioprine) that allowed human organ transplantation; the first drug to induce remission of childhood leukaemia; pivotal anti-cancer treatments; an anti-malarial; an anti-bacterial; and a treatment for gout.

Cloning of human proteins made possible the screening of large libraries of compounds against specific targets thought to be linked to specific diseases. This approach is known as reverse pharmacology and is the most frequently used approach today.

Drug Targets

The definition of "target" itself is something argued within the pharmaceutical industry. Generally, the "target" is the naturally existing cellular or molecular structure involved in the pathology of interest that the drug-in-development is meant to act on. However, the distinction between a "new" and "established" target can be made without a full understanding of just what a "target" is. This distinction is typically made by pharmaceutical companies engaged in discovery and development of therapeutics. In an estimate from 2011, 435 human genome products were identified as therapeutic drug targets of FDA-approved drugs.

"Established targets" are those for which there is a good scientific understanding, supported by a lengthy publication history, of both how the target functions in normal physiology and how it is involved in human pathology. This does not imply that the mechanism of action of drugs that are thought to act through a particular established target is fully understood. Rather, "established" relates directly to the amount of background information available on a target, in particular functional information. The more such information is available, the less investment is (generally) required to develop a therapeutic directed against the target. The process of gathering such functional information is called "target validation" in pharmaceutical industry parlance. Established targets also include those that the pharmaceutical industry has had experience mounting drug discovery campaigns against in the past; such a history provides information on the chemical feasibility of developing a small molecular therapeutic against the target and can provide licensing opportunities and freedom-to-operate indicators with respect to small-molecule therapeutic candidates.

In general, "new targets" are all those targets that are not "established targets" but which have been or are the subject of drug discovery campaigns. These typically include newly discovered proteins, or proteins whose function has now become clear as a result of basic scientific research.

The majority of targets currently selected for drug discovery efforts are proteins. Two classes predominate: G-protein-coupled receptors (or GPCRs) and protein kinases.

Screening and Design

The process of finding a new drug against a chosen target for a particular disease usually involves high-throughput screening (HTS), wherein large libraries of chemicals are tested for their ability to modify the target. For example, if the target is a novel GPCR, compounds will be screened for their ability to inhibit or stimulate that receptor: if the target is a protein kinase, the chemicals will be tested for their ability to inhibit that kinase.

Another important function of HTS is to show how selective the compounds are for the chosen target. The ideal is to find a molecule which will interfere with only the chosen target, but not other, related targets. To this end, other screening runs will be made to see whether the "hits" against the chosen target will interfere with other related targets – this is the process of cross-screening. Cross-screening is important, because the more unrelated targets a compound hits, the more likely that off-target toxicity will occur with that compound once it reaches the clinic.

It is very unlikely that a perfect drug candidate will emerge from these early screening runs. It is more often observed that several compounds are found to have some degree of activity, and if these compounds share common chemical features, one or more pharmacophores can then be developed. At this point, medicinal chemists will attempt to use structure-activity relationships (SAR) to improve certain features of the lead compound:

- increase activity against the chosen target

- reduce activity against unrelated targets

- improve the druglikeness or ADME properties of the molecule.

This process will require several iterative screening runs, during which, it is hoped, the properties of the new molecular entities will improve, and allow the favoured compounds to go forward to in vitro and in vivo testing for activity in the disease model of choice.

Amongst the physico-chemical properties associated with drug absorption include ionization (pKa), and solubility; permeability can be determined by PAMPA and Caco-2. PAMPA is attractive as an early screen due to the low consumption of drug and the low cost compared to tests such as Caco-2, gastrointestinal tract (GIT) and Blood–brain barrier (BBB) with which there is a high correlation.

A range of parameters can be used to assess the quality of a compound, or a series of compounds, as proposed in the Lipinski's Rule of Five. Such parameters include calculated properties such as cLogP to estimate lipophilicity, molecular weight, polar surface area and measured properties, such as potency, in-vitro measurement of enzymatic clearance etc. Some descriptors such as ligand efficiency (LE) and lipophilic efficiency (LiPE) combine such parameters to assess druglikeness.

While HTS is a commonly used method for novel drug discovery, it is not the only method. It is often possible to start from a molecule which already has some of the desired properties. Such a molecule might be extracted from a natural product or even be a drug on the market which could be improved upon (so-called "me too" drugs). Other methods, such as virtual high throughput screening, where screening is done using computer-generated models and attempting to "dock" virtual libraries to a target, are also often used.

Another important method for drug discovery is *de novo* drug design, in which a prediction is made of the sorts of chemicals that might (e.g.) fit into an active site of the target enzyme. For example, virtual screening and computer-aided drug design are often used to identify new chemical moieties that may interact with a target protein. Molecular modelling and molecular dynamics simulations can be used as a guide to improve the potency and properties of new drug leads.

There is also a paradigm shift in the drug discovery community to shift away from HTS, which is expensive and may only cover limited chemical space, to the screening of smaller libraries (maximum a few thousand compounds). These include fragment-based lead discovery (FBDD) and protein-directed dynamic combinatorial chemistry. The ligands in these approaches are usually much smaller, and they bind to the target protein with weaker binding affinity than those hits that are identified from HTS. Further modified through organic synthesis into lead compounds are often required. Such modifications are often guided by protein X-ray crystallography of the protein-fragment complex. The advantages of these approaches are that they allow more efficient screening and the compound library, although small, typically covers a large chemical space when compared to HTS.

Once a lead compound series has been established with sufficient target potency and selectivity and favourable drug-like properties, one or two compounds will then be proposed for drug development. The best of these is generally called the lead compound, while the other will be designated as the "backup".

Nature as Source of Drugs

Traditionally many drugs and other chemicals with biological activity have been discovered by studying allelopathy – chemicals that organisms create that affect the activity of other organisms in the fight for survival.

Despite the rise of combinatorial chemistry as an integral part of lead discovery process, natural products still play a major role as starting material for drug discovery. A 2007 report found that of the 974 small molecule new chemical entities developed between 1981 and 2006, 63% were natural derived or semisynthetic derivatives of natural products. For certain therapy areas, such as antimicrobials, antineoplastics, antihypertensive and anti-inflammatory drugs, the numbers were higher. In many cases, these products have been used traditionally for many years.

Natural products may be useful as a source of novel chemical structures for modern techniques of development of antibacterial therapies.

Despite the implied potential, only a fraction of Earth's living species has been tested for bioactivity.

Plant-derived

Prior to Paracelsus, the vast majority of traditionally used crude drugs in Western medicine were plant-derived extracts. This has resulted in a pool of information about the potential of plant species as an important source of starting material for drug discovery. A different set of metabolites is sometimes produced in the different anatomical parts of the plant (e.g. root, leaves and flower), and botanical knowledge is crucial also for the correct identification of bioactive plant materials.

Microbial Metabolites

Microbes compete for living space and nutrients. To survive in these conditions, many microbes have developed abilities to prevent competing species from proliferating. Microbes are the main source of antimicrobial drugs. *Streptomyces* species have been a valuable source of antibiotics. The classical example of an antibiotic discovered as a defense mechanism against another microbe is the discovery of penicillin in bacterial cultures contaminated by *Penicillium* fungi in 1928.

Marine Invertebrates

Marine environments are potential sources for new bioactive agents. Arabinose nucleosides discovered from marine invertebrates in 1950s, demonstrating for the first time that sugar moieties other than ribose and deoxyribose can yield bioactive nucleoside structures. However, it was 2004 when the first marine-derived drug was approved. The cone snail toxin ziconotide, also known as Prialt, was approved by the Food and Drug Administration to treat severe neuropathic pain. Several other marine-derived agents are now in clinical trials for indications such as cancer, anti-inflammatory use and pain. One class of these agents are bryostatin-like compounds, under investigation as anti-cancer therapy.

Chemical Diversity of Natural Products

As above mentioned, combinatorial chemistry was a key technology enabling the efficient generation of large screening libraries for the needs of high-throughput screening. However, now, after two decades of combinatorial chemistry, it has been pointed out that despite the increased efficiency in chemical synthesis, no increase in lead or drug candidates has been reached. This has led to analysis of chemical characteristics of combinatorial chemistry products, compared to existing drugs or natural products. The chemoinformatics concept chemical diversity, depicted as distribution of compounds in the chemical space based on their physicochemical characteristics, is often used to describe the difference between the combinatorial chemistry libraries and natural products. The synthetic, combinatorial library compounds seem to cover only a limited and quite uniform chemical space, whereas existing drugs and particularly natural products, exhibit much greater chemical diversity, distributing more evenly to the chemical space. The most prominent differences between natural products and compounds in combinatorial chemistry libraries is the number of chiral centers (much higher in natural compounds), structure rigidity (higher in natural compounds) and number of aromatic moieties (higher in combinatorial chemistry libraries). Other chemical differences between these two groups include the nature of heteroatoms (O and N enriched in natural products, and S and halogen atoms more often present in synthetic compounds), as well as level of non-aromatic unsaturation (higher in natural products). As both structure rigidity and chirality are both well-established factors in medicinal chemistry known to enhance compounds specificity and efficacy as a drug, it has been suggested that natural products compare favourable to today's combinatorial chemistry libraries as potential lead molecules.

Natural Product

Screening

Two main approaches exist for the finding of new bioactive chemical entities from natural sources.

The first is sometimes referred to as random collection and screening of material, but in fact the collection is often far from random in that biological (often botanical) knowledge is used about which families show promise, based on a number of factors, including past screening. This approach is based on the fact that only a small part of earth's biodiversity has ever been tested for pharmaceutical activity. It is also based on the fact that organisms living in a species-rich environment need to evolve defensive and competitive mechanisms to survive, mechanisms which might usefully be exploited in the development of drugs that can cure diseases affecting humans. A collection of plant, animal and microbial samples from rich ecosystems can potentially give rise to novel biological activities worth exploiting in the drug development process. One example of a successful use of this strategy is the screening for antitumour agents by the National Cancer Institute, started in the 1960s. Paclitaxel was identified from Pacific yew tree *Taxus brevifolia*. Paclitaxel showed anti-tumour activity by a previously undescribed mechanism (stabilization of microtubules) and is now approved for clinical use for the treatment of lung, breast and ovarian cancer, as well as for Kaposi's sarcoma. Early in the 21st century, Cabazitaxel (made by Sanofi, a French firm), another relative of taxol has been shown effective against prostate cancer, also because it works by preventing the formation of microtubules, which pull the chromosomes apart in dividing cells (such as cancer cells). Other examples are: 1. Camptotheca (Camptothecin · Topotecan · Irinotecan · Rubitecan · Belotecan); 2. Podophyllum (Etoposide · Teniposide); 3a. Anthracyclines (Aclarubicin · Daunorubicin · Doxorubicin · Epirubicin · Idarubicin · Amrubicin · Pirarubicin · Valrubicin · Zorubicin); 3b. Anthracenediones (Mitoxantrone · Pixantrone).

The second main approach involves ethnobotany, the study of the general use of plants in society, and ethnopharmacology, an area inside ethnobotany, which is focused specifically on medicinal uses.

Both of these two main approaches can be used in selecting starting materials for future drugs. Artemisinin, an antimalarial agent from sweet wormtree *Artemisia annua*, used in Chinese medicine since 200BC is one drug used as part of combination therapy for multiresistant *Plasmodium falciparum*.

Structural Elucidation

The elucidation of the chemical structure is critical to avoid the re-discovery of a chemical agent that is already known for its structure and chemical activity. Mass spectrometry is a method in which individual compounds are identified based on their mass/charge ratio, after ionization. Chemical compounds exist in nature as mixtures, so the combination of liquid chromatography and mass spectrometry (LC-MS) is often used to separate the individual chemicals. Databases of mass spectras for known compounds are available, and can be used to assign a structure to an unknown mass spectrum. Nuclear magnetic resonance spectroscopy is the primary technique for determining chemical structures of natural products. NMR yields information about individual hydrogen and carbon atoms in the structure, allowing detailed reconstruction of the molecule's architecture.

New Chemical Entity

A new chemical entity (NCE) is, according to the U.S. Food and Drug Administration, a drug that contains no active moiety that has been approved by the FDA in any other application submitted under section 505(b) of the Federal Food, Drug, and Cosmetic Act.

A new molecular entity (NME) is a drug that contains an active moiety that has never been approved by the FDA or marketed in the US.

Definition

An active moiety is a molecule or ion, excluding those appended portions of the molecule that cause the drug to be an ester, salt (including a salt with hydrogen or coordination bonds), or other noncovalent derivative (such as a complex, chelate, or clathrate) of the molecule, responsible for the physiological or pharmacological action of the drug substance.

An NCE is a molecule developed by the innovator company in the early drug discovery stage, which after undergoing clinical trials could translate into a drug that could be a treatment for some disease. Synthesis of an NCE is the first step in the process of drug development. Once the synthesis of the NCE has been completed, companies have two options before them. They can either go for clinical trials on their own or license the NCE to another company. In the latter option, companies can avoid the expensive and lengthy process of clinical trials, as the licensee company would be conducting further clinical trials and subsequently launching the drug. Companies adopting this model of business would be able to generate high margins as they get a huge one-time payment for the NCE as well as entering into a revenue sharing agreement with the licensee company.

Under the Food and Drug Administration Amendments Act of 2007, all new chemical entities must first be reviewed by an advisory committee before the FDA can approve these products.

High-throughput Screening

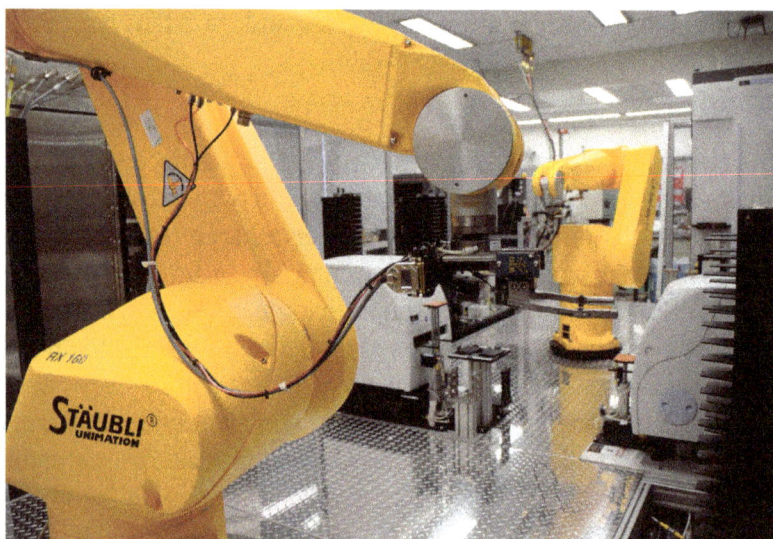

High-throughput screening robots

High-throughput screening (HTS) is a method for scientific experimentation especially used in drug discovery and relevant to the fields of biology and chemistry. Using robotics, data processing and control software, liquid handling devices, and sensitive detectors, High-throughput screening allows a researcher to quickly conduct millions of chemical, genetic, or pharmacological tests.

Through this process one can rapidly identify active compounds, antibodies, or genes that modulate a particular biomolecular pathway. The results of these experiments provide starting points for drug design and for understanding the interaction or role of a particular biochemical process in biology.

Assay Plate Preparation

The key labware or testing vessel of HTS is the microtiter plate: a small container, usually disposable and made of plastic, that features a grid of small, open divots called *wells*. In general, modern (circa 2013) microplates for HTS have either 384, 1536, or 3456 wells. These are all multiples of 96, reflecting the original 96-well microplate with spaced wells of 8 x 12 9 mm . Most of the wells contain test items, depending on the nature of the experiment. These could be different chemical compounds dissolved e.g. in an aqueous solution of dimethyl sulfoxide (DMSO). The wells could also contain cells or enzymes of some type. (The other wells may be empty or contain pure solvent or untreated samples, intended for use as experimental controls.)

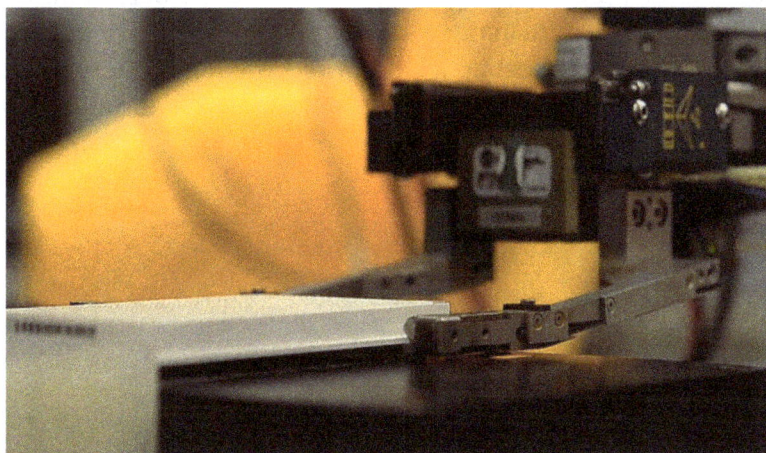

A robot arm handles an assay plate

A screening facility typically holds a library of *stock plates*, whose contents are carefully catalogued, and each of which may have been created by the lab or obtained from a commercial source. These stock plates themselves are not directly used in experiments; instead, separate *assay plates* are created as needed. An assay plate is simply a copy of a stock plate, created by pipetting a small amount of liquid (often measured in nanoliters) from the wells of a stock plate to the corresponding wells of a completely empty plate.

Reaction Observation

To prepare for an assay, the researcher fills each well of the plate with some biological entity that they wish to conduct the experiment upon, such as a protein, cells, or an animal embryo. After some incubation time has passed to allow the biological matter to absorb, bind to, or otherwise react (or fail to react) with the compounds in the wells, measurements are taken across all the plate's wells, either manually or by a machine. Manual measurements are often necessary when the researcher is using microscopy to (for example) seek changes or defects in embryonic development caused by the wells' compounds, looking for effects that a computer could not easily determine by itself. Otherwise, a specialized automated analysis machine can run a number of experiments on the wells (such as shining polarized light on them and measuring reflectivity, which can be an indication of protein binding). In this case, the machine outputs the result of each experiment as a grid of numeric values, with each number mapping to the value obtained from a single well. A high-capacity analysis machine can measure dozens of plates in the space of a few minutes like this, generating thousands of experimental datapoints very quickly.

Depending on the results of this first assay, the researcher can perform follow up assays within the same screen by "cherrypicking" liquid from the source wells that gave interesting results (known as "hits") into new assay plates, and then re-running the experiment to collect further data on this narrowed set, confirming and refining observations.

Automation Systems

Automation is an important element in HTS's usefulness. Typically, an integrated robot system consisting of one or more robots transports assay-microplates from station to station for sample and reagent addition, mixing, incubation, and finally readout or detection. An HTS system can usually prepare, incubate, and analyze many plates simultaneously, further speeding the data-collection process. HTS robots that can test up to 100,000 compounds per day currently exist. Automatic colony pickers pick thousands of microbial colonies for high throughput genetic screening. The term uHTS or *ultra-high-throughput screening* refers (circa 2008) to screening in excess of 100,000 compounds per day.

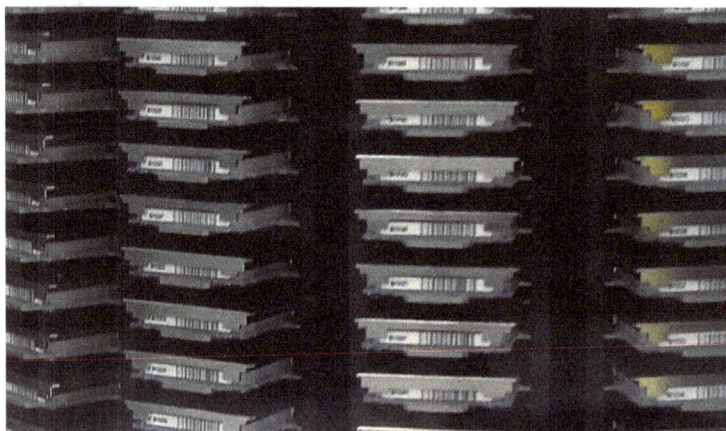

A carousel system to store assay plates for high storage capacity and high speed access

Experimental Design and Data Analysis

With the ability of rapid screening of diverse compounds (such as small molecules or siRNAs) to identify active compounds, HTS has led to an explosion in the rate of data generated in recent years . Consequently, one of the most fundamental challenges in HTS experiments is to glean biochemical significance from mounds of data, which relies on the development and adoption of appropriate experimental designs and analytic methods for both quality control and hit selection . HTS research is one of the fields that have a feature described by John Blume, Chief Science Officer for Applied Proteomics, Inc., as follows: Soon, if a scientist does not understand some statistics or rudimentary data-handling technologies, he or she may not be considered to be a true molecular biologist and, thus, will simply become "a dinosaur."

Quality Control

High-quality HTS assays are critical in HTS experiments. The development of high-quality HTS assays requires the integration of both experimental and computational approaches for quality control (QC). Three important means of QC are (i) good plate design, (ii) the selection of effective positive and negative chemical/biological controls, and (iii) the development of effective QC metrics to measure the degree of differentiation so that assays with inferior data quality can be identified. A good plate design helps to identify systematic errors (especially those linked with well position) and determine what normalization should be used to remove/reduce the impact of systematic errors on both QC and hit selection.

Effective analytic QC methods serve as a gatekeeper for excellent quality assays. In a typical HTS experiment, a clear distinction between a positive control and a negative reference such as a negative control is an index for good quality. Many quality-assessment measures have been proposed to measure the degree of differentiation between a positive control and a negative reference. Signal-to-background ratio, signal-to-noise ratio, signal window, assay variability ratio, and Z-factor have been adopted to evaluate data quality. Strictly standardized mean difference (SSMD) has recently been proposed for assessing data quality in HTS assays.

Hit Selection

A compound with a desired size of effects in an HTS is called a hit. The process of selecting hits is called hit selection. The analytic methods for hit selection in screens without replicates (usually in primary screens) differ from those with replicates (usually in confirmatory screens). For example, the z-score method is suitable for screens without replicates whereas the t-statistic is suitable for screens with replicates. The calculation of SSMD for screens without replicates also differs from that for screens with replicates .

For hit selection in primary screens without replicates, the easily interpretable ones are average fold change, mean difference, percent inhibition, and percent activity. However, they do not capture data variability effectively. The z-score method or SSMD, which can capture data variability based on an assumption that every compound has the same variability as a negative reference in the screens. However, outliers are common in HTS experiments, and methods such as z-score are sensitive to outliers and can be problematic. As a consequence, robust methods such as the z*-score method, SSMD*, B-score method, and quantile-based method have been proposed and adopted for hit selection.

In a screen with replicates, we can directly estimate variability for each compound; as a consequence, we should use SSMD or t-statistic that does not rely on the strong assumption that the z-score and z*-score rely on. One issue with the use of t-statistic and associated p-values is that they are affected by both sample size and effect size. They come from testing for no mean difference, and thus are not designed to measure the size of compound effects. For hit selection, the major interest is the size of effect in a tested compound. SSMD directly assesses the size of effects. SSMD has also been shown to be better than other commonly used effect sizes . The population value of SSMD is comparable across experiments and, thus, we can use the same cutoff for the population value of SSMD to measure the size of compound effects .

Techniques for Increased Throughput and Efficiency

Unique distributions of compounds across one or many plates can be employed either to increase the number of assays per plate or to reduce the variance of assay results, or both. The simplifying assumption made in this approach is that any N compounds in the same well will not typically interact with each other, or the assay target, in a manner that fundamentally changes the ability of the assay to detect true hits.

For example, imagine a plate wherein compound A is in wells 1-2-3, compound B is in wells 2-3-4, and compound C is in wells 3-4-5. In an assay of this plate against a given target, a hit in wells 2, 3, and 4 would indicate that compound B is the most likely agent, while also providing three measurements of compound B's efficacy against the specified target. Commercial applications of this approach involve combinations in which no two compounds ever share more than one well, to reduce the (second-order) possibility of interference between pairs of compounds being screened.

Recent Advances

In March 2010, research was published demonstrating an HTS process allowing 1,000 times faster screening (100 million reactions in 10 hours) at 1-millionth the cost (using 10^{-7} times the reagent volume) than conventional techniques using drop-based microfluidics. Drops of fluid separated by oil replace microplate wells and allow analysis and hit sorting while reagents are flowing through channels.

In 2010, researchers developed a silicon sheet of lenses that can be placed over microfluidic arrays to allow the fluorescence measurement of 64 different output channels simultaneously with a single camera. This process can analyze 200,000 drops per second.

Whereby traditional HTS drug discovery uses purified proteins or intact cells, very interesting recent development of the technology is associated with the use of intact living organisms, like the nematode *Caenorhabditis elegans* and zebrafish (*Danio rerio*).

Increasing Utilization of HTS in Academia for Biomedical Research

HTS is a relatively recent innovation, made feasible largely through modern advances in robotics and high-speed computer technology. It still takes a highly specialized and expensive screening lab to run an HTS operation, so in many cases a small- to moderate-size research institution will use the services of an existing HTS facility rather than set up one for itself.

There is a trend in academia for universities to be their own drug discovery enterprise. These facilities, which normally are found only in industry, are now increasingly found at universities as well. UCLA, for example, features an open access HTS laboratory Molecular Screening Shared Resources (MSSR, UCLA), which can screen more than 100,000 compounds a day on a routine basis. The open access policy ensures that researchers from all over the world can take advantage of this facility without lengthy intellectual property negotiations. With a compound library of over 200,000 small molecules, the MSSR has one of the largest compound deck of all universities on the west coast. Also, the MSSR features full functional genomics capabilities (genome wide siRNA, shRNA, cDNA and CRISPR) which are complementary to small molecule efforts: Functional genomics leverages HTS capabilities to execute genome wide screens which examine the function of each gene in the context of interest by either knocking each gene out or overexpressing it. Parallel access to high-throughput small molecule screen and a genome wide screen enables researcher to perform target identification and validation for given disease or the mode of action determination on a small molecule. The most accurate results can be obtained by use of "arrayed" functional genomics libraries, i.e. each library contains a single construct such as a single siRNA or cDNA. Functional genomics is typically paired with high content screening using e.g. epifluorescent miscroscopy or laser scanning cytometry. The University of Illinois also has a facility for HTS, as does the University of Minnesota. The Life Sciences Institute at the University of Michigan houses the HTS facility in the Center for Chemical Genomics. The Rockefeller University has an open-access HTS Resource Center HTSRC (The Rockefeller University, HTSRC), which offers a library of over 165,000 compounds. Northwestern University's High Throughput Analysis Laboratory supports target identification, validation, assay development, and compound screening. The non-profit Sanford Burnham Prebys Medical Discovery Institute also has a long-standing HTS facility in the Conrad Prebys Center for Chemical Genomics which was part of the MLPCN.

In the United States, the National Institutes of Health or NIH has created a nationwide consortium of small-molecule screening centers to produce innovative chemical tools for use in biological research. The Molecular Libraries Probe Production Centers Network, or MLPCN, performs HTS on assays provided by the research community, against a large library of small molecules maintained in a central molecule repository.

Structure–activity Relationship

The structure–activity relationship (SAR) is the relationship between the chemical or 3D structure of a molecule and its biological activity. The analysis of SAR enables the determination of the chemical groups responsible for evoking a target biological effect in the organism. This allows modification of the effect or the potency of a bioactive compound (typically a drug) by changing its chemical structure. Medicinal chemists use the techniques of chemical synthesis to insert new chemical groups into the biomedical compound and test the modifications for their biological effects.

This method was refined to build mathematical relationships between the chemical structure and the biological activity, known as quantitative structure–activity relationships (QSAR). A related term is structure affinity relationship (SAFIR).

Structure-biodegradability Relationship

The large number of synthetic organic chemicals currently in production presents a huge challenge for timely collection of detailed environmental data on each compound. The concept of structure biodegradability relationships (SBR) has been applied to explain variability in persistence among organic chemicals in the environment. Early attempts generally consisted of examining the degradation of a homologous series of structurally related compounds under identical conditions with a complex "universal" inoculum, typically derived from numerous sources. This approach revealed that the nature and positions of substituents affected the apparent biodegradability of several chemical classes, with resulting general themes, such as halogens generally conferring persistence under aerobic conditions. Subsequently, more quantitative approaches have been developed using principles of QSAR and often accounting for the role of sorption (bioavailability) in chemical fate.

Drug Development

Drug development is the process of bringing a new pharmaceutical drug to the market once a lead compound has been identified through the process of drug discovery. It includes pre-clinical research on microorganisms and animals, filing for regulatory status, such as via the United States Food and Drug Administration for an investigational new drug to initiate clinical trials on humans, and may include the step of obtaining regulatory approval with a new drug application to market the drug.

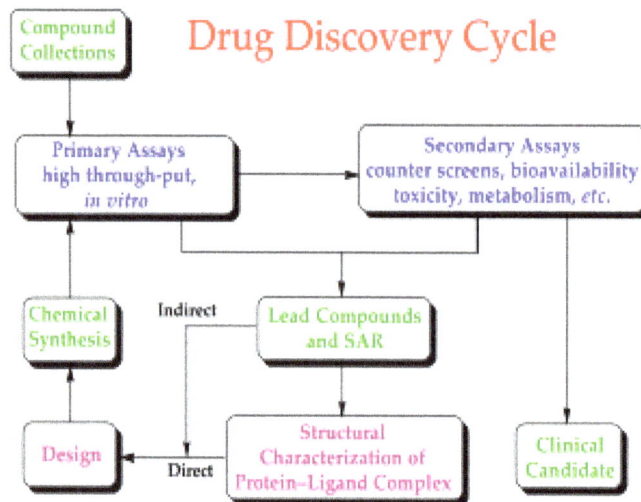

New Chemical Entity Development

Broadly, the process of drug development can be divided into pre-clinical and clinical work.

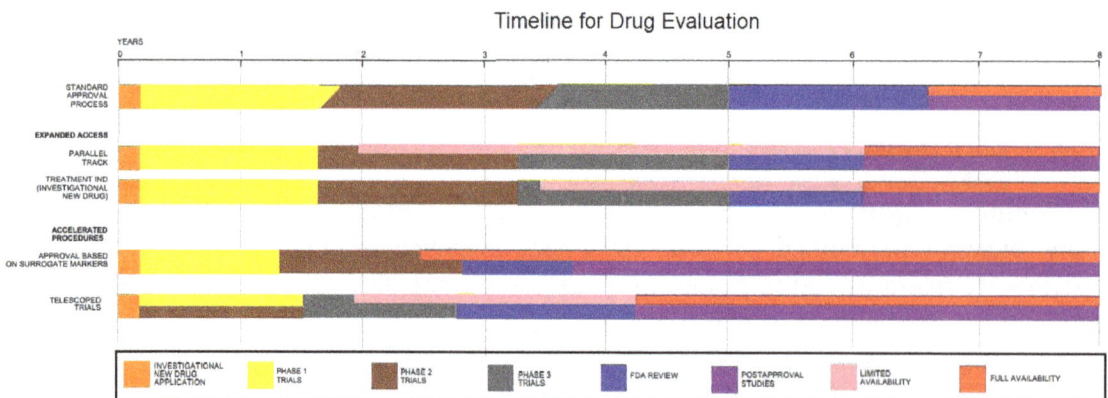

Timeline showing the various drug approval tracks and research phases

Pre-clinical

New chemical entities (NCEs, also known as new molecular entities or NMEs) are compounds that emerge from the process of drug discovery. These have promising activity against a particular biological target that is important in disease. However, little is known about the safety, toxicity, pharmacokinetics, and metabolism of this NCE in humans. It is the function of drug development to assess all of these parameters prior to human clinical trials. A further major objective of drug development is to recommend the dose and schedule for the first use in a human clinical trial ("first-in-man" [FIM] or First Human Dose [FHD]).

In addition, drug development must establish the physicochemical properties of the NCE: its chemical makeup, stability, and solubility. Manufacturers must optimize the process they use to make the chemical so they can scale up from a medicinal chemist producing milligrams, to manufacturing on the kilogram and ton scale. They further examine the product for suitability to package as capsules, tablets, aerosol, intramuscular injectable, subcutaneous injectable, or intravenous formulations. Together, these processes are known in preclinical development as *chemistry, manufacturing, and control* (CMC).

Many aspects of drug development focus on satisfying the regulatory requirements of drug licensing authorities. These generally constitute a number of tests designed to determine the major toxicities of a novel compound prior to first use in humans. It is a legal requirement that an assessment of major organ toxicity be performed (effects on the heart and lungs, brain, kidney, liver and digestive system), as well as effects on other parts of the body that might be affected by the drug (e.g., the skin if the new drug is to be delivered through the skin). Increasingly, these tests are made using *in vitro* methods (e.g., with isolated cells), but many tests can only be made by using experimental animals to demonstrate the complex interplay of metabolism and drug exposure on toxicity.

The information is gathered from this pre-clinical testing, as well as information on CMC, and submitted to regulatory authorities (in the US, to the FDA), as an Investigational New Drug application or IND. If the IND is approved, development moves to the clinical phase.

Clinical Phase

Clinical trials involve three or four steps:

- Phase I trials, usually in healthy volunteers, determine safety and dosing.

- Phase II trials are used to get an initial reading of efficacy and further explore safety in small numbers of patients having the disease targeted by the NCE.

- Phase III trials are large, pivotal trials to determine safety and efficacy in sufficiently large numbers of patients with the targeted disease. If safety and efficacy are adequately proved, clinical testing may stop at this step and the NCE advances to the new drug application (NDA) stage.

- Phase IV trials are post-approval trials that are sometimes a condition attached by the FDA, also called post-market surveillance studies.

The process of defining characteristics of the drug does not stop once an NCE begins human clinical trials. In addition to the tests required to move a novel drug into the clinic for the first time, manufacturers must ensure that any long-term or chronic toxicities are well-defined, including effects on systems not previously monitored (fertility, reproduction, immune system, among others). They must also test the compound for its potential to cause cancer (carcinogenicity testing).

If a compound emerges from these tests with an acceptable toxicity and safety profile, and the company can further show it has the desired effect in clinical trials, then the NCE portfolio of evidence can be submitted for marketing approval in the various countries where the manufacturer plans to sell it. In the United States, this process is called a "new drug application" or NDA.

Most NCEs fail during drug development, either because they have unacceptable toxicity or because they simply do not have the intended effect on the targeted disease as shown in clinical trials.

Cost

The full cost of bringing a new drug (i.e., new chemical entity) to market – from discovery through clinical trials to approval – is complex and controversial. Typically, companies spend tens to hundreds of millions of U.S. dollars. One element of the complexity is that the much-publicized final numbers often not only include the out-of-pocket expenses for conducting a series of Phase I-III clinical trials, but also the *capital costs* of the long period (10 or more years) during which the company must cover out-of-pocket costs for preclinical drug discovery. Additionally, companies often do not report whether a given figure includes the capitalized cost or comprises only out-of-pocket expenses, or both.

Another element of complexity is that all estimates are based on confidential information controlled by drug companies, released by them voluntarily, leading to inability to verify costs. The numbers are controversial, as drug companies use them to justify the prices of their drugs and various advocates for lower drug prices have challenged them. The controversy is not only between "high" and "low", but also the high numbers may vary considerably for the manifold factors in drug development.

One study assessed both capitalized and out-of-pocket costs as about US$1.8 billion and $870 million, respectively.

In an analysis of the drug development costs for 98 companies over a decade, the average cost per drug developed and approved by a single-drug company was $350 million. But for companies that approved between eight and 13 drugs over 10 years, the cost per drug went as high as $5.5 billion, due mainly to geographic expansion for marketing and ongoing costs for Phase IV trials and continuous monitoring for safety.

Alternatives to conventional drug development have the objective for universities, governments and pharmaceutical industry to collaborate and optimize resources.

Valuation

The nature of a drug development project is characterised by high attrition rates, large capital expenditures, and long timelines. This makes the valuation of such projects and companies a challenging task. Not all valuation methods can cope with these particularities. The most commonly used valuation methods are risk-adjusted net present value (rNPV), decision trees, real options, or comparables.

The most important value drivers are the cost of capital or discount rate that is used, phase attributes such as duration, success rates, and costs, and the forecasted sales, including cost of goods and marketing and sales expenses. Less objective aspects like quality of the management or novelty of the technology should be reflected in the cash flows estimation.

Success Rate

Candidates for a new drug to treat a disease might, theoretically, include from 5,000 to 10,000 chemical compounds. On average about 250 of these show sufficient promise for further evaluation using laboratory tests, mice and other test animals. Typically, about ten of these qualify for tests on humans. A study conducted by the Tufts Center for the Study of Drug Development covering the 1980s and 1990s found that only 21.5 percent of drugs that started Phase I trials were eventually approved for marketing. In the time period of 2006 to 2015, the success rate was 9.6%. The high failure rates associated with pharmaceutical development are referred to as the "attrition rate" problem. Careful decision making during drug development is essential to avoid costly failures. In many cases, intelligent programme and clinical trial design can prevent false negative results. Well designed dose-finding studies and comparisons against both a placebo and a gold-standard treatment arm play a major role in achieving reliable data.

Novel Initiatives to Boost Development

Novel initiatives include partnering between governmental organizations and industry. The world's largest such initiative is the Innovative Medicines Initiative (IMI), and examples of major national initiatives are Top Institute Pharma in the Netherlands and Biopeople in Denmark. In 2004, the FDA created the "Critical Path Initiative" to guide the new drug development process.

Pre-clinical Development

In drug development, preclinical development, also named preclinical studies and nonclinical studies, is a stage of research that begins before clinical trials (testing in humans) can begin, and during which important feasibility, iterative testing and drug safety data are collected.

The main goals of pre-clinical studies are to determine the safe dose for first-in-man study and assess a product's safety profile. Products may include new medical devices, drugs, gene therapy solutions and diagnostic tools.

On average, only one in every 5,000 compounds that enters drug discovery to the stage of preclinical development becomes an approved drug.

Types of Preclinical Research

Each class of product may undergo different types of preclinical research. For instance, drugs may undergo pharmacodynamics (what the drug does to the body) (PD), pharmacokinetics (what the body does to the drug) (PK), ADME, and toxicology testing. This data allows researchers to allometrically estimate a safe starting dose of the drug for clinical trials in humans. Medical devices that do not have drug attached will not undergo these additional tests and may go directly to good laboratory practices (GLP) testing for safety of the device and its components. Some medical devices will also undergo biocompatibility testing which helps to show whether a component of the device or all components are sustainable in a living model. Most preclinical studies must adhere to GLPs in ICH Guidelines to be acceptable for submission to regulatory agencies such as the Food & Drug Administration in the United States.

Typically, both *in vitro* and *in vivo* tests will be performed. Studies of a drug's toxicity include which organs are targeted by that drug, as well as if there are any long-term carcinogenic effects or toxic effects on mammalian reproduction.

Animal Testing

The information collected from these studies is vital so that safe human testing can begin. Typically, in drug development studies animal testing involves two species. The most commonly used models are murine and canine, although primate and porcine are also used.

Choice of Species

The choice of species is based on which will give the best correlation to human trials. Differences in the gut, enzyme activity, circulatory system, or other considerations make certain models more appropriate based on the dosage form, site of activity, or noxious metabolites. For example, canines may not be good models for solid oral dosage forms because the characteristic carnivore intestine is underdeveloped compared to the omnivore's, and gastric emptying rates are increased. Also, rodents can not act as models for antibiotic drugs because the resulting alteration to their intestinal flora causes significant adverse effects. Depending on a drug's functional groups, it may be metabolized in similar or different ways between species, which will affect both efficacy and toxicology.

Medical device studies also use this basic premise. Most studies are performed in larger species such as dogs, pigs and sheep which allow for testing in a similar sized model as that of a human. In addition, some species are used for similarity in specific organs or organ system physiology (swine for dermatological and coronary stent studies; goats for mammary implant studies; dogs for gastric and cancer studies; etc.).

Importantly, the regulatory guidelines of FDA, EMA, and other similar international and regional authorities usually require safety testing in at least two mammalian species, including one non-rodent species, prior to human trials authorization.

Ethical Issues

Animal testing in the research-based pharmaceutical industry has been reduced in recent years both for ethical and cost reasons. However, most research will still involve animal based testing for the need of similarity in anatomy and physiology that is required for diverse product development.

No Observable Effect Levels

Based on preclinical trials, No Observable Adverse Effect Levels (NOAEL) on drugs are established, which are used to determine initial phase 1 clinical trial dosage levels on a mass API per mass patient basis. Generally a 1/100 uncertainty factor or "safety margin" is included to account for interspecies (1/10) and inter-individual (1/10) differences.

Clinical Trial

Clinical trials are experiments done in clinical research. Such prospective biomedical or behavioral research studies on human participants are designed to answer specific questions about biomedical or behavioral interventions, including new treatments (such as novel vaccines, drugs, dietary choices, dietary supplements, and medical devices) and known interventions that warrant further study and comparison. Clinical trials generate data on safety and efficacy. They are conducted only after they have received health authority/ethics committee approval in the country where approval of the therapy is sought. These authorities are responsible for vetting the risk/benefit ratio of the trial - their approval does not mean that the therapy is 'safe' or effective, only that the trial may be conducted.

Depending on product type and development stage, investigators initially enroll volunteers and/or patients into small pilot studies, and subsequently conduct progressively larger scale comparative studies. Clinical trials can vary in size and cost, and they can involve a single research center or multiple centers, in one country or in multiple countries. Clinical study design aims to ensure the scientific validity and reproducibility of the results.

Trials can be quite costly, depending on a number of factors. The sponsor may be a governmental organization or a pharmaceutical, biotechnology or medical device company. Certain functions necessary to the trial, such as monitoring and lab work, may be managed by an outsourced partner, such as a contract research organization or a central laboratory.

Only 10 percent of all drugs started in human clinical trials become an approved drug.

Overview

Trials of Drugs

Some clinical trials involve healthy subjects with no pre-existing medical conditions. Other clinical trials pertain to patients with specific health conditions who are willing to try an experimental treatment.

When participants are healthy volunteers who receive financial incentives, the goals are different than when the participants are sick. During dosing periods, study subjects typically remain under supervision for one to 40 nights.

Usually pilot experiments are conducted to gain insights for design of the clinical trial to follow.

There are two goals to testing medical treatments: to learn whether they work well enough, called "efficacy" or "effectiveness"; and to learn whether they are safe enough, called "safety". Neither is an absolute criterion; both safety and efficacy are evaluated relative to how the treatment is intended to be used, what other treatments are available, and the severity of the disease or condition. The benefits must outweigh the risks. For example, many drugs to treat cancer have severe side effects that would not be acceptable for an over-the-counter pain medication, yet the cancer drugs have been approved since they are used under a physician's care, and are used for a life-threatening condition.

In the US, the elderly constitute only 14 percent of the population, while they consume over one-third of drugs. People over 55 (or a similar cutoff age) are often excluded from trials because their greater health issues and drug use complicate data interpretation, and because they have different physiological capacity than younger people. Women, children and people with unrelated medical conditions are also frequently excluded. For women, a major reason for exclusion is the possibility of pregnancy and the unknown risks to the fetus.

The sponsor designs the trial in coordination with a panel of expert clinical investigators, including what alternative and/or existing treatments to compare to the new drug and what type(s) of patients might benefit. If the sponsor cannot obtain enough test subjects at one location investigators at other locations are recruited to join the study.

During the trial, investigators recruit subjects with the predetermined characteristics, administer the treatment(s) and collect data on the subjects' health for a defined time period. Data include measurements such as vital signs, concentration of the study drug in the blood and/or tissues, changes to symptoms, and whether improvement or worsening of the condition targeted by the study drug occurs. The researchers send the data to the trial sponsor, who then analyzes the pooled data using statistical tests.

Examples of clinical trial goals include assessing the safety and relative effectiveness of a medication or device:

- On a specific kind of patient, for example, a patient who has been diagnosed with Alzheimer's disease

- At varying dosages, for example, a 10 milligram dose instead of a 5 milligram dose

- For a new indication

- Evaluation for improved efficacy in treating a patient's condition as compared to the standard therapy for that condition

- Evaluation of the study drug or device relative to two or more already approved/common interventions for that condition, for example, device A versus device B, or therapy A versus therapy B)

While most clinical trials test one alternative to the novel intervention, some expand to three or four and may include a placebo].

Except for small, single-location trials, the design and objectives are specified in a document called a clinical trial protocol. The protocol is the trial's "operating manual" and ensures that all researchers perform the trial in the same way on similar subjects and that the data is comparable across all subjects.

As a trial is designed to test hypotheses and rigorously monitor and assess outcomes, it can be seen as an application of the scientific method, specifically the experimental step.

The most common clinical trials evaluate new pharmaceutical products, medical devices (such as a new catheter), biologics, psychological therapies, or other interventions. Clinical trials may be required before a national regulatory authority approves marketing of the innovation.

Trials of Devices

Similarly to drugs, medical devices are sometimes subjected to clinical trials. Device trials may compare a new device to an established therapy, or may compare similar devices to each other. An example of the former in the field of vascular surgery is the Open versus Endovascular Repair (OVER trial) for the treatment of abdominal aortic aneurysm, which compared the older open aortic repair technique to the newer endovascular aneurysm repair device. An example of the latter is the LEOPARD trial, which compares EVAR devices.

Trials of Procedures

Similarly to drugs, medical or surgical procedures may be subjected to clinical trials, such as case-controlled studies for surgical interventions.

History

The concepts behind clinical trials are ancient. The Book of Daniel chapter 1, verses 12 through 15, for instance, describes a planned experiment with both baseline and follow-up observations of two groups who either partook of, or did not partake of, "the King's meat" over a trial period of ten days. Persian physician Avicenna, in *The Canon of Medicine* (1025) gave similar advice for determining the efficacy of medical drugs and substances.

Development

Although early medical experimentation was often performed, the use of a control group to provide an accurate comparison for the demonstration of the intervention's efficacy, was generally lacking. For instance, Lady Mary Wortley Montagu, who campaigned for the introduction of inoculation (then called variolation) to prevent smallpox, arranged for seven prisoners who had been sentenced to death to undergo variolation in exchange for their life. Although they survived and did not contract smallpox, there was no control group to assess whether this result was due to the inoculation or some other factor. Similar experiments performed by Edward Jenner over his smallpox vaccine were equally conceptually flawed.

The first proper clinical trial was conducted by the physician James Lind. The disease scurvy, now known to be caused by a Vitamin C deficiency, would often have terrible effects on the welfare of the crew of long distance ocean voyages. In 1740, the catastrophic result of Anson's circumnavigation attracted much attention in Europe; out of 1900 men, 1400 had died, most of them allegedly from having contracted scurvy. John Woodall, an English military surgeon of the British East India Company, had recommended the consumption of citrus fruit (it has an antiscorbutic effect) from the 17th century, but their use did not become widespread.

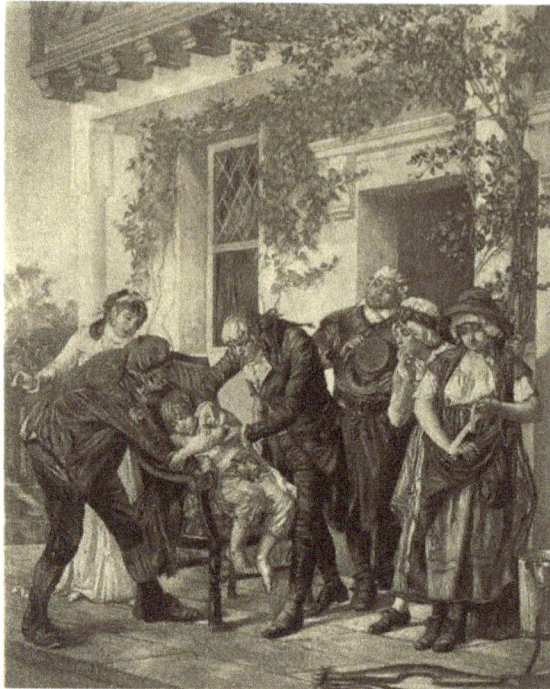

Edward Jenner vaccinating James Phipps, a boy of eight, on 14 May 1796. Jenner failed to use a control group.

Lind conducted the first systematic clinical trial in 1747. He included a dietary supplement of an acidic quality in the experiment after two months at sea, when the ship was already afflicted with scurvy. He divided twelve scorbutic sailors into six groups of two. They all received the same diet but, in addition, group one was given a quart of cider daily, group two twenty-five drops of elixir of vitriol (sulfuric acid), group three six spoonfuls of vinegar, group four half a pint of seawater, group five received two oranges and one lemon, and the last group a spicy paste plus a drink of barley water. The treatment of group five stopped after six days when they ran out of fruit, but by that time one sailor was fit for duty while the other had almost recovered. Apart from that, only group one also showed some effect of its treatment.

After 1750 the discipline began to take its modern shape. John Haygarth demonstrated the importance of a control group for the correct identification of the placebo effect in his celebrated study of the ineffective remedy called *Perkin's tractors*. Further work in that direction was carried out by the eminent physician Sir William Gull, 1st Baronet in the 1860s.

Frederick Akbar Mahomed (d. 1884), who worked at Guy's Hospital in London, made substantial contributions to the process of clinical trials, where "he separated chronic nephritis with secondary hypertension from what we now term essential hypertension. He also founded the Collective Investigation Record for the British Medical Association; this organization collected data from physicians practicing outside the hospital setting and was the precursor of modern collaborative clinical trials."

Modern Trials

Sir Ronald A. Fisher, while working for the Rothamsted experimental station in the field of agriculture, developed his *Principles of experimental design* in the 1920s as an accurate methodology for the proper design of experiments. Among his major ideas, was the importance of randomization - the random assignment of individuals to different groups for the experiment; replication - to reduce uncertainty, measurements should be repeated and experiments replicated to identify sources of variation; blocking - to arrange experimental units into groups of units that are similar to each other, and thus reducing irrelevant sources of variation; use of factorial experiments - efficient at evaluating the effects and possible interactions of several independent factors.

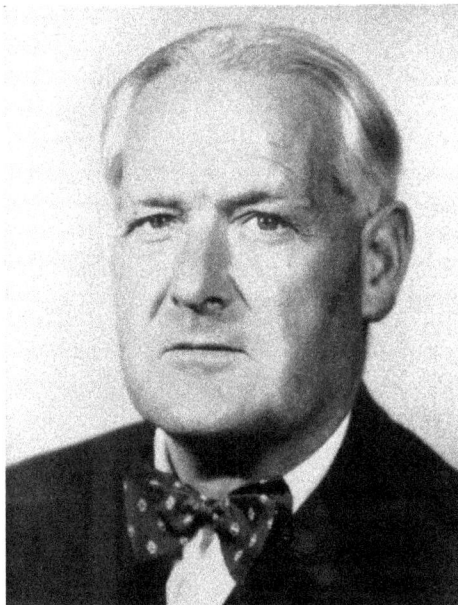

Austin Bradford Hill was a pivotal figure in the modern development of clinical trials.

The British Medical Research Council officially recognized the importance of clinical trials from the 1930s. The Council established the *Therapeutic Trials Committee* to advise and assist in the arrangement of properly controlled clinical trials on new products that seem likely on experimental grounds to have value in the treatment of disease.

The first randomised curative trial was carried out at the MRC Tuberculosis Research Unit by Sir Geoffrey Marshall (1887–1982). The trial, carried out between 1946-1947, aimed to test the efficacy of the chemical streptomycin for curing pulmonary tuberculosis. The trial was both double-blind and placebo-controlled.

The methodology of clinical trials was further developed by Sir Austin Bradford Hill, who had been involved in the streptomcyin trials. From the 1920s, Hill applied statistics to medicine, attending the lectures of renowned mathematician Karl Pearson, amongst others. He became famous for a landmark study carried out in collaboration with Richard Doll on the correlation between smoking and lung cancer. They carried out a case-control study in 1950, which compared lung cancer patients with matched control and also began a sustained long-term prospective study into the broader issue of smoking and health, which involved studying the smoking habits and health of over 30,000 doctors over a period of several years. His certificate for election to the Royal Society called him "...the leader in the development in medicine of the precise experimental methods now used nationally and internationally in the evaluation of new therapeutic and prophylactic agents."

International clinical trials day is celebrated on 20 May.

Types

One way of classifying clinical trials is by the way the researchers behave.

- In a clinical observational study, the investigators observe the subjects and measure their outcomes. The researchers do not actively manage the study.

- In an interventional study, the investigators give the research subjects a particular medicine or other intervention to compare the treated subjects with those receiving no treatment or the standard treatment. Then the researchers measure how the subjects' health changes.

Another way of classifying trials is by their purpose. The U.S. National Institutes of Health (NIH) organizes trials into five different types:

- Prevention trials look for better ways to prevent disease in people who have never had the disease or to prevent a disease from returning. These approaches may include medicines, vitamins, vaccines, minerals, or lifestyle changes.

- Screening trials test the best way to detect certain diseases or health conditions.

- Diagnostic trials are conducted to find better tests or procedures for diagnosing a particular disease or condition.

- Treatment trials test experimental treatments, new combinations of drugs, or new approaches to surgery or radiation therapy.

- Quality of life trials (supportive care trials) explore ways to improve comfort and the quality of life for individuals with a chronic illness.

- Compassionate use trials or expanded access trials provide partially tested, unapproved therapeutics to a small number of patients who have no other realistic options. Usually, this involves a disease for which no effective therapy has been approved, or a patient who has already failed all standard treatments and whose health is too compromised to qualify for participation in randomized clinical trials. Usually, case-by-case approval must be granted by both the United States Food and Drug Administration and the pharmaceutical company for such exceptions.

A third classification is whether the trial design allows changes based on data accumulated during the trial.

- Fixed trials consider existing data only during the trial's design, do not modify the trial after it begins and do not assess the results until the study is complete.

- Adaptive clinical trials use existing data to design the trial, and then use interim results to modify the trial as it proceeds. Modifications include dosage, sample size, drug undergoing trial, patient selection criteria and "cocktail" mix. Adaptive trials often employ a Bayesian experimental design to assess the trial's progress. In some cases, trials have become an ongoing process that regularly adds and drops therapies and patient groups as more information is gained. The aim is to more quickly identify drugs that have a therapeutic effect and to zero in on patient populations for whom the drug is appropriate.

Finally, a common way of distinguishing trials is by phase, which in simple terms, relates to how close the drug is to being clinically proven both effective for its stated purpose and accepted by the regulatory authorities for use for that purpose.

Phases

Clinical trials involving new drugs are commonly classified into five phases. Each phase of the drug approval process is treated as a separate clinical trial. The drug-development process will normally proceed through all four phases over many years. If the drug successfully passes through phases 0, 1, 2, and 3, it will usually be approved by the national regulatory authority for use in the general population. Before pharmaceutical companies start clinical trials on a drug, they will also have conducted extensive preclinical studies. Each phase has a different purpose and helps scientists answer a different question.

Phase	Aim	Notes
Phase 0	Pharmacodynamics and pharmacokinetics in humans	Phase 0 trials are the first-in-human trials. Single subtherapeutic doses of the study drug or treatment are given to a small number of subjects (10 to 15) to gather preliminary data on the agent's pharmacodynamics (what the drug does to the body) and pharmacokinetics (what the body does to the drugs). For a test drug, the trial documents the absorption, distribution, metabolization, and removal (excretion) of the drug, and the drug's interactions within the body, to confirm that these appear to be as expected.
Phase 1	Screening for safety.	Testing within a small group of people (20–80) to evaluate safety, determine safe dosage ranges, and begin to identify side effects. A drug's side effects could be subtle or long term, or may only happen with a few people, so phase 1 trials are not expected to identify all side effects.
Phase 2	Establishing the efficacy of the drug, usually against a placebo.	Testing with a larger group of people (100–300) to determine efficacy and to further evaluate its safety. The gradual increase in test group size allows for the evocation of less-common side effects.
Phase 3	Final confirmation of safety and efficacy.	Testing with large groups of people (1,000–3,000) to confirm its efficacy, evaluate its effectiveness, monitor side effects, compare it to commonly used treatments, and collect information that will allow it to be used safely.
Phase 4	Safety studies during sales.	Postmarketing studies delineate additional information, including the treatment's risks, benefits, and optimal use. As such, they are ongoing during the drug's lifetime of active medical use. (Particularly relevant after approval under FDA Accelerated Approval Program)

Trial Design

A fundamental distinction in evidence-based practice is between observational studies and randomized controlled trials. Types of observational studies in epidemiology, such as the cohort study and the case-control study, provide less compelling evidence than the randomized controlled trial. In observational studies, the investigators only observe associations (correlations) between the treatments experienced by participants and their health status. However, under certain conditions, causal effects can be inferred from observational studies.

A randomized controlled trial can provide compelling evidence that the study treatment causes an effect on human health.

Currently, some phase 2 and most phase 3 drug trials are designed as randomized, double-blind, and placebo-controlled.

- Randomized: Each study subject is randomly assigned to receive either the study treatment or a placebo.

- Blind: The subjects involved in the study do not know which study treatment they receive. If the study is double-blind, the researchers also do not know which treatment a subject receives. This intent is to prevent researchers from treating the two groups differently. A form of double-blind study called a "double-dummy" design allows additional insurance against bias. In this kind of study, all patients are given both placebo and active doses in alternating periods.

- Placebo-controlled: The use of a placebo (fake treatment) allows the researchers to isolate the effect of the study treatment from the placebo effect.

Although the term "clinical trials" is most commonly associated with the large, randomized studies typical of phase 3, many clinical trials are small. They may be "sponsored" by single researchers or a small group of researchers, and are designed to test simple questions. In the field of rare diseases, sometimes the number of patients is the limiting factor for the size of a clinical trial.

Active Comparator Studies

Of note, during the last 10 years or so, it has become a common practice to conduct "active comparator" studies (also known as "active control" trials). In other words, when a treatment is clearly better than doing nothing for the subject (*i.e.* giving them the placebo), the alternate treatment would be a standard-of-care therapy. The study would compare the 'test' treatment to standard-of-care therapy.

A growing trend in the pharmacology field involves the use of third-party contractors to obtain the required comparator compounds. Such third parties provide expertise in the logistics of obtaining, storing, and shipping the comparators. As an advantage to the manufacturer of the comparator compounds, a well-established comparator sourcing agency can alleviate the problem of parallel importing (importing a patented compound for sale in a country outside the patenting agency's sphere of influence).

Master Protocol

In such studies, multiple experimental treatments are tested in a single trial. Genetic testing enables researchers to group patients according to their genetic profile, deliver drugs based on that profile to that group and compare the results. Multiple companies can participate, each bringing a different drug. The first such approach targets squamous cell cancer, which includes varying genetic disruptions from patient to patient. Amgen, AstraZeneca and Pfizer are involved, the first time they have worked together in a late-stage trial. Patients whose genomic profiles do not match any of the trial drugs receive a drug designed to stimulate the immune system to attack cancer.

Clinical Trial Protocol

A clinical trial protocol is a document used to define and manage the trial. It is prepared by a panel of experts. All study investigators are expected to strictly observe the protocol.

The protocol describes the scientific rationale, objective(s), design, methodology, statistical considerations and organization of the planned trial. Details of the trial are provided in documents referenced in the protocol, such as an investigator's brochure.

The protocol contains a precise study plan to assure safety and health of the trial subjects and to provide an exact template for trial conduct by investigators. This allows data to be combined across all investigators/sites. The protocol also informs the study administrators (often a contract research organization).

The format and content of clinical trial protocols sponsored by pharmaceutical, biotechnology or medical device companies in the United States, European Union, or Japan have been standardized to follow Good Clinical Practice guidance issued by the International Conference on Harmonization of Technical Requirements for Registration of Pharmaceuticals for Human Use (ICH). Regulatory authorities in Canada and Australia also follow ICH guidelines. Journals such as *Trials*, encourage investigators to publish their protocols.

Design Features

Informed Consent

Clinical trials recruit study subjects to sign a document representing their "informed consent". The document includes details such as its purpose, duration, required procedures, risks, potential benefits, key contacts and institutional requirements. The participant then decides whether to sign the document. The document is not a contract, as the participant can withdraw at any time without penalty.

Example of informed consent document from the PARAMOUNT trial

Informed consent is a legal process in which a recruit is instructed about key facts before deciding whether to participate. Researchers explain the details of the study in terms the subject can understand. The information is presented in the subject's native language. Generally, children cannot autonomously provide informed consent, but depending on their age and other factors, may be required to provide informed assent.

Statistical Power

The number of subjects has a large impact on the ability to reliably detect and measure effects of the intervention. This is described as its "power". The larger the number of participants, the greater the statistical power and the greater the cost.

The statistical power estimates the ability of a trial to detect a difference of a particular size (or larger) between the treatment and control groups. For example, a trial of a lipid-lowering drug versus placebo with 100 patients in each group might have a power of 0.90 to detect a difference between placebo and trial groups receiving dosage of 10 mg/dL or more, but only 0.70 to detect a difference of 6 mg/dL.

Placebo Groups

Merely giving a treatment can have nonspecific effects. These are controlled for by the inclusion of patients who receive only a placebo. Subjects are assigned randomly without informing them to which group they belonged. Many trials are doubled-blinded so that researchers do not know to which group a subject is assigned.

Assigning a subject to a placebo group can pose an ethical problem if it violates his or her right to receive the best available treatment. The Declaration of Helsinki provides guidelines on this issue.

Duration

Clinical trials are only a small part of the research that goes into developing a new treatment. Potential drugs, for example, first have to be discovered, purified, characterized, and tested in labs (in cell and animal studies) before ever undergoing clinical trials. In all, about 1,000 potential drugs are tested before just one reaches the point of being tested in a clinical trial. For example, a new cancer drug has, on average, six years of research behind it before it even makes it to clinical trials. But the major holdup in making new cancer drugs available is the time it takes to complete clinical trials themselves. On average, about eight years pass from the time a cancer drug enters clinical trials until it receives approval from regulatory agencies for sale to the public. Drugs for other diseases have similar timelines.

Some reasons a clinical trial might last several years:

- For chronic conditions such as cancer, it takes months, if not years, to see if a cancer treatment has an effect on a patient.

- For drugs that are not expected to have a strong effect (meaning a large number of patients must be recruited to observe 'any' effect), recruiting enough patients to test the drug's effectiveness (i.e., getting statistical power) can take several years.

- Only certain people who have the target disease condition are eligible to take part in each clinical trial. Researchers who treat these particular patients must participate in the trial. Then they must identify the desirable patients and obtain consent from them or their families to take part in the trial.

The biggest barrier to completing studies is the shortage of people who take part. All drug and many device trials target a subset of the population, meaning not everyone can participate. Some drug trials require patients to have unusual combinations of disease characteristics. It is a challenge to find the appropriate patients and obtain their consent, especially when they may receive no direct benefit (because they are not paid, the study drug is not yet proven to work, or the patient may receive a placebo). In the case of cancer patients, fewer than 5% of adults with cancer will participate in drug trials. According to the Pharmaceutical Research and Manufacturers of America (PhRMA), about 400 cancer medicines were being tested in clinical trials in 2005. Not all of these will prove to be useful, but those that are may be delayed in getting approved because the number of participants is so low.

For clinical trials involving a seasonal indication (such as airborne allergies, seasonal affective disorder, influenza, and others), the study can only be done during a limited part of the year (such as spring for pollen allergies), when the drug can be tested. This can be an additional complication on the length of the study, yet proper planning and the use of trial sites in the Southern, as well as the Northern Hemisphere allows for year-round trials, which can reduce the length of the studies.

Clinical trials that do not involve a new drug usually have a much shorter duration. (Exceptions are epidemiological studies, such as the Nurses' Health Study).

Administration

Clinical trials designed by a local investigator, and (in the US) federally funded clinical trials, are almost always administered by the researcher who designed the study and applied for the grant. Small-scale device studies may be administered by the sponsoring company. Clinical trials of new drugs are usually administered by a contract research organization (CRO) hired by the sponsoring company. The sponsor provides the drug and medical oversight. A CRO is contracted to perform all the administrative work on a clinical trial. For phases 2, 3 and 4, the CRO recruits participating researchers, trains them, provides them with supplies, coordinates study administration and data collection, sets up meetings, monitors the sites for compliance with the clinical protocol, and ensures the sponsor receives data from every site. Specialist site management organizations can also be hired to coordinate with the CRO to ensure rapid IRB/IEC approval and faster site initiation and patient recruitment. Phase 1 clinical trials of new medicines are often conducted in a specialist clinical trial clinic, with dedicated pharmacologists, where the subjects can be observed by full-time staff. These clinics are often run by a CRO which specialises in these studies.

At a participating site, one or more research assistants (often nurses) do most of the work in conducting the clinical trial. The research assistant's job can include some or all of the following: providing the local institutional review board (IRB) with the documentation necessary to obtain its permission to conduct the study, assisting with study start-up, identifying eligible patients, obtaining consent from them or their families, administering study treatment(s), collecting and statistically analyzing data, maintaining and updating data files during followup, and communicating with the IRB, as well as the sponsor and CRO.

Marketing

Janet Yang uses the Interactional Justice Model to test the effects of willingness to talk with a doctor and clinical trial enrollment. Results found that potential clinical trial candidates were less likely to enroll in clinical trials if the patient is more willing to talk with their doctor. The reasoning behind this discovery may be patients are happy with their current care. Another reason for the negative relationship between perceived fairness and clinical trial enrollment is the lack of independence from the care provider. Results found that there is a positive relationship between a lack of willingness to talk with their doctor and clinical trial enrollment. Lack of willingness to talk about clinical trials with current care providers may be due to patients' independence from the doctor. Patients who are less likely to talk about clinical trials are more willing to use other sources of information to gain a better insight of alternative treatments. Clinical trial enrollment should be motivated to utilize websites and television advertising to inform the public about clinical trial enrollment.

Information Technology

The last decade has seen a proliferation of information technology use in the planning and conduct of clinical trials. Clinical trial management systems are often used by research sponsors or CROs to help plan and manage the operational aspects of a clinical trial, particularly with respect to investigational sites. Advanced analytics for identifying researchers and research sites with expertise in a given area utilize public and private information about ongoing research. Web-based electronic data capture (EDC) and clinical data management systems are used in a majority of clinical trials to collect case report data from sites, manage its quality and prepare it for analysis. Interactive voice response systems are used by sites to register the enrollment of patients using a phone and to allocate patients to a particular treatment arm (although phones are being increasingly replaced with web-based (IWRS) tools which are sometimes part of the EDC system). While patient-reported outcome were often paper based in the past, measurements are increasingly being collected using web portals or hand-held ePRO (or eDiary) devices, sometimes wireless. Statistical software is used to analyze the collected data and prepare them for regulatory submission. Access to many of these applications are increasingly aggregated in web-based clinical trial portals. In 2011, the FDA approved a phase 1 trial that used telemonitoring, also known as remote patient monitoring, to collect biometric data in patients' homes and transmit it electronically to the trial database. This technology provides many more data points and is far more convenient for patients, because they have fewer visits to trial sites.

Ethical Aspects

Clinical trials are closely supervised by appropriate regulatory authorities. All studies involving a medical or therapeutic intervention on patients must be approved by a supervising ethics committee before permission is granted to run the trial. The local ethics committee has discretion on how it will supervise noninterventional studies (observational studies or those using already collected data). In the US, this body is called the Institutional Review Board (IRB); in the EU, they are called Ethics committees. Most IRBs are located at the local investigator's hospital or institution, but some sponsors allow the use of a central (independent/for profit) IRB for investigators who work at smaller institutions.

To be ethical, researchers must obtain the full and informed consent of participating human subjects. (One of the IRB's main functions is to ensure potential patients are adequately informed about the clinical trial.) If the patient is unable to consent for him/herself, researchers can seek consent from the patient's legally authorized representative. In California, the state has prioritized the individuals who can serve as the legally authorized representative.

In some US locations, the local IRB must certify researchers and their staff before they can conduct clinical trials. They must understand the federal patient privacy (HIPAA) law and good clinical practice. The International Conference of Harmonisation Guidelines for Good Clinical Practice is a set of standards used internationally for the conduct of clinical trials. The guidelines aim to ensure the "rights, safety and well being of trial subjects are protected".

The notion of informed consent of participating human subjects exists in many countries all over the world, but its precise definition may still vary.

Informed consent is clearly a 'necessary' condition for ethical conduct but does not 'ensure' ethical conduct. In compassionate use trials the latter becomes a particularly difficult problem. The final objective is to serve the community of patients or future patients in a best-possible and most responsible way. However, it may be hard to turn this objective into a well-defined, quantified, objective function. In some cases this can be done, however, for instance, for questions of when to stop sequential treatments, and then quantified methods may play an important role.

Additional ethical concerns are present when conducting clinical trials on children (pediatrics), and in emergency or epidemic situations.

Conflicts of Interest and Unfavorable Studies

In response to specific cases in which unfavorable data from pharmaceutical company-sponsored research were not published, the Pharmaceutical Research and Manufacturers of America published new guidelines urging companies to report all findings and limit the financial involvement in drug companies by researchers. The US Congress signed into law a bill which requires phase II and phase III clinical trials to be registered by the sponsor on the the clinical trials website compiled by the National Institutes of Health.

Drug researchers not directly employed by pharmaceutical companies often seek grants from manufacturers, and manufacturers often look to academic researchers to conduct studies within networks of universities and their hospitals, e.g., for translational cancer research. Similarly, competition for tenured academic positions, government grants and prestige create conflicts of interest among academic scientists. According to one study, approximately 75% of articles retracted for misconduct-related reasons have no declared industry financial support. Seeding trials are particularly controversial.

In the United States, all clinical trials submitted to the FDA as part of a drug approval process are independently assessed by clinical experts within the Food and Drug Administration, including inspections of primary data collection at selected clinical trial sites.

In 2001, the editors of 12 major journals issued a joint editorial, published in each journal, on the control over clinical trials exerted by sponsors, particularly targeting the use of contracts which allow sponsors to review the studies prior to publication and withhold publication. They strengthened editorial restrictions to counter the effect. The editorial noted that contract research organizations had, by 2000, received 60% of the grants from pharmaceutical companies in the US. Researchers may be restricted from contributing to the trial design, accessing the raw data, and interpreting the results.

Safety

Responsibility for the safety of the subjects in a clinical trial is shared between the sponsor, the local site investigators (if different from the sponsor), the various IRBs that supervise the study, and (in some cases, if the study involves a marketable drug or device), the regulatory agency for the country where the drug or device will be sold.

For safety reasons, many clinical trials of drugs are designed to exclude women of childbearing age, pregnant women, and/or women who become pregnant during the study. In some cases, the male partners of these women are also excluded or required to take birth control measures.

Sponsor

Throughout the clinical trial, the sponsor is responsible for accurately informing the local site investigators of the true historical safety record of the drug, device or other medical treatments to be tested, and of any potential interactions of the study treatment(s) with already approved treatments. This allows the local investigators to make an informed judgment on whether to participate in the study or not. The sponsor is also responsible for monitoring the results of the study as they come in from the various sites, as the trial proceeds. In larger clinical trials, a sponsor will use the services of a data monitoring committee (DMC, known in the US as a data safety monitoring board). This independent group of clinicians and statisticians meets periodically to review the unblinded data the sponsor has received so far. The DMC has the power to recommend termination of the study based on their review, for example if the study treatment is causing more deaths than the standard treatment, or seems to be causing unexpected and study-related serious adverse events.The sponsor is responsible for collecting adverse event reports from all site investigators in the study, and for informing all the investigators of the sponsor's judgment as to whether these adverse events were related or not related to the study treatment. This is an area where sponsors can slant their judgment to favor the study treatment.

The sponsor and the local site investigators are jointly responsible for writing a site-specific informed consent that accurately informs the potential subjects of the true risks and potential benefits of participating in the study, while at the same time presenting the material as briefly as possible and in ordinary language. FDA regulations and ICH guidelines both require "the information that is given to the subject or the representative shall be in language understandable to the subject or the representative." If the participant's native language is not English, the sponsor must translate the informed consent into the language of the participant.

Local Site Investigators

The ethical principle of *primum non nocere* ("first, do no harm") guides the trial, and if an investigator believes the study treatment may be harming subjects in the study, the investigator can stop participating at any time. On the other hand, investigators often have a financial interest in recruiting subjects, and could act unethically to obtain and maintain their participation.

The local investigators are responsible for conducting the study according to the study protocol, and supervising the study staff throughout the duration of the study. The local investigator or his/her study staff are also responsible for ensuring the potential subjects in the study understand the risks and potential benefits of participating in the study. In other words, they (or their legally authorized representatives) must give truly informed consent.

Local investigators are responsible for reviewing all adverse event reports sent by the sponsor. These adverse event reports contain the opinion of both the investigator at the site where the adverse event occurred, and the sponsor, regarding the relationship of the adverse event to the study treatments. Local investigators also are responsible for making an independent judgment of these reports, and promptly informing the local IRB of all serious and study treatment-related adverse events.

When a local investigator is the sponsor, there may not be formal adverse event reports, but study staff at all locations are responsible for informing the coordinating investigator of anything unexpected. The local investigator is responsible for being truthful to the local IRB in all communications relating to the study.

Institutional Review Boards (IRBs)

Approval by an Institutional Review Board (IRB), or ethics board, is necessary before all but the most informal research can begin. In commercial clinical trials, the study protocol is not approved by an IRB before the sponsor recruits sites to conduct the trial. However, the study protocol and procedures have been tailored to fit generic IRB submission requirements. In this case, and where there is no independent sponsor, each local site investigator submits the study protocol, the consent(s), the data collection forms, and supporting documentation to the local IRB. Universities and most hospitals have in-house IRBs. Other researchers (such as in walk-in clinics) use independent IRBs.

The IRB scrutinizes the study for both medical safety and protection of the patients involved in the study, before it allows the researcher to begin the study. It may require changes in study procedures or in the explanations given to the patient. A required yearly "continuing review" report from the investigator updates the IRB on the progress of the study and any new safety information related to the study.

Regulatory Agencies

In the US, the FDA can audit the files of local site investigators after they have finished participating in a study, to see if they were correctly following study procedures. This audit may be random, or for cause (because the investigator is suspected of fraudulent data). Avoiding an audit is an incentive for investigators to follow study procedures.

Alternatively, many American pharmaceutical companies have moved some clinical trials overseas. Benefits of conducting trials abroad include lower costs (in some countries) and the ability to run larger trials in shorter timeframes. Critics have argued that clinical trials performed outside the U.S. allow companies to avoid many of the FDA's regulations, since the FDA audits these trials less frequently than U.S. studies. For drug applications approved by the FDA in 2008, 0.7 percent of foreign clinical study sites were audited by the FDA compared to 1.9 percent domestically. Other criticisms of foreign clinical studies, especially in developing countries, relate to the rights and welfare of study participants, integrity of study data, and relevance of data to the U.S. population.

Different countries have different regulatory requirements and enforcement abilities. An estimated 40% of all clinical trials now take place in Asia, Eastern Europe, and Central and South America. "There is no compulsory registration system for clinical trials in these countries and many do not follow European directives in their operations", says Jacob Sijtsma of the Netherlands-based WEMOS, an advocacy health organisation tracking clinical trials in developing countries.

Beginning in the 1980s, harmonization of clinical trial protocols was shown as feasible across countries of the European Union. At the same time, coordination between Europe, Japan and the United States led to a joint regulatory-industry initiative on international harmonization named after 1990 as the International Conference on Harmonisation of Technical Requirements for Registration of Pharmaceuticals for Human Use (ICH) Currently, most clinical trial programs follow ICH guidelines, aimed at "ensuring that good quality, safe and effective medicines are developed and registered in the most efficient and cost-effective manner. These activities are pursued in the interest of the consumer and public health, to prevent unnecessary duplication of clinical trials in humans and to minimize the use of animal testing without compromising the regulatory obligations of safety and effectiveness."

Economics

Sponsor

The cost of a study depends on many factors, especially the number of sites conducting the study, the number of patients required, and whether the study treatment is already approved for medical use. Clinical trials follow a standardized process.

The expenses incurred by a pharmaceutical company in administering a phase 3 or 4 clinical trial may include, among others:

- production of the drug(s) or device(s) being evaluated
- staff salaries for the designers and administrators of the trial
- payments to the contract research organization, the site management organization (if used) and any outside consultants
- payments to local researchers and their staffs for their time and effort in recruiting test subjects and collecting data for the sponsor
- the cost of study materials and the charges incurred to ship them
- communication with the local researchers, including on-site monitoring by the CRO before and (in some cases) multiple times during the study
- one or more investigator training meetings

- expense incurred by the local researchers, such as pharmacy fees, IRB fees and postage

- any payments to subjects enrolled in the trial (all payments are strictly overseen by the IRBs to ensure the amount of remuneration offered to test subjects does not entice anyone to participate in the trial)

- the expense of treating a test subject who develops a medical condition unrelated to that being targeted by the study drug, but caused by the study drug

These expenses are incurred over several years.

In the USA, sponsors may receive a 50 percent tax credit for clinical trials conducted on drugs being developed for the treatment of orphan diseases. National health agencies, such as the US National Institutes of Health, offer grants to investigators who design clinical trials that attempt to answer research questions of interest to the agency. In these cases, the investigator who writes the grant and administers the study acts as the sponsor, and coordinates data collection from any other sites. These other sites may or may not be paid for participating in the study, depending on the amount of the grant and the amount of effort expected from them.

Clinical trials are traditionally expensive and difficult to undertake. Using internet resources can, in some cases, reduce the economic burden. New technologies enable sponsors and CRO's to reduce trial costs by executing online feasibility assessments and better collaborate with research centers such as ViS Research Institute.

Investigators

Many clinical trials do not involve any money. However, when the sponsor is a private company or a national health agency, investigators are almost always paid to participate. These amounts can be small, just covering a partial salary for research assistants and the cost of any supplies (usually the case with national health agency studies), or be substantial and include 'overhead' that allows the investigator to pay the research staff during times between clinical trials.

Subjects

Participants in phase 1 drug trials do not gain any direct benefit from taking part. They are generally paid an inconvenience allowance because they give up their time (sometimes away from their homes); the amounts paid are regulated and are not related to the level of risk involved. In most other trials, subjects are not paid to ensure their motivation for participating is the hope of getting better or contributing to medical knowledge, without their judgment being skewed by financial considerations. However, they are often given small payments for study-related expenses such as travel or as compensation for their time in providing follow-up information about their health after they are discharged from medical care.

Participation as Labour

It has been suggested that clinical trial participants be considered to be performing 'experimental' or 'clinical labour'. Re-classifying clinical trials as labour is supported by the fact that information gained from clinical trials contributes to biomedical knowledge, and thus increases the profits of pharmaceutical companies. The labour performed by those participants in clinical trials includes the provision of tissue samples and information, the performance of other tasks, such as adhering to a special diet, or (in the case of phase I trials particularly) exposing themselves to risk. The participants in exchange are offered potential access to medical treatment. For some, this may be a treatment with the potential to succeed where other treatments have failed. For other individuals, particularly those situated in countries such as China or India, they may be given access to healthcare which they otherwise would be unable to afford, for the duration of the trial. Thus, the exchange which exists may serve to classify clinical trials as a form of labour.

Participant Recruitment and Participation

Phase 0 and phase 1 drug trials seek healthy volunteers. Most other clinical trials seek patients who have a specific disease or medical condition. The diversity observed in society, by consensus, should be reflected in clinical trials through the appropriate inclusion of ethnic minority populations. Patient recruitment or participant recruitment (as some participants in clinical trials are considered 'healthy' and not patients) plays a significant role in the activities and responsibilities of sites conducting clinical trials.

Newspaper advertisements seeking patients and healthy volunteers to participate in clinical trials

Locating Trials

Depending on the kind of participants required, sponsors of clinical trials, or contract research organizations working on their behalf, try to find sites with qualified personnel as well as access to patients who could participate in the trial. Working with those sites, they may use various recruitment strategies, including patient databases, newspaper and radio advertisements, flyers, posters in places the patients might go (such as doctor's offices), and personal recruitment of patients by investigators.

Volunteers with specific conditions or diseases have additional online resources to help them locate clinical trials. For example, the Fox Trial Finder connects Parkinson's disease trials around the world to volunteers who have a specific set of criteria such as location, age, and symptoms. Other disease-specific services exist for volunteers to find trials related to their condition. Volunteers may search directly on ClinicalTrials.gov to locate trials using a registry run by the U.S. National Institutes of Health and National Library of Medicine.

However, many clinical trials will not accept participants who contact them directly to volunteer, as it is believed this may bias the characteristics of the population being studied. Such trials typically recruit via networks of medical professionals who ask their individual patients to consider enrollment.

Steps for Volunteers

Before participating in a clinical trial, interested volunteers should speak with their doctors, family members, and others who have participated in trials in the past. After locating a trial, volunteers will often have the opportunity to speak or e-mail the clinical trial coordinator for more information and to answer any questions. After receiving consent from their doctors, volunteers then arrange an appointment for a screening visit with the trial coordinator.

All volunteers being considered for a trial are required to undertake a medical screening. Requirements differ according to the trial needs, but typically volunteers would be screened in a medical laboratory for:

- Measurement of the electrical activity of the heart (ECG)

- Measurement of blood pressure, heart rate and body temperature

- Blood sampling

- Urine sampling

- Weight and height measurement

- Drug abuse testing

- Pregnancy testing

Volunteers have the right to know and understand the details of what will happen during a clinical trial, a process called informed consent.

Research

In 2012, Z. Janet Yang, Katherine A. McComas, Geri K. Gay, John P. Leonard, Andrew J. Dannenberg, and Hildy Dillon conducted research on the attitudes towards clinical trial treatment and the decision making of signing up for such trials by cancer patients and the general population. They used the risk information seeking and processing (RISP) model to analyze the social implications that affect attitudes and decision making pertaining to clinical trials. People who hold a higher stake or interest in clinical trial treatment showed a greater likelihood of seeking information about clinical trials. Those with networks that stress the importance of learning about clinical trials are also more likely to seek and process information more deeply. People with more knowledge about clinical trials tend to have to a greater likelihood of signing up. In the study, cancer patients reported more optimistic attitudes towards clinical trials than the general population. Having a more optimistic outlook on clinical trials also leads to greater likelihood of enrolling.

Regulation of Therapeutic Goods

The regulation of therapeutic goods, that is drugs and therapeutic devices, varies by jurisdiction. In some countries, such as the United States, they are regulated at the national level by a single agency. In other jurisdictions they are regulated at the state level, or at both state and national levels by various bodies, as is the case in Australia.

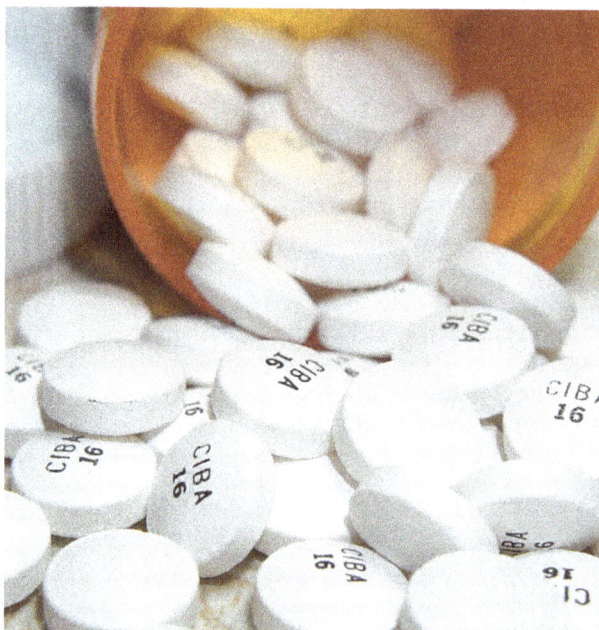
Methylphenidate, in the form of Ritalin pills.

The role of therapeutic goods regulation is designed mainly to protect the health and safety of the population. Regulation is aimed at ensuring the safety, quality, and efficacy of the therapeutic goods which are covered under the scope of the regulation. In most jurisdictions, therapeutic goods must be registered before they are allowed to be marketed. There is usually some degree of restriction of the availability of certain therapeutic goods depending on their risk to consumers.

Regulation by Country

Australia

Therapeutic goods in Australia are regulated by the Therapeutic Goods Administration (TGA). The availability of drugs and poisoperuns is regulated by scheduling under individual state legislation, but is generally under the guidance of the national Standard for the Uniform Scheduling of Drugs and Poisons (SUSDP).

Under the SUSDP, medicinal agents generally belong to one of five categories:

- Unscheduled/exempt

- Schedule 2 (S2) - Pharmacy Medicines

- Schedule 3 (S3) - Pharmacist Only Medicines

- Schedule 4 (S4) - Prescription Only Medicines

- Schedule 8 (S8) - Controlled Drugs

Brazil

Therapeutic goods in Brazil are regulated by the Brazilian Health Ministry, through its National Health Surveillance Agency (equivalent to USA's FDA). There are 5 main categories:

- Normal Medicines - Cough, cold and fever medicines, antiseptics, vitamins and others. Sold freely in pharmacies and some large supermarkets.

- Red Stripe Medicines - These medicines are sold only with medical prescription. Antibiotics, Anti allergenics, Anti inflammatories, and other medicines. In Brazil, governmental control is loose on this type; it is not uncommon to buy this type of prescription medicine over the counter without a prescription.

- Red Stripe Psychoactive Medicines - These medicines are sold only with a "Special Control" white medical prescription with carbon copy, which is valid for 30 days. The original must be retained by the pharmacist after the sale and the patient keeps the carbon copy. Drugs include anti-depressants, anti-convulsants, some sleep aids, anti-psychotics and other non-habit-inducing controlled medicines. Though some consider them habit inducing, anabolic steroids are also regulated under this category.

- Black Stripe Medicines - These medicines are sold only with the "Blue B Form" medical prescription, which is valid for 30 days and must be retained by the pharmacist after the sale. Includes sedatives (benzodiazepines), some anorexic inducers and other habit-inducing controlled medicines.

- "Yellow A Form" prescription medicines - These medicines are sold only with the "Yellow A Form" medical prescription - the most tightly controlled, which is valid for 30 days and must be retained by the pharmacist after the sale. Includes amphetamines and other stimulants (such as methylphenidate), opioids (such as morphine and oxycodone) and other strong habit-forming controlled medicines.

Canada

In Canada, regulation of therapeutic goods are governed by the Food and Drug Act and associated regulations. In addition, the Controlled Drugs and Substances Act requires additional regulatory requirements for controlled drugs and drug precursors.

Burma (Myanmar)

The regulation of drugs in Burma is governed by the Food and Drug Administration (Burma) and Food and Drug Board of Authority.

China

The regulation of drugs in China is governed by the China Food and Drug Administration.

Europe

United Kingdom

Medicines for Human Use in the United Kingdom are regulated by the Medicines and Healthcare products Regulatory Agency (MHRA). The availability of drugs is regulated by classification by the MHRA as part of marketing authorisation of a product.

The United Kingdom has a three-tiered classification system:

- General Sale List (GSL)

- Pharmacy medicines (P)

- Prescription Only Medicines (POM)

Within POM, certain agents with a high abuse/addiction liability are also separately scheduled under the Misuse of Drugs Act 1971 (amended with the Misuse of Drugs Regulations 2001); and are commonly known as Controlled Drugs (CD).

Norway

Medicines in Norway are divided into five groups:

Class A Narcotics, sedative-hypnotics, and amphetamines in this class require a special prescription form:

- morphine and its immediate family, heroin, desomorphine, nicomorphine;

- codeine and its immediate family, dihydrocodeine, ethylmorphine, nicocodeine;

- morphine relatives: hydromorphone and oxymorphone;

- codeine relatives: hydrocodone and oxycodone;

- synthetic opioids: pethidine, methadone, fentanyl, and levorphanol;

- various sedative-hypnotics: temazepam, methaqualone, pentobarbital, and secobarbital;

- various stimulants: amphetamines and methylphenidate;

- flunitrazepam (moved from class B)

Class B Restricted substances which easily lead to addiction like:

- co-codamol

- diazepam

- nitrazepam

- all other benzodiazepines (with the exception of temazepam and flunitrazepam)

- phentermine

Class C - All prescription-only substances

Class F - Substances and package-sizes not requiring a prescription

Unclassifieds - Brands and packages not actively marketed in Norway

Iceland

Medicines in Iceland are regulated by the Icelandic Medicines Control Agency.

Ireland

Medicines in the Republic of Ireland are regulated according to the Misuse of Drugs Regulations 1988. Controlled drugs (CD's) are divided into five categories based on their potential for misuse and therapeutic effectiveness.

- CD1: cannabis, lysergamide, coca leaf, etc. Use prohibited except in limited circumstances where a license has been granted.

- CD2: amphetamine, methadone, morphine, fentanyl, oxycodone, tapentadol, etc. Prescriptions must be handwritten and are only valid for 14 days. Repeat prescriptions are not permitted. Drugs must comply with safe custody and destruction of unsold/unused medication must be witnessed. Must be registered in a Controlled Drugs register.

- CD3: temazepam, flunitrazepam, etc. As CD2, except witnessed destruction and CD register are not required.

- CD4: benzodiazepines, e.g. diazepam, nitrazepam, low dose (methyl)phenobarbitone

- CD5: low-dose codeine, etc.

Switzerland

Medicines in Switzerland are regulated by Swissmedic. The country is not part of the European Union, and is regarded by many as one of the easiest places to conduct clinical trials on new drug compounds.

There are 5 categories from A to E to cover different types of delivery category:

- A: Supply once with a prescription from a doctor or veterinarian

- B: Supply with a prescription from a doctor or veterinarian

- C: Supply on technical advice from medical staff

- D: Supply on technical advice

- E: Supply without technical advice

India

Medicines in India are regulated by CDSCO - Central Drugs Standard Control Organization Under Ministry of Health and Family Welfare. Headed by Directorate General of Health Services CDSCO regulates the Pharmaceutical Products through DCGI - Drugs Controller General of India at Chair. Under Retail and Distribution:- Drugs classified under 5 heads 1. Schedule X drugs – Narcotics 2. Schedule H and L – Injectables, Antibiotics, Antibacterials 3. Schedule C and C1- Biological Products-example Serums and Vaccines

Under Manufacturing Practice 1. Schedule N List of the equipment for the efficient running of manufacturing wing, Qualified personnel 2. Schedule M

United States

Therapeutic goods in the United States are regulated by the U.S. Food and Drug Administration (FDA), which makes some drugs available over the counter (OTC) at retail outlets and others by prescription only.

The prescription or possession of some substances is controlled or prohibited by scheduling in the Controlled Substances Act, under the joint jurisdiction of the FDA and the Drug Enforcement Administration (DEA). Some US states apply more stringent limits on the prescription of certain controlled substances and OTC drugs such as pseudoephedrine.

References

- Madsen U, Krogsgaard-Larsen P, Liljefors T (2002). Textbook of Drug Design and Discovery. Washington, DC: Taylor & Francis. ISBN 0-415-28288-8.

- Reynolds CH, Merz KM, Ringe D, eds. (2010). Drug Design: Structure- and Ligand-Based Approaches (1 ed.). Cambridge, UK: Cambridge University Press. ISBN 978-0521887236.

- Wu-Pong S, Rojanasakul Y (2008). Biopharmaceutical drug design and development (2nd ed.). Totowa, NJ Humana Press: Humana Press. ISBN 978-1-59745-532-9.

- Hopkins AL (2011). "Chapter 25: Pharmacological space". In Wermuth CG. The Practice of Medicinal Chemistry (3 ed.). Academic Press. pp. 521–527. ISBN 978-0-12-374194-3.

- Kirchmair J (2014). Drug Metabolism Prediction. Wiley's Methods and Principles in Medicinal Chemistry. 63. Wiley-VCH. ISBN 978-3-527-67301-8.

- Guner OF (2000). Pharmacophore Perception, Development, and use in Drug Design. La Jolla, Calif: International University Line. ISBN 0-9636817-6-1.

- Timmerman H, Gubernator K, Böhm H, Mannhold R, Kubinyi H (1998). Structure-based Ligand Design (Methods and Principles in Medicinal Chemistry). Weinheim: Wiley-VCH. ISBN 3-527-29343-4.

- Folkers G, Jahnke W, Erlanson DA, Mannhold R, Kubinyi H (2006). Fragment-based Approaches in Drug Discovery (Methods and Principles in Medicinal Chemistry). Weinheim: Wiley-VCH. ISBN 3-527-31291-9.

- Roger MJ, Reigosa MJ, Pedrol N, González L (2006), Allelopathy: a physiological process with ecological implications, Springer, p. 1, ISBN 1-4020-4279-5

- Curtis L. Meinert; Susan Tonascia (1986). Clinical trials: design, conduct, and analysis. Oxford University Press, USA. p. 3. ISBN 978-0-19-503568-1.

- Simon, Harvey B. (2002). The Harvard Medical School guide to men's health. New York: Free Press. p. 31. ISBN 0-684-87181-5.

Pharmaceutical Drug and its Types

4

Pharmaceutical drugs are used to diagnose and cure diseases. Some of the different types of drug classes are antiplatelet drugs, anticoagulants, prescription drugs, anti-diabetic medications and generic drugs. Pharmaceutical drugs are best understood in confluence with the major topics listed in the following section.

Pharmaceutical Drug

A pharmaceutical drug (also referred to as medication and drug) is a drug used to diagnose, cure, treat, or prevent disease. Drug therapy (pharmacotherapy) is an important part of the medical field and relies on the science of pharmacology for continual advancement and on pharmacy for appropriate management.

Drugs are classified in various ways. One of the key divisions is by level of control, which distinguishes prescription drugs (those that a pharmacist dispenses only on the order of a physician, physician assistant, or qualified nurse) from over-the-counter drugs (those that consumers can order for themselves). Another key distinction is between traditional small-molecule drugs, usually derived from chemical synthesis, and biopharmaceuticals, which include recombinant proteins, vaccines, blood products used therapeutically (such as IVIG), gene therapy, monoclonal antibodies and cell therapy (for instance, stem-cell therapies). Other ways to classify medicines are by mode of action, route of administration, biological system affected, or therapeutic effects. An elaborate and widely used classification system is the Anatomical Therapeutic Chemical Classification System (ATC system). The World Health Organization keeps a list of essential medicines.

Drug discovery and drug development are complex and expensive endeavors undertaken by pharmaceutical companies, academic scientists, and governments. Governments generally regulate what drugs can be marketed, how drugs are marketed, and in some jurisdictions, drug pricing. Controversies have arisen over drug pricing and disposal of used drugs.

Definition

In Europe, the term is "medicinal product", and it is defined by EU law as: "(a) Any substance or combination of substances presented as having properties for treating or preventing disease in human beings; or

(b) Any substance or combination of substances which may be used in or administered to human beings either with a view to restoring, correcting or modifying physiological functions by exerting a pharmacological, immunological or metabolic action, or to making a medical diagnosis."

In the US, a "drug" is:

- A substance recognized by an official pharmacopoeia or formulary.

- A substance intended for use in the diagnosis, cure, mitigation, treatment, or prevention of disease.

- A substance (other than food) intended to affect the structure or any function of the body.

- A substance intended for use as a component of a medicine but not a device or a component, part or accessory of a device.

- Biological products are included within this definition and are generally covered by the same laws and regulations, but differences exist regarding their manufacturing processes (chemical process versus biological process.)

Usage

Drug use among elderly Americans has been studied; in a group of 2377 people with average age of 71 surveyed between 2005 and 2006, 84% took at least one prescription drug, 44% took at least one over-the-counter (OTC) drug, and 52% took at least one dietary supplement; in a group of 2245 elderly Americans (average age of 71) surveyed over the period 2010 - 2011, those percentages were 88%, 38%, and 64%.

Classification

Pharmaceutical or a drug is classified on the basis of their origin.

1. Drug from natural origin: Herbal or plant or mineral origin, some drug substances are of marine origin.

2. Drug from chemical as well as natural origin: Derived from partial herbal and partial chemical synthesis Chemical, example steroidal drugs

3. Drug derived from chemical synthesis.

4. Drug derived from animal origin: For example, hormones, and enzymes.

5. Drug derived from microbial origin: Antibiotics

6. Drug derived by biotechnology genetic-engineering, hybridoma technique for example

7. Drug derived from radioactive substances.

One of the key classifications is between traditional small molecule drugs, usually derived from chemical synthesis, and biologic medical products, which include recombinant proteins, vaccines, blood products used therapeutically (such as IVIG), gene therapy, and cell therapy (for instance, stem cell therapies).

Pharmaceutical or drug or medicines are classified in various other groups besides their origin on the basis of pharmacological properties like mode of action and their pharmacological action or activity, such as by chemical properties, mode or route of administration, biological system affected, or therapeutic effects. An elaborate and widely used classification system is the Anatomical

Therapeutic Chemical Classification System (ATC system). The World Health Organization keeps a list of essential medicines.

A sampling of classes of medicine includes:

1. Antipyretics: reducing fever (pyrexia/pyresis)

2. Analgesics: reducing pain (painkillers)

3. Antimalarial drugs: treating malaria

4. Antibiotics: inhibiting germ growth

5. Antiseptics: prevention of germ growth near burns, cuts and wounds

6. Mood stabilizers: lithium and valpromide

7. Hormone replacements: Premarin

8. Oral contraceptives: Enovid, "biphasic" pill, and "triphasic" pill

9. Stimulants: methylphenidate, amphetamine

10. Tranquilizers: meprobamate, chlorpromazine, reserpine, chlordiazepoxide, diazepam, and alprazolam

11. Statins: lovastatin, pravastatin, and simvastatin

Pharmaceuticals may also be described as "specialty", independent of other classifications, which is an ill defined class of drugs that might be difficult to administer, require special handling during administration, require patient monitoring during and immediately after administration, have particular regulatory requirements restricting their use, and are generally expensive relative to other drugs.

Types of Medicines

For the Digestive System

- Upper digestive tract: antacids, reflux suppressants, antiflatulents, antidopaminergics, proton pump inhibitors (PPIs), H_2-receptor antagonists, cytoprotectants, prostaglandin analogues

- Lower digestive tract: laxatives, antispasmodics, antidiarrhoeals, bile acid sequestrants, opioid

For the Cardiovascular System

- General: β-receptor blockers ("beta blockers"), calcium channel blockers, diuretics, cardiac glycosides, antiarrhythmics, nitrate, antianginals, vasoconstrictors, vasodilators.

- Affecting blood pressure/(antihypertensive drugs): ACE inhibitors, angiotensin receptor blockers, beta-blockers, α blockers, calcium channel blockers, thiazide diuretics, loop diuretics, aldosterone inhibitors

- Coagulation: anticoagulants, heparin, antiplatelet drugs, fibrinolytics, anti-hemophilic factors, haemostatic drugs

- HMG-CoA reductase inhibitors (statins) for lowering LDL cholesterol inhibitors: hypolipidaemic agents.

For the Central Nervous System

Drugs affecting the central nervous system include: Psychedelics, hypnotics, anaesthetics, antipsychotics, eugeroics, antidepressants (including tricyclic antidepressants, monoamine oxidase inhibitors, lithium salts, and selective serotonin reuptake inhibitors (SSRIs)), antiemetics, Anticonvulsants/antiepileptics, anxiolytics, barbiturates, movement disorder (e.g., Parkinson's disease) drugs, stimulants (including amphetamines), benzodiazepines, cyclopyrrolones, dopamine antagonists, antihistamines, cholinergics, anticholinergics, emetics, cannabinoids, and 5-HT (serotonin) antagonists.

For pain

The main classes of painkillers are NSAIDs, opioids and Local anesthetics.

For Consciousness (Anesthetic Drugs)

Some anesthetics include Benzodiazepines ande Barbiturates

For Musculo-skeletal Disorders

The main categories of drugs for musculoskeletal disorders are: NSAIDs (including COX-2 selective inhibitors), muscle relaxants, neuromuscular drugs, and anticholinesterases.

For the Eye

- General: adrenergic neurone blocker, astringent, ocular lubricant

- Diagnostic: topical anesthetics, sympathomimetics, parasympatholytics, mydriatics, cycloplegics

- Antibacterial: antibiotics, topical antibiotics, sulfa drugs, aminoglycosides, fluoroquinolones

- Antiviral drug

- Anti-fungal: imidazoles, polyenes

- Anti-inflammatory: NSAIDs, corticosteroids

- Anti-allergy: mast cell inhibitors

- Anti-glaucoma: adrenergic agonists, beta-blockers, carbonic anhydrase inhibitors/hyperosmotics, cholinergics, miotics, parasympathomimetics, prostaglandin agonists/prostaglandin inhibitors. nitroglycerin

For the Ear, Nose and Oropharynx

Antibiotics, sympathomimetics, antihistamines, anticholinergics, NSAIDs, corticosteroids, antiseptics, local anesthetics, antifungals, cerumenolytic

For the Respiratory System

bronchodilators, antitussives, mucolytics, decongestants inhaled and systemic corticosteroids, Beta2-adrenergic agonists, anticholinergics, Mast cell stabilizers. Leukotriene antagonists

For Endocrine Problems

androgens, antiandrogens, estrogens, gonadotropin, corticosteroids, human growth hormone, insulin, antidiabetics (sulfonylureas, biguanides/metformin, thiazolidinediones, insulin), thyroid hormones, antithyroid drugs, calcitonin, diphosponate, vasopressin analogues

For the Reproductive System or Urinary System

antifungal, alkalinizing agents, quinolones, antibiotics, cholinergics, anticholinergics, antispasmodics, 5-alpha reductase inhibitor, selective alpha-1 blockers, sildenafils, fertility medications

For Contraception

- Hormonal contraception

- Ormeloxifene

- Spermicide

For Obstetrics and Gynecology

NSAIDs, anticholinergics, haemostatic drugs, antifibrinolytics, Hormone Replacement Therapy (HRT), bone regulators, beta-receptor agonists, follicle stimulating hormone, luteinising hormone, LHRH gamolenic acid, gonadotropin release inhibitor, progestogen, dopamine agonists, oestrogen, prostaglandins, gonadorelin, clomiphene, tamoxifen, Diethylstilbestrol

For the Skin

Emollients, anti-pruritics, antifungals, disinfectants, scabicides, pediculicides, tar products, vitamin A derivatives, vitamin D analogues, keratolytics, abrasives, systemic antibiotics, topical antibiotics, hormones, desloughing agents, exudate absorbents, fibrinolytics, proteolytics, sunscreens, antiperspirants, corticosteroids, immune modulators

For Infections and Infestations

Antibiotics, antifungals, antileprotics, antituberculous drugs, antimalarials, anthelmintics, amoebicides, antivirals, antiprotozoals, probiotics, prebiotics, antitoxins and antivenoms.

For the Immune System

Vaccines, immunoglobulins, immunosuppressants, interferons, monoclonal antibodies

For Allergic Disorders

Anti-allergics, antihistamines, NSAIDs, Corticosteroids

For Nutrition

Tonics, electrolytes and mineral preparations (including iron preparations and magnesium preparations), parenteral nutritions, vitamins, anti-obesity drugs, anabolic drugs, haematopoietic drugs, food product drugs

For Neoplastic Disorders

Cytotoxic drugs, therapeutic antibodies, sex hormones, aromatase inhibitors, somatostatin inhibitors, recombinant interleukins, G-CSF, erythropoietin

For Diagnostics

Contrast media

For Euthanasia

A euthanaticum is used for euthanasia and physician-assisted suicide. Euthanasia is not permitted by law in many countries, and consequently medicines will not be licensed for this use in those countries.

Administration

Administration is the process by which a patient takes a medicine. There are three major categories of drug administration; enteral (by mouth), parenteral (into the blood stream), and other (which includes giving a drug through intranasal, topical, inhalation, and rectal means).

It can be performed in various dosage forms such as pills, tablets, or capsules.

There are many variations in the routes of administration, including intravenous (into the blood through a vein) and oral administration (through the mouth).

They can be administered all at once as a bolus, at frequent intervals or continuously. Frequencies are often abbreviated from Latin, such as *every 8 hours* reading Q8H from *Quaque VIII Hora*.

Drug Discovery

In the fields of medicine, biotechnology and pharmacology, drug discovery is the process by which new candidate drugs are discovered.

Historically, drugs were discovered through identifying the active ingredient from traditional remedies or by serendipitous discovery. Later chemical libraries of synthetic small molecules, natural products or extracts were screened in intact cells or whole organisms to identify substances that have a desirable therapeutic effect in a process known as classical pharmacology. Since sequencing of the human genome which allowed rapid cloning and synthesis of large quantities of purified proteins, it has become common practice to use high throughput screening of large compounds libraries against isolated biological targets which are hypothesized to be disease modifying in a process known as reverse pharmacology. Hits from these screens are then tested in cells and then in animals for efficacy. Even more recently, scientists have been able to understand the shape of biological molecules at the atomic level, and to use that knowledge to design drug candidates.

Modern drug discovery involves the identification of screening hits, medicinal chemistry and optimization of those hits to increase the affinity, selectivity (to reduce the potential of side effects), efficacy/potency, metabolic stability (to increase the half-life), and oral bioavailability. Once a compound that fulfills all of these requirements has been identified, it will begin the process of drug development prior to clinical trials. One or more of these steps may, but not necessarily, involve computer-aided drug design.

Despite advances in technology and understanding of biological systems, drug discovery is still a lengthy, "expensive, difficult, and inefficient process" with low rate of new therapeutic discovery. In 2010, the research and development cost of each new molecular entity (NME) was approximately US$1.8 billion. Drug discovery is done by pharmaceutical companies, with research assistance from universities. The "final product" of drug discovery is a patent on the potential drug. The drug requires very expensive Phase I, II and III clinical trials, and most of them fail. Small companies have a critical role, often then selling the rights to larger companies that have the resources to run the clinical trials.

Development

Drug development is a blanket term used to define the process of bringing a new drug to the market once a lead compound has been identified through the process of drug discovery. It includes pre-clinical research (microorganisms/animals) and clinical trials (on humans) and may include the step of obtaining regulatory approval to market the drug.

Regulation

The regulation of drugs varies by jurisdiction. In some countries, such as the United States, they are regulated at the national level by a single agency. In other jurisdictions they are regulated at the state level, or at both state and national levels by various bodies, as is the case in Australia. The role of therapeutic goods regulation is designed mainly to protect the health and safety of the population. Regulation is aimed at ensuring the safety, quality, and efficacy of the therapeutic goods which are covered under the scope of the regulation. In most jurisdictions, therapeutic goods must be registered before they are allowed to be marketed. There is usually some degree of restriction of the availability of certain therapeutic goods depending on their risk to consumers.

Depending upon the jurisdiction, drugs may be divided into over-the-counter drugs (OTC) which may be available without special restrictions, and prescription drugs, which must be prescribed by a licensed medical practitioner. The precise distinction between OTC and prescription depends on the legal jurisdiction. A third category, "behind-the-counter" drugs, is implemented in some jurisdictions. These do not require a prescription, but must be kept in the dispensary, not visible to the public, and only be sold by a pharmacist or pharmacy technician. Doctors may also prescribe prescription drugs for off-label use - purposes which the drugs were not originally approved for by the regulatory agency. The Classification of Pharmaco-Therapeutic Referrals helps guide the referral process between pharmacists and doctors.

The International Narcotics Control Board of the United Nations imposes a world law of prohibition of certain drugs. They publish a lengthy list of chemicals and plants whose trade and consumption (where applicable) is forbidden. OTC drugs are sold without restriction as they are considered safe enough that most people will not hurt themselves accidentally by taking it as instructed. Many countries, such as the United Kingdom have a third category of "pharmacy medicines", which can only be sold in registered pharmacies by or under the supervision of a pharmacist.

Drug Pricing

In many jurisdictions drug prices are regulated.

United Kingdom

In the UK the Pharmaceutical Price Regulation Scheme is intended to ensure that the National Health Service is able to purchase drugs at reasonable prices.

Canada

In Canada, the Patented Medicine Prices Review Board examines drug pricing, compares the proposed Canadian price to that of seven other countries and determines if a price is excessive or not. In these circumstances, drug manufacturers must submit a proposed price to the appropriate regulatory agency.

Brazil

In Brazil, the prices are regulated through a legislation under the name of *Medicamento Genérico* (generic drugs) since 1999.

India

In India, drug prices are regulated by the National Pharmaceutical Pricing Authority.

United States

In the United States, drug costs are unregulated, but instead are the result of negotiations between drug companies and insurance companies. High prices have been attributed to monopolies given to manufacturers by the government and a lack of ability for organizations to negotiate prices.

Blockbuster Drug

A blockbuster drug is a drug generating more than $1 billion of revenue for the pharmaceutical company that sells it each year. Cimetidine was the first drug ever to reach more than $1 billion a year in sales, thus making it the first blockbuster drug.

"In the pharmaceutical industry, a blockbuster drug is one that achieves acceptance by prescribing physicians as a therapeutic standard for, most commonly, a highly prevalent chronic (rather than acute) condition. Patients often take the medicines for long periods."

History

Prescription Drug History

Antibiotics first arrived on the medical scene in 1932 thanks to Gerhard Domagk; and coined the "wonder drugs". The introduction of the sulfa drugs led to a decline in the U.S. mortality rate from pneumonia to drop from 0.2% each year to 0.05% by 1939. Antibiotics inhibit the growth or the metabolic activities of bacteria and other microorganisms by a chemical substance of microbial origin. Penicillin, introduced a few years later, provided a broader spectrum of activity compared to sulfa drugs and reduced side effects. Streptomycin, found in 1942, proved to be the first drug effective against the cause of tuberculosis and also came to be the best known of a long series of important antibiotics. A second generation of antibiotics was introduced in the 1940s: aureomycin and chloramphenicol. Aureomycin was the best known of the second generation.

Lithium was discovered in the 19th century for nervous disorders and its possible mood-stabilizing or prophylactic effect; it was cheap and easily produced. As lithium fell out of favor in France, valpromide came into play. This antibiotic was the origin of the drug that eventually created the mood stabilizer category. Valpromide had distinct psychotrophic effects that were of benefit in both the treatment of acute manic states and in the maintenance treatment of manic depression illness. Psychotropics can either be sedative or stimulant; sedatives aim at damping down the extremes of behavior. Stimulants aim at restoring normality by increasing tone. Soon arose the notion of a tranquilizer which was quite different from any sedative or stimulant. The term tranquilizer took over the notions of sedatives and became the dominant term in the West through the 1980s. In Japan, during this time, the term tranquilizer produced the notion of a psyche-stabilizer and the term mood stabilizer vanished.

Premarin (conjugated estrogens, introduced in 1942) and Prempro (a combination estrogen-progestin pill, introduced in 1995) dominated the hormone replacement therapy (HRT) during the 1990s. HRT is not a life-saving drug, nor does it cure any disease. HRT has been prescribed to improve one's quality of life. Doctors prescribe estrogen for their older female patients both to treat short-term menopausal symptoms and to prevent long-term diseases. In the 1960s and early 1970s more and more physicians began to prescribe estrogen for their female patients. between 1991 and 1999, Premarin was listed as the most popular prescription and best-selling drug in America.

The first oral contraceptive, Enovid, was approved by FDA in 1960. Oral contraceptives inhibit ovulation and so prevent conception. Enovid was known to be much more effective than alternatives including the condom and the diaphragm. As early as 1960, oral contraceptives were available in several different strengths by every manufacturer. In the 1980s and 1990s an increasing number of options arose including, most recently, a new delivery system for the oral contraceptive via a transdermal patch. In 1982, a new version of the Pill was introduced, known as the "biphasic" pill. By 1985, a new triphasic pill was approved. Physicians began to think of the Pill as an excellent means of birth control for young women.

Stimulants such as Ritalin (methylphenidate) came to be pervasive tools for behavior management and modification in young children. Ritalin was first marketed in 1955 for narcolepsy; its potential users were middle-aged and the elderly. It wasn't until some time in the 1980s along with hyperactivity in children that Ritalin came onto the market. Medical use of methlyphanidate is predominately for symptoms of attention deficit/hyperactivity disorder (ADHD). Consumption of methylphenidate in the U.S. out-paced all other countries between 1991 and 1999. Significant growth in consumption was also evident in Canada, New Zealand, Australia, and Norway. Currently, 85% of the world's methylphanidate is consumed in America.

The first minor tranquilizer was Meprobamate. Only fourteen months after it was made available, meprobamate had become the country's largest-selling prescription drug. By 1957, meprobamate had become the fastest-growing drug in history. The popularity of meprobamate paved the way for Librium and Valium, two minor tranquilizers that belonged to a new chemical class of drugs called the benzodiazepines. These were drugs that worked chiefly as anti-anxiety agents and muscle relaxants. The first benzodiazepine was Librium. Three months after it was approved, Librium had become the most prescribed tranquilizer in the nation. Three years later, Valium hit the shelves and was ten times more effective as a muscle relaxant and anti-convulsant. Valium was the most versatile of the minor tranquilizers. Later came the widespread adoption of major tranquilizers such as chlorpromazine and the drug reserpine. In 1970 sales began to decline for Valium and Librium, but sales of new and improved tranquilizers, such as Xanax, introduced in 1981 for the newly created diagnosis of panic disorder, soared.

Mevacor (lovastatin) is the first and most influential statin in the American market. The 1991 launch of Pravachol (pravastatin), the second available in the United States, and the release of Zocor (simvastatin) made Mevacor no longer the only statin on the market. In 1998, Viagra was released as a treatment for erectile dysfunction.

Ancient Pharmacology

Using plants and plant substances to treat all kinds of diseases and medical conditions is believed to date back to prehistoric medicine.

The Kahun Gynaecological Papyrus, the oldest known medical text of any kind, dates to about 1800 BC and represents the first documented use of any kind of drug. It and other medical papyri describe Ancient Egyptian medical practices, such as using honey to treat infections and the legs of bee-eaters to treat neck pains.

Ancient Babylonian medicine demonstrate the use of prescriptions in the first half of the 2nd millennium BC. Medicinal creams and pills were employed as treatments.

On the Indian subcontinent, the Atharvaveda, a sacred text of Hinduism whose core dates from the 2nd millennium BC, although the hymns recorded in it are believed to be older, is the first Indic text dealing with medicine. It describes plant-based drugs to counter diseases. The earliest foundations of ayurveda were built on a synthesis of selected ancient herbal practices, together with a massive addition of theoretical conceptualizations, new nosologies and new therapies dating from about 400 BC onwards. The student of Āyurveda was expected to know ten arts that were indispensable in the preparation and application of his medicines: distillation, operative skills, cooking, horticulture, metallurgy, sugar manufacture, pharmacy, analysis and separation of minerals, compounding of metals, and preparation of alkalis.

The Hippocratic Oath for physicians, attributed to 5th century BC Greece, refers to the existence of "deadly drugs", and ancient Greek physicians imported drugs from Egypt and elsewhere.

Medieval Pharmacology

Al-Kindi's 9th century AD book, *De Gradibus* and Ibn Sina (Avicenna)'s *The Canon of Medicine* cover a range of drugs known to Medicine in the medieval Islamic world.

Medieval medicine saw advances in surgery, but few truly effective drugs existed, beyond opium (found in such extremely popular drugs as the "Great Rest" of the Antidotarium Nicolai at the time) and quinine. Folklore cures and potentially poisonous metal-based compounds were popular treatments. Theodoric Borgognoni, (1205–1296), one of the most significant surgeons of the medieval period, responsible for introducing and promoting important surgical advances including basic antiseptic practice and the use of anaesthetics. Garcia de Orta described some herbal treatments that were used.

Modern Pharmacology

For most of the 19th century, drugs were not highly effective, leading Oliver Wendell Holmes, Sr. to famously comment in 1842 that "if all medicines in the world were thrown into the sea, it would be all the better for mankind and all the worse for the fishes".

During the First World War, Alexis Carrel and Henry Dakin developed the Carrel-Dakin method of treating wounds with an irrigation, Dakin's solution, a germicide which helped prevent gangrene.

In the inter-war period, the first anti-bacterial agents such as the sulpha antibiotics were developed. The Second World War saw the introduction of widespread and effective antimicrobial therapy with the development and mass production of penicillin antibiotics, made possible by the pressures of the war and the collaboration of British scientists with the American pharmaceutical industry.

Medicines commonly used by the late 1920s included aspirin, codeine, and morphine for pain; digitalis, nitroglycerin, and quinine for heart disorders, and insulin for diabetes. Other drugs included antitoxins, a few biological vaccines, and a few synthetic drugs. In the 1930s antibiotics emerged: first sulfa drugs, then penicillin and other antibiotics. Drugs increasingly became "the center of medical practice". In the 1950s other drugs emerged including corticosteroids for inflammation, rauwolfia alkaloids as tranquilizers and antihypertensives, antihistamines for nasal allergies, xanthines for asthma, and typical antipsychotics for psychosis. As of 2007, thousands of approved drugs have been developed. Increasingly, biotechnology is used to discover biopharmaceuticals. Recently, multi-disciplinary approaches have yielded a wealth of new data on the development of novel antibiotics and antibacterials and on the use of biological agents for antibacterial therapy.

In the 1950s new psychiatric drugs, notably the antipsychotic chlorpromazine, were designed in laboratories and slowly came into preferred use. Although often accepted as an advance in some ways, there was some opposition, due to serious adverse effects such as tardive dyskinesia. Patients often opposed psychiatry and refused or stopped taking the drugs when not subject to psychiatric control.

Governments have been heavily involved in the regulation of drug development and drug sales. In the U.S., the Elixir Sulfanilamide disaster led to the establishment of the Food and Drug Administration, and the 1938 Federal Food, Drug, and Cosmetic Act required manufacturers to file new drugs with the FDA. The 1951 Humphrey-Durham Amendment required certain drugs to be sold by prescription. In 1962 a subsequent amendment required new drugs to be tested for efficacy and safety in clinical trials.

Until the 1970s, drug prices were not a major concern for doctors and patients. As more drugs became prescribed for chronic illnesses, however, costs became burdensome, and by the 1970s nearly every U.S. state required or encouraged the substitution of generic drugs for higher-priced brand names. This also led to the 2006 U.S. law, Medicare Part D, which offers Medicare coverage for drugs.

As of 2008, the United States is the leader in medical research, including pharmaceutical development. U.S. drug prices are among the highest in the world, and drug innovation is correspondingly high. In 2000 U.S. based firms developed 29 of the 75 top-selling drugs; firms from the second-largest market, Japan, developed eight, and the United Kingdom contributed 10. France, which imposes price controls, developed three. Throughout the 1990s outcomes were similar.

Controversies

Controversies concerning pharmaceutical drugs include patient access to drugs under development and not yet approved, pricing, and environmental issues.

Access to Unapproved Drugs

Governments worldwide have created provisions for granting access to drugs prior to approval for patients who have exhausted all alternative treatment options and do not match clinical trial entry criteria. Often grouped under the labels of compassionate use, expanded access, or named patient supply, these programs are governed by rules which vary by country defining access criteria, data collection, promotion, and control of drug distribution.

Within the United States, pre-approval demand is generally met through treatment IND (investigational new drug) applications (INDs), or single-patient INDs. These mechanisms, which fall under the label of expanded access programs, provide access to drugs for groups of patients or individuals residing in the US. Outside the US, Named Patient Programs provide controlled, pre-approval access to drugs in response to requests by physicians on behalf of specific, or "named", patients before those medicines are licensed in the patient's home country. Through these programs, patients are able to access drugs in late-stage clinical trials or approved in other countries for a genuine, unmet medical need, before those drugs have been licensed in the patient's home country.

Patients who have not been able to get access to drugs in development have organized and advocated for greater access. In the United States, ACT UP formed in the 1980s, and eventually formed its Treatment Action Group in part to pressure the US government to put more resources into discovering treatments for AIDS and then to speed release of drugs that were under development.

The Abigail Alliance was established in November 2001 by Frank Burroughs in memory of his daughter, Abigail. The Alliance seeks broader availability of investigational drugs on behalf of terminally ill patients.

In 2013, BioMarin Pharmaceutical was at the center of a high-profile debate regarding expanded access of cancer patients to experimental drugs.

Access to Medicines and Drug Pricing

Essential medicines as defined by the World Health Organization (WHO) are "those drugs that satisfy the health care needs of the majority of the population; they should therefore be available at all times in adequate amounts and in appropriate dosage forms, at a price the community can afford." Recent studies have found that most of the medicines on the WHO essential medicines list, outside of the field of HIV drugs, are not patented in the developing world, and that lack of widespread access to these medicines arise from issues fundamental to economic development - lack of infrastructure and poverty. Médecins Sans Frontières also runs a Campaign for Access to Essential Medicines campaign, which includes advocacy for greater resources to be devoted to currently untreatable diseases that primarily occur in the developing world. The Access to Medicine Index tracks how well pharmaceutical companies make their products available in the developing world.

World Trade Organization negotiations in the 1990s, including the TRIPS Agreement and the Doha Declaration, have centered on issues at the intersection of international trade in pharmaceuticals and intellectual property rights, with developed world nations seeking strong intellectual property rights to protect investments made to develop new drugs, and developing world nations seeking to promote their generic pharmaceuticals industries and their ability to make medicine available to their people via compulsory licenses.

Some have raised ethical objections specifically with respect to pharmaceutical patents and the high prices for drugs that they enable their proprietors to charge, which poor people in the developed world, and developing world, cannot afford. Critics also question the rationale that exclusive patent rights and the resulting high prices are required for pharmaceutical companies to recoup the large investments needed for research and development. One study concluded that marketing expenditures for new drugs often doubled the amount that was allocated for research and development. Other critics claim that patent settlements would be costly for consumers, the health care system, and state and federal governments because it would result in delaying access to lower cost generic medicines.

Novartis fought a protracted battle with the government of India over the patenting of its drug, Gleevec, in India, which ended up in India's Supreme Court in a case known as Novartis v. Union of India & Others. The Supreme Court ruled narrowly against Novartis, but opponents of patenting drugs claimed it as a major victory.

Environmental Issues

The environmental impact of pharmaceuticals and personal care products is controversial. PPCPs are substances used by individuals for personal health or cosmetic reasons and the products used by agribusiness to boost growth or health of livestock. PPCPs comprise a diverse collection of thousands of chemical substances, including prescription and over-the-counter therapeutic drugs, veterinary drugs, fragrances, and cosmetics. PPCPs have been detected in water bodies throughout the world and ones that persist in the environment are called Environmental Persistent Pharmaceutical Pollutants. The effects of these chemicals on humans and the environment are not yet known, but to date there is no scientific evidence that they affect human health.

Drug Class

A drug class is a set of medications that have similar chemical structures, the same mechanism of action (i.e., bind to the same biological target), a related mode of action, and/or are used to treat the same disease.

In several dominant drug classification systems, these four types of classifications form a hierarchy. For example, the fibrates are a chemical class of drugs (amphipathic carboxylic acids) that share the same mechanism of action (PPAR agonist), mode of action (reducing blood triglycerides), and are used to prevent and to treat the same disease (atherosclerosis). Conversely not all PPAR agonists are fibrates, not all triglyceride lowering agents are PPAR agonists, and not all drugs that are used to treat atherosclerosis are triglyceride lowering agents.

The most widely used drug classification system is the Anatomical Therapeutic Chemical Classification System (ATC). The Systematized Nomenclature of Medicine (SNOMED) also includes a section devoted to drug classification.

Chemical Class

Examples of drug classes that are based on chemical structures include:

- β-lactam antibiotic
- Benzodiazepine
- Cardiac glycoside
- Fibrate
- Thiazide diuretic

Mechanism of Action

Drug classes that share a common molecular mechanism of action by modulating the activity of a specific biological target. The definition of a mechanism of action also includes the type of activity at that biological target. For receptors, these activities include agonist, antagonist, inverse agonist, or modulator. Enzyme target mechanisms include activator or inhibitor. Ion channel modulators include opener or blocker. The following are specific examples of drug classes whose definition is based on a specific mechanism of action:

- 5-Alpha-reductase inhibitor
- Angiotensin II receptor antagonist
- ACE inhibitor
- Alpha-adrenergic agonist
- Beta blocker
- Dopamine agonist
- Dopamine antagonist
- Incretin mimetic
- Nonsteroidal anti-inflammatory drug – cyclooxygenase inhibitor
- Proton-pump inhibitor
- Renin inhibitor
- Selective glucocorticoid receptor modulator
- Selective serotonin reuptake inhibitor
- Statin – HMG-CoA reductase inhibitor

Mode of Action

Drug classes that are defined by common cellular mode of action include:

- Diuretic
- Cholinergic
- Dopaminergic
- GABAergic
- Serotonergic

Therapeutic Class

Drug classes that are defined by their therapeutic use include:

- Analgesic
- Antibiotic
- Anticoagulant
- Antidepressant
- Anticancer

- Antiepileptic

- Antipsychotic

- Antiviral

- Sedative

Amalgamated Classes

Some drug classes have been amalgamated from these three principles to meet practical needs. The class of non-steroidal anti-inflammatory drugs (NSAIDs) is one such example. Strictly speaking, and also historically, the wider class of anti-inflammatory drugs also comprises *steroidal* anti-inflammatory drugs. These drugs were in fact the predominant anti-inflammatories during the decade leading up to the introduction of the term "non-steroidal anti-inflammatory drugs". Because of the disastrous reputation that the corticosteroids had got in the 1950s, the new term, which offered to signal that an anti-inflammatory drug was not a steroid, rapidly gained currency. The drug class of "non-steroidal anti-inflammatory drugs" (NSAIDs) is thus composed by one element ("anti-inflammatory") that designates the mechanism of action, and one element ("non-steroidal") that separates it from other drugs with that same mechanism of action. Similarly, one might argue that the class of disease-modifying anti-rheumatic drugs (DMARD) is composed by one element ("disease-modifying") that albeit vaguely designates a mechanism of action, and one element ("anti-rheumatic drug") that indicates its therapeutic use.

- Nonsteroidal anti-inflammatory drug (NSAID)

- Disease-modifying antirheumatic drug (DMARD)

Antiplatelet Drug

An antiplatelet drug (antiaggregant) is a member of a class of pharmaceuticals that decrease platelet aggregation   and inhibit thrombus formation. They are effective in the arterial circulation, where anticoagulants have little effect.

They are widely used in primary and secondary prevention of thrombotic cerebrovascular or cardiovascular disease.

Antiplatelet drug decreases the ability of blood clot to form by interfering with platelet activation process in primary haemostasis. Antiplatelet drugs can reversibly or irreversibly inhibit the process involved in platelet activation resulting in decreased tendency of platelets to adhere to one another and to damaged blood vessels endothelium.

Choice of Antiplatelet Drug

A 2006 review states: "...low-dose aspirin increases the risk of major bleeding 2-fold compared with placebo. However, the annual incidence of major bleeding due to low-dose aspirin is modest—only 1.3 patients per thousand higher than what is observed with placebo treatment. Treatment of approximately 800 patients with low-dose aspirin annually for cardiovascular prophylaxis will result in only 1 additional major bleeding episode."

Classification

The class of antiplatelet drugs include:

- Irreversible cyclooxygenase inhibitors
    - Aspirin
    - Triflusal (Disgren)
- Adenosine diphosphate (ADP) receptor inhibitors
    - Clopidogrel (Plavix)
    - Prasugrel (Effient)
    - Ticagrelor (Brilinta)
    - Ticlopidine (Ticlid)
- Phosphodiesterase inhibitors
    - Cilostazol (Pletal)
- Protease-activated receptor-1 (PAR-1) antagonists
    - Vorapaxar (Zontivity)
- Glycoprotein IIB/IIIA inhibitors (intravenous use only)
    - Abciximab (ReoPro)
    - Eptifibatide (Integrilin)
    - Tirofiban (Aggrastat)
- Adenosine reuptake inhibitors
    - Dipyridamole (Persantine)
- Thromboxane inhibitors
    - Thromboxane synthase inhibitors
    - Thromboxane receptor antagonists
        - Terutroban

Usage

Prevention and Treatment of Arterial Thrombosis

Prevention and treatment of arterial thrombosis is essential in patients with certain medical conditions whereby the risk of thrombosis or thromboembolism may result in disastrous consequences such as heart attack, pulmonary embolism or stroke. Patients who require the use of antiplatelet drugs are: stroke with or without atrial fibrillation, any heart surgery (especially prosthetic replacement heart valve), Coronary Heart Disease such as stable angina, unstable angina and heart attack, patients with coronary stent, Peripheral Vascular Disease/Peripheral Arterial Disease and apical/ventricular/mural thrombus.

Treatment of established arterial thrombosis includes the use of antiplatelet drugs and thrombolytic therapy. Antiplatelet drugs alter the platelet activation at the site of vascular damage crucial to the development of arterial thrombosis.

- Aspirin and Triflusal irreversibly inhibits the enzyme COX, resulting in reduced platelet production of TXA_2 (thromboxane - powerful vasoconstrictor that lowers cyclic AMP and initiates the platelet release reaction).

- Dipyridamole inhibits platelet phosphodiesterase, causing an increase in cyclic AMP with potentiation of the action of PGI_2 – opposes actions of TXA_2

- Clopidogrel affects the ADP-dependent activation of IIb/IIIa complex

- Glycoprotein IIb/IIIa receptor antagonists block a receptor on the platelet for fibrinogen and von Willebrand factor. 3 classes:

    o Murine-human chimeric antibodies (e.g., abciximab)

    o Synthetic peptides (e.g., eptifibatide)

    o Synthetic non-peptides (e.g., tirofiban)

- Epoprostenol is a prostacyclin that is used to inhibit platelet aggregation during renal dialysis (with or without heparin) and is also used in primary pulmonary hypertension.

Thrombolytic therapy is used in myocardial infarction, cerebral infarction, and, on occasion, in massive pulmonary embolism. The main risk is bleeding. Treatment should not be given to patients having had recent bleeding, uncontrolled hypertension or a hemorrhagic stroke, or surgery or other invasive procedures within the previous 10 days.

- Streptokinase forms a complex with plasminogen, resulting in a conformational change that activates other plasminogen molecules to form plasmin.

- Plasminogen activators (PA), tissue-type plasminogen activators (alteplase, tenecteplase) are produced by recombinant technology.

Drug Toxicity

Drug toxicity may be increased when multiple antiplatelet drugs are used. Gastrointestinal bleeding is a common adverse event seen in many patients.

Anticoagulant

Anticoagulants are a class of drugs that work to prevent blood coagulation or which prolong the clotting time. Such substances occur naturally in leeches and blood-sucking insects. A group of pharmaceuticals called anticoagulants can be used as an injection as a medication for thrombotic disorders. Oral anticoagulants are also available. Some anticoagulants are used in medical equipment, such as test tubes, blood transfusion bags, and renal dialysis equipment.

Anticoagulants are closely related to antiplatelet drugs and thrombolytic drugs by manipulating the various pathways of blood coagulation. Specifically, anticoagulants manipulate the coagulation cascade that builds upon the initial platelet thrombus.

Medical Uses

The use of anticoagulants is a decision based upon the risks and benefits of anticoagulation. The biggest risk of anticoagulation therapy is the increased risk of bleeding. In otherwise healthy people, the increased risk of bleeding is minimal, but those who have had recent surgery, cerebral aneurysms, and other conditions may have too great of risk of bleeding. Generally, the benefit of anticoagulation is prevention of or reduction of progression of a disease. Some indications for anticoagulant therapy that are known to have benefit from therapy include:

- Atrial fibrillation — commonly forms an atrial appendage clot
- Coronary artery disease
- Deep vein thrombosis — can lead to pulmonary embolism
- Ischemic stroke
- Hypercoagulable states (e.g., Factor V Leiden) — can lead to deep vein thrombosis
- Myocardial infarction
- Pulmonary embolism
- Restenosis from stents

In these cases, anticoagulation therapy can prevent formation of dangerous clots or prevent growth of clots.

The decision to begin therapeutic anticoagulation often involves the use of multiple bleeding risk predictable outcome tools as non-invasive pre-test stratifications due to the potential for bleeds while on blood thinning agents. Among these tools are HAS-BLED, ATRIA, and CHA2DS2-VASc.

Adverse Effects

Patients aged 80 years or more may be especially susceptible to bleeding complications, with a rate of 13 bleeds per 100 person-years. Depletion of vitamin K by coumarin therapy increases risk of arterial calcification and heart valve calcification, especially if too much vitamin D is present.

Interactions

Foods and food supplements with blood-thinning effects include nattokinase, lumbrokinase, beer, bilberry, celery, cranberries, fish oil, garlic, ginger, ginkgo, ginseng, green tea, horse chestnut, licorice, niacin, onion, papaya, pomegranate, red clover, soybean, St. John's wort, turmeric, wheatgrass, and willow bark. Many herbal supplements have blood-thinning properties, such as danshen and feverfew. Multivitamins that do not interact with clotting are available for patients on anticoagulants.

However, some foods and supplements encourage clotting. These include alfalfa, avocado, cat's claw, coenzyme Q10, and dark leafy greens such as spinach. Their intake should be avoided whilst taking anticoagulants or, if coagulability is being monitored, their intake should be kept approximately constant so that anticoagulant dosage can be maintained at a level high enough to counteract this effect without fluctuations in coagulability.

Grapefruit interferes with some anticoagulant drugs, increasing the amount of time it takes for them to be metabolized out of the body, and so should be eaten only with caution when on anticoagulant drugs.

Anticoagulants are often used to treat acute deep vein thrombosis. People using anticoagulants to treat this condition should avoid using bed rest as a complementary treatment because there are clinical benefits to continuing to walk and remaining mobile while using anticoagulants in this way. Bed rest while using anticoagulants can harm patients in circumstances in which it is not medically necessary.

Types

A number of anticoagulants are available. The traditional ones (warfarin, other coumarins and heparins) are in widespread use. Since the 2000s a number of new agents have been introduced that are collectively referred to as the novel oral anticoagulants (NOACs) or directly acting oral anticoagulants (DOACs). These agents include inhibitors of factor IIa (dabigatran) and factor Xa (rivaroxaban, apixaban and edoxaban) and they have been shown to be as good or possibly better than the coumarins with less serious side effects. The newer anticoagulants (NOACs/DOACs), are more expensive than the traditional ones and should be used with care in patients with kidney problems. Additionally, there is no antidote for the factor Xa inhibitors, so it is difficult to stop their effects in the body in cases of emergency (accidents, urgent surgery). Idarucizumab was FDA approved for the reversal of dabigatran in 2015.

Novel Oral Anticoagulants

Novel oral anticoagulants (NOACs) are a new class of anticoagulant drugs that, like warfarin, can help inhibit clot formation. The most commonly prescribed NOACs are dabigatran, rivaroxaban, and apixaban.

Compared to warfarin, NOACs have a rapid onset action and relatively short half-lives, hence they carry out their function more rapidly and effectively, and allow for drugs to quickly reduce their anticoagulation effects. Routine monitoring and dose adjustments of NOACs is less important than for warfarin, as they have better predictable anticoagulation activity. Both NOACs and warfarin are equivalently effect, but NOACs are less influenced by diet and medications compared to warfarin. However, there is presently no countermeasure for most NOACs unlike in warfarin; nonetheless, the short half-lives of NOACs will result in its effects to swiftly recede. A reversal agent for dabigatran, idarucizumab, is currently the only NOAC reversal agent approved for use by the FDA.

NOACs are a lot costlier compared to warfarin, after having taken into consideration the cost of frequent blood testing associated with warfarin.

Relevance to Dental Treatments

With regards to NOAC medication and invasive dental treatments, there has not been enough clinical evidence and experience to prove any reliable side-effects, relevance or interaction between these two. Further clinical prospective studies on NOACs are required to investigate the bleeding risk and haemostasis associated to surgical dental procedures.

Recommendations of modifications to use/dosage of NOACs prior to dental treatments are made based on the balance of likely effects of each option of each procedure, and also the individual's bleeding risks and renal functionality. With low bleeding risk of dental procedures, it is recommended that NOAC medicine is still taken by patient as per normal, so as to avoid increase in the risk of thromboembolic event. For dental procedures with a higher risk of bleeding complications, the recommended practice is for patient to miss or delay a dose of their NOAC before such procedures so as to minimize the effect on thromboembolic risk.

Coumarins (Vitamin K Antagonists)

These oral anticoagulants are derived from coumarin, which is found in many plants. A prominent member of this class is warfarin (Coumadin). It takes at least 48 to 72 hours for the anticoagulant effect to develop. Where an immediate effect is required, heparin must be given concomitantly. These anticoagulants are used to treat patients with deep-vein thrombosis (DVT), pulmonary embolism (PE) and to prevent emboli in patients with atrial fibrillation (AF), and mechanical prosthetic heart valves. Other examples are acenocoumarol, phenprocoumon, atromentin, and phenindione.

The coumarins brodifacoum and difenacoum are used as rodenticides, but are not used medically.

Heparin and Derivative Substances

Heparin is a biological substance, usually made from pig intestines. It works by activating antithrombin III, which blocks thrombin from clotting blood. Heparin can be used *in vivo* (by injection), and also *in vitro* to prevent blood or plasma clotting in or on medical devices. In venipuncture, Vacutainer brand blood collecting tubes containing heparin usually have a green cap.

Low Molecular Weight Heparin

Low molecular weight heparin, a more highly processed product, is useful as it does not require monitoring of the APTT coagulation parameter (it has more predictable plasma levels) and has fewer side effects.

Synthetic Pentasaccharide Inhibitors of Factor Xa

- Fondaparinux is a synthetic sugar composed of the five sugars (pentasaccharide) in heparin that bind to antithrombin. It is a smaller molecule than low molecular weight heparin.

- Idraparinux

Direct Factor Xa Inhibitors

Drugs such as rivaroxaban, apixaban and edoxaban work by inhibiting factor Xa directly (unlike the heparins and fondaparinux, which work via antithrombin activation). Also betrixaban from Portola Pharmaceuticals, darexaban (YM150) from Astellas, and more recently letaxaban (TAK-442) from Takeda and eribaxaban (PD0348292) from Pfizer. The development of darexaban was discontinued in September 2011: in a trial for prevention of recurrences of myocardial infarction in top of dual antiplatelet therapy, the drug did not demonstrate effectiveness and the risk of bleeding was increased by approximately 300%. The development of letaxaban was discontinued for acute coronary syndrome in May 2011 following negative results from a Phase II study.

Direct Thrombin Inhibitors

Another type of anticoagulant is the direct thrombin inhibitor. Current members of this class include the bivalent drugs hirudin, lepirudin, and bivalirudin; and the monovalent drugs argatroban and dabigatran. An oral direct thrombin inhibitor, ximelagatran (Exanta) was denied approval by the Food and Drug Administration (FDA) in September 2004 and was pulled from the market entirely in February 2006 after reports of severe liver damage and heart attacks. In November 2010, dabigatran was approved by the FDA to treat atrial fibrillation.

Antithrombin Protein Therapeutics

The antithrombin protein itself is used as a protein therapeutic that can be purified from human plasma or produced recombinantly (for example, Atryn, which is produced in the milk of genetically modified goats.)

Antithrombin is approved by the FDA as an anticoagulant for the prevention of clots before, during, or after surgery or birthing in patients with hereditary antithrombin deficiency.

Other Types of Anticoagulants

Many other anticoagulants exist, for use in research and development, diagnostics, or as drug candidates.

- Batroxobin, a toxin from a snake venom, clots platelet-rich plasma without affecting platelet functions (lyses fibrinogen).

- Hementin is an anticoagulant protease from the salivary glands of the giant Amazon leech, *Haementeria ghilianii*.

- Vitamin E

Society and Culture

Warfarin (Coumadin) is the main agent used in the US and UK. Acenocoumarol and phenprocoumon are used more commonly outside the US and the UK.

Laboratory Use

Laboratory instruments, blood transfusion bags, and medical and surgical equipment will get clogged up and become non-operational if blood is allowed to clot. In addition, test tubes used for laboratory blood tests will have chemicals added to stop blood clotting. Apart from heparin, most of these chemicals work by binding calcium ions, preventing the coagulation proteins from using them.

- Ethylenediaminetetraacetic acid (EDTA) strongly and irreversibly chelates (binds) calcium ion to prevent blood from clotting.

- Citrate is in liquid form in the tube and is used for coagulation tests, as well as in blood transfusion bags. It binds the calcium, but not as strongly as EDTA. Correct proportion of this anticoagulant to blood is crucial because of the dilution, and it can be reversed with the addition of calcium. It can be in the form of sodium citrate or acid-citrate-dextrose.

- Oxalate has a mechanism similar to that of citrate. It is the anticoagulant used in fluoride oxalate tubes used to determine glucose and lactate levels.

Prescription Drug

A prescription drug (also prescription medication or prescription medicine) is a pharmaceutical drug that legally requires a medical prescription to be dispensed. In contrast, over-the-counter drugs can be obtained without a prescription. The reason for this difference in substance control is the potential scope of misuse, from drug abuse to practicing medicine without a license and without sufficient education. Different jurisdictions have different definitions of what constitutes a prescription drug.

"Rx" (℞) is often used as a short form for prescription drug in North America- a contraction of the Latin word "*recipe*" (an imperative form of "recipere") meaning "take". Prescription drugs are often dispensed together with a monograph (in Europe, a Patient Information Leaflet or PIL) that gives detailed information about the drug.

The use of prescription drugs has been increasing since the 1960s. In the U.S., 88% of older adults (62–85 years) use at least 1 prescription drug, while 36% take at least 5 prescription medicines concurrently.

Regulation in Australia

In Australia the Standard for the Uniform Scheduling of Medicines and Poisons, abbreviated SUSMP, governs the manufacture and supply of drugs:

The categories defined by the SUSMP are:

- Schedule 1 - Defunct

- Schedule 2 - Pharmacy Medicine

- Schedule 3 - Pharmacist-Only Medicine

- Schedule 4 - Prescription-Only Medicine/Prescription Animal Remedy

- Schedule 5 - Caution

- Schedule 6 - Poison

- Schedule 7 - Dangerous Poison

- Schedule 8 - Controlled Drug (Possession without authority illegal)

- Schedule 9 - Prohibited Substance

- Unscheduled Substances

Similar to the UK, the patient visits a health practitioner, such as a doctor, nurse, dentist, podiatrist, etc., who is able to prescribe the drug.

Many prescriptions issued by health practitioners in Australia are covered by the Pharmaceutical Benefits Scheme, a scheme that provides subsidised prescription drugs to residents of Australia to ensure that all Australians have affordable and reliable access to a wide range of necessary medicines. When purchasing a drug under the PBS the maximum price a consumer pays is the patient co-payment contribution, which, as of January 1, 2014, is A$36.90 for general patients. Those covered by government entitlements (low-income earners, welfare recipients, Health Care Card holders, etc.) and those covered under the Repatriation Pharmaceutical Benefits Scheme (RPBS) have a reduced co-payment, which is $6.00 in 2014. The table below indicates the changes in co-payments over the years. These co-payments are compulsory and cannot be discounted by pharmacies under any circumstances.

Private prescriptions are issued for medicines not covered on the PBS, or being used off-label, for indications other than those covered by the PBS. The patient pays the pharmacy for medicines privately prescribed.

Regulation in United Kingdom

In the United Kingdom the Medicines Act 1968 and Prescription Only Medicines (Human Use) Order 1997 contain regulations that cover the supply of sale, use and production of medicines. Prescribing is also covered by this legislation. There are three categories of medicine:

- Prescription-only medicines (POM), which can be sold by a pharmacist if prescribed by a prescriber

- Pharmacy medicines (P), which may be sold by a pharmacist without prescription

- General sales list (GSL) medicines that may be sold without a prescription in any shop

Possession of prescription-only medicines without a prescription is not a criminal offence unless it falls under the Misuse of Drugs Act 1971.

A patient visits a medical practitioner or dentist authorised to prescribe drugs and certain other medical items, such as blood glucose-testing equipment for diabetics. Also, suitably qualified and experienced nurses and pharmacists may be independent prescribers. Both can prescribe all

POMs but pharmacists are not allowed to prescribe schedule 1 controlled drugs. District nurses and health visitors have had limited prescribing rights since the mid-nineties, before which prescriptions for dressings and simple medicines would have had to have been signed by a doctor. Once issued, a prescription is taken by the patient to a pharmacy, which dispenses the medicine.

Most prescriptions in the UK are NHS prescriptions, subject to a standard charge unrelated to what is dispensed. The NHS prescription fee was increased to £8.40 per item in England on 1 April 2016; prescriptions are free of charge if prescribed and dispensed in Scotland, Wales or Northern Ireland.

The pharmacy charges the NHS the actual cost of the medicine; the patient pays a set prescription charge in England to the pharmacy. Most of the prescriptions dispensed on the NHS are exempt from charges even in England, as there are many exceptions on grounds such as age and chronic disease, and "season tickets" may be purchased to cover an unlimited amount of medication during a set period. The fee for each item does not depend upon the quantity prescribed by the doctor (which is subject to a maximum of three months' supply), or the cost of the medicine to the NHS, which may vary from a few pence to hundreds of pounds.

Outside the NHS, private prescriptions are issued by private medical practitioners, and sometimes under the NHS for medicines not covered by the NHS. NHS supply beyond three months' worth is not covered, and must be purchased privately. A patient pays the pharmacy the normal price for medicine prescribed outside the NHS.

Survey results published by Ipsos MORI in 2008 found that around 800,000 people in England were not collecting prescriptions or getting them dispensed due to the cost, a figure which was the same as in 2001.

Regulation in United States

In the United States, the Federal Food, Drug, and Cosmetic Act defines what requires a prescription. In general, prescription drugs are authorized by physicians, physician assistants, nurse practitioners, and other APRNs, veterinarians, dentists, and optometrists. In general, it is required that an MD, DO, PA, OD, DPM, NMD, ND, DVM, DDS, or DMD, some psychologists, clinical pharmacists, nurse practitioners, and other APRNs write the prescription; basic-level registered nurses, medical assistants, emergency medical technicians, most psychologists, and social workers as examples, do not have the authority to prescribe drugs.

The Controlled Substances Act (CSA) was enacted into law by the Congress of the United States in 1970. The CSA is the federal U.S. drug policy under which the manufacture, importation, possession, use and distribution of certain substances is regulated. The legislation created five Schedules (classifications), with varying qualifications for a substance to be included in each.

The safety and effectiveness of prescription drugs in the US is regulated by the federal Prescription Drug Marketing Act of 1987. The Food and Drug Administration (FDA) is charged with implementing this law. Misuse or abuse of prescription drugs can lead to adverse drug events, including those due to dangerous drug interactions. Fifteen percent of older American adults are at risk of potential major drug-drug interactions.

The package insert for a prescription drug contains information about the intended effect of the drug and how it works in the body. It also contains information about side-effects, how a patient should take the drug, and cautions for its use, including warnings about allergies.

As a general rule, *over-the-counter drugs* (OTC) are used to treat conditions not necessarily requiring care from a healthcare professional and have been proven to meet higher safety standards for self-medication by patients. Often a lower strength of a drug will be approved for OTC use, whereas higher strengths require a prescription to be obtained; a notable case is ibuprofen, which has been widely available as an OTC pain killer since the mid-1980s but is still available by prescription in doses up to four times the OTC dose for use in cases of severe pain not adequately controlled by the lower, OTC strength.

Herbal preparations, amino acids, vitamins, minerals, and other food supplements are regulated by the FDA as dietary supplements. Because specific health claims cannot be made, the consumer must make informed decisions when purchasing such products.

In the United States, the term "prescription drug" is most commonly used, but they are also called Rx-only drugs or legend drugs, after the Federal and State laws that mandate that all such drugs bear a "legend" prohibiting sale without a prescription; though more complex legends have been used, on most original drug packaging today the legend simply states "Rx only". Some of the more controlled medications, such as amphetamines, are usually almost impossible to obtain without a prescription. However, they are often the most abused, especially by college students. Students use them as study aids or "energy boosts" to gain more focus and "drive" to study and complete assignments. The loophole that students use to obtain these drugs without a prescription is still unresolved due to a lack of concrete evidence of if students actually have the attention deficit disorder, ADD, but more extensive studies will be most likely be conducted in the near future to avoid this particular issue. .

Although this may seem as beneficial to the student, studies have shown that these types of drugs are extremely addictive. Another setback that has been observed is that, after prolonged use, students may strive towards finishing tasks or irrelevant goals that the drug causes them to feel like they need to finish. . The physiological aspects of these types of drugs on the human body are mainly due to the stimulation of the β-Adrenergic receptor. Symptoms from this stimulation includes increased heart rate, stroke volume, and skeletal muscle blood flow. This drug can be diagnosed and detected in the human body from stomach content, vomit, or positive results found in urine tests that identify illicit drug use.

Also, pharmacies operated by membership clubs, such as Costco and Sam's Club, by law must allow non-members to use their pharmacy services and must charge the same prices as to members.

Physicians may legally prescribe drugs for uses other than those specified in the FDA approval; this is known as off-label use. Drug companies may not promote or market drugs for off-label uses.

Large U.S. retailers that operate pharmacies and pharmacy chains use inexpensive generic drugs as a way to attract customers into stores. Several chains, including Walmart, Kroger (including subsidiaries such as Dillons), Target, and others, offer $4 monthly prescriptions on select generic drugs as a customer draw. Publix Supermarkets, which has pharmacies in many of their stores, offers free prescriptions on a few older but still effective medications to their customers. The maximum supply is for 30 days.

A number of prescription drugs are commonly abused, including fentanyl (Duragesic), hydroco-done (Vicodin), oxycodone (OxyContin), oxymorphone (Opana), propoxyphene (Darvon), hydro-morphone (Dilaudid), meperidine (Demerol), and diphenoxylate (Lomotil).

Regulation in European Union

In European Union (EU), there are two main routes for authorising medicines:

- Centralised Route
- National Route

Expiration Date

The expiration date, required in several countries, specifies the date up to which the manufacturer guarantees the full potency and safety of a drug. In the United States, expiration dates are deter-mined by regulations established by the FDA. The FDA advises consumers not to use products after their expiration dates.

A study conducted by the U.S. Food and Drug Administration covered over 100 drugs, prescription and over-the-counter. The results showed that about 85% of them were safe and effective as far as 15 years past their expiration date. Joel Davis, a former FDA expiration-date compliance chief, said that with a handful of exceptions—notably nitroglycerin, insulin, some liquid antibiotics; out-dated tetracyclines can cause Fanconi syndrome—most expired drugs are probably effective.

The American Medical Association (AMA) issued a report and statement on Pharmaceutical Expi-ration Dates. The Harvard Medical School Family Health Guide notes that, with rare exceptions, "it's true the effectiveness of a drug may decrease over time, but much of the original potency still remains even a decade after the expiration date".

The expiration date is the final day that the manufacturer guarantees the full potency and safety of a medication. Drug expiration dates exist on most medication labels, including prescription, over-the-counter (OTC) and dietary (herbal) supplements. U.S. pharmaceutical manufacturers are required by law to place expiration dates on prescription products prior to marketing. For legal and liability reasons, manufacturers will not make recommendations about the stability of drugs past the original expiration date.

Cost

Prices for prescription drugs vary widely around the world. Prescription costs for biosimilar and generic drugs are usually less than brand names, but the cost is different from one pharmacy to another.

Prescription drug prices including generic prices are rising faster than the average rate of inflation

Environment

Traces of prescription drugs — including antibiotics, anti-convulsants, mood stabilizers and sex hormones — have been detected in drinking water.

Anti-obesity Medication

Anti-obesity medication or weight loss drugs are all pharmacological agents that reduce or control weight. These drugs alter one of the fundamental processes of the human body, weight regulation, by altering either appetite, or absorption of calories. The main treatment modalities for overweight and obese individuals remain dieting and physical exercise.

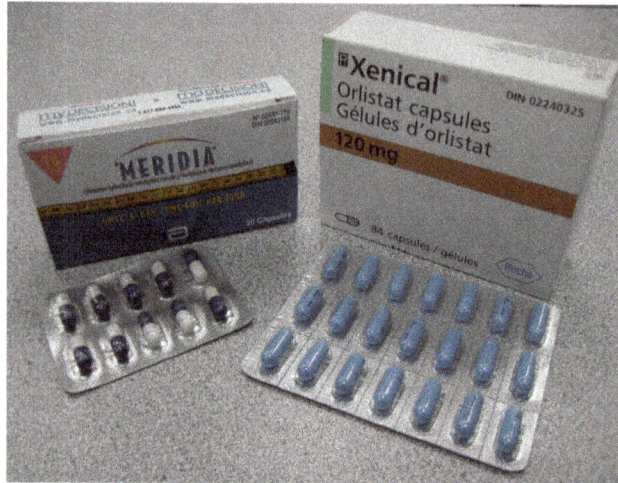

Orlistat (Xenical) the most commonly used medication to treat obesity and sibutramine (Meridia) a medication that was recently withdrawn due to cardiovascular side effects

In the United States orlistat (Xenical) is currently approved by the FDA for long-term use. It reduces intestinal fat absorption by inhibiting pancreatic lipase. Rimonabant (Acomplia), a second drug, works via a specific blockade of the endocannabinoid system. It has been developed from the knowledge that cannabis smokers often experience hunger, which is often referred to as "the munchies". It had been approved in Europe for the treatment of obesity but has not received approval in the United States or Canada due to safety concerns. The European Medicines Agency in October 2008 recommended the suspension of the sale of rimonabant as the risks seem to be greater than the benefits. Sibutramine (Meridia), which acts in the brain to inhibit deactivation of the neurotransmitters, thereby decreasing appetite was withdrawn from the United States and Canadian markets in October 2010 due to cardiovascular concerns.

Because of potential side effects, and limited evidence of small benefits in weight reduction especially in obese children and adolescents, it is recommended that anti-obesity drugs only be prescribed for obesity where it is hoped that the benefits of the treatment outweigh its risks.

Mechanisms of Action

Current and potential anti-obesity drugs may operate through one or more of the following mechanisms:

- Appetite suppression-Catecholamines and their derivatives (such as phentermine and other amphetamine-based drugs) are the main tools used for this, although other classes of drugs such as anti-depressants and mood stabilizers have been anecdotally used for appetite suppression. Drugs blocking the cannabinoid receptors may be a future strategy for appetite suppression.

- Increase of the body's metabolism.

- Interference with the body's ability to absorb specific nutrients in food. For example, Orlistat (also known as Xenical and Alli) blocks fat breakdown and thereby prevents fat absorption. The OTC fiber supplements glucomannan and guar gum have been used for the purpose of inhibiting digestion and lowering caloric absorption

Anorectics are primarily intended to suppress the appetite, but most of the drugs in this class also act as stimulants (e.g., dexedrine), and patients have abused drugs "off label" to suppress appetite (e.g. digoxin).

History

The first described attempts at producing weight loss are those of Soranus of Ephesus, a Greek physician, in the second century AD. He prescribed elixirs of laxatives and purgatives, as well as heat, massage, and exercise. This remained the mainstay of treatment for well over a thousand years. It was not until the 1920s and 1930s that new treatments began to appear. Based on its effectiveness for hypothyroidism, thyroid hormone became a popular treatment for obesity in euthyroid people. It had a modest effect but produced the symptoms of hyperthyroidism as a side effect, such as palpitations and difficulty sleeping. 2,4-Dinitrophenol (DNP) was introduced in 1933; this worked by uncoupling the biological process of oxidative phosphorylation in mitochondria, causing them to produce heat instead of ATP. The most significant side effect was a sensation of warmth, frequently with sweating. Overdose, although rare, lead to a rise in body temperature and, ultimately, fatal hyperthermia. By the end of 1938 DNP had fallen out of use because the FDA had become empowered to put pressure on manufacturers, who voluntarily withdrew it from the market.

Amphetamines (marketed as Benzedrine) became popular for weight loss during the late 1930s. They worked primarily by suppressing appetite, and had other beneficial effects such as increased alertness. Use of amphetamines increased over the subsequent decades, including Obetrol and culminating in the "rainbow pill" regime. This was a combination of multiple pills, all thought to help with weight loss, taken throughout the day. Typical regimens included stimulants, such as amphetamines, as well as thyroid hormone, diuretics, digitalis, laxatives, and often a barbiturate to suppress the side effects of the stimulants. In 1967/1968 a number of deaths attributed to diet pills triggered a Senate investigation and the gradual implementation of greater restrictions on the market.

Meanwhile, phentermine had been FDA approved in 1959 and fenfluramine in 1973. The two were no more popular than other drugs until in 1992 a researcher reported that when combined the two caused a 10% weight loss which was maintained for more than two years. *Fen-phen* was born and rapidly became the most commonly prescribed diet medication. Dexfenfluramine (Redux) was developed in the mid-1990s as an alternative to fenfluramine with less side-effects, and received regulatory approval in 1996. However, this coincided with mounting evidence that the combination could cause valvular heart disease in up to 30% of those who had taken it, leading to withdrawal of Fen-phen and dexfenfluramine from the market in September 1997.

Ephedra was removed from the US market in 2004 over concerns that it raises blood pressure and could lead to strokes and death.

Contemporary Anti-obesity Drugs

Some patients find that diet and exercise is not a viable option; for these patients, anti-obesity drugs can be a last resort. Some prescription weight loss drugs are stimulants, which are recommended only for short-term use, and thus are of limited usefulness for extremely obese patients, who may need to reduce weight over months or years.

Orlistat

Orlistat (Xenical) reduces intestinal fat absorption by inhibiting pancreatic lipase. Some side-effects of using Orlistat include frequent, oily bowel movements (steatorrhea). But if fat in the diet is reduced, symptoms often improve. Originally available only by prescription, it was approved by the FDA for over-the-counter sale in February 2007. On 26 May 2010, the U.S. Food and Drug Administration (FDA) has approved a revised label for Xenical to include new safety information about cases of severe liver injury that have been reported rarely with the use of this medication. Of the 40 million users of Orlistat worldwide, 13 cases of severe liver damage have been reported.

Lorcaserin

Lorcaserin (Belviq) was approved June 28, 2012 for obesity with other co-morbidities. The average weight loss by study participants was modest, but the most common side effects of the drug are considered benign.

Sibutramine

Sibutramine (Reductil or Meridia) is an anorectic or appetite suppressant, reducing the desire to eat. Sibutramine may increase blood pressure and may cause dry mouth, constipation, headache, and insomnia.

In the past, it was noted by the US that Meridia was a harmless drug for fighting obesity. The US District Court of the Northern District of Ohio rejected 113 cases complaining about the negative effects of the drug, stating that the clients lacked supporting facts and that the representatives involved were not qualified enough.

Sibutramine has been withdrawn from the market in the United States, the UK, the EU, Australia, Canada, Hong Kong and Colombia. Its risks (non-life-threatening myocardial infarction and stroke) have been shown to outweigh the benefits.

Rimonabant

Rimonabant (Acomplia) is a recently developed anti-obesity medication. It is a cannabinoid (CB1) receptor antagonist that acts centrally on the brain thus decreasing appetite. It may also act peripherally by increasing thermogenesis and therefore increasing energy expenditure.

Weight loss with Rimonabant however has not been shown to be greater than other available weight-loss medication. Due to safety concerns, primarily psychiatric in nature, the drug has not received approval in the United States or Canada, either as an anti-obesity treatment or as a smoking-cessation drug.

Sanofi-Aventis has received approval to market Rimonabant as a prescription anti-obesity drug in the European Union, subject to some restrictions. However, in October 2008, the European Medicines Agency (EMEA) recommended that Acomplia no longer be available in UK. One month later, Sanofi-Aventis decided it would no longer study rimonabant for any indication.

Metformin

In people with Diabetes mellitus type 2, the drug metformin (Glucophage) can reduce weight. Metformin limits the amount of glucose that is produced by the liver as well as increases muscle consumption of glucose. It also helps in increasing our body's response to insulin.

Exenatide / Liraglutide

Exenatide (Byetta) is a long-acting analogue of the hormone GLP-1, which the intestines secrete in response to the presence of food. Among other effects, GLP-1 delays gastric emptying and promotes a feeling of satiety. Some obese people are deficient in GLP-1, and dieting reduces GLP-1 further. Byetta is currently available as a treatment for Diabetes mellitus type 2. Some, but not all, patients find that they lose substantial weight when taking Byetta. Drawbacks of Byetta include that it must be injected subcutaneously twice daily, and that it causes severe nausea in some patients, especially when therapy is initiated. Byetta is recommended only for patients with Type 2 Diabetes. A somewhat similar drug, Symlin, is currently available for treating diabetes and is in testing for treating obesity in non-diabetics.Template:Horm Metab Res; 47(8): 560-4, 2015 Jul.

Liraglutide (Saxenda) is another GLP-1 analogue.

Pramlintide

Pramlintide (Symlin) is a synthetic analogue of the hormone Amylin, which in normal people is secreted by the pancreas in response to eating. Among other effects, Amylin delays gastric emptying and promotes a feeling of satiety. Many diabetics are deficient in Amylin. Currently, Symlin is only approved to be used along with insulin by Type 1 and Type 2 diabetics. However, Symlin is currently being tested in non-diabetics as a treatment for obesity. A drawback is that Symlin must be injected at mealtimes.

Phentermine/Topiramate

The combination of phentermine and topiramate, brand name Qsymia (formerly Qnexa) was approved by the U.S. FDA on July 17, 2012, as an obesity treatment complementary to a diet and exercise regimen. The European Medicines Agency, by contrast, rejected the combination as a treatment for obesity, citing concerns about long-term effects on the heart and blood vessels, mental health and cognitive side-effects.

Naltrexone / Bupropion

The combination of naltrexone and bupropion, brand name Contrave is another option.

Other Drugs

Other weight loss drugs have also been associated with medical complications, such as fatal pulmonary hypertension and heart valve damage due to Redux and Fen-phen, and hemorrhagic stroke due phenylpropanolamine. Many of these substances are related to amphetamine.

Unresearched nonprescription products or programs for weight loss are heavily promoted by mail and print advertising and on the internet. The US Food and Drug Administration recommends caution with use of these products, since many of the claims of safety and effectiveness are unsubstantiated. Individuals with anorexia nervosa and some athletes try to control body weight with laxatives, diet pills or diuretic drugs, although these generally have no impact on body fat. Products that work as a laxative can cause the blood's potassium level to drop, which may cause heart and/or muscle problems. Pyruvate is a popular product that may result in a small amount of weight loss. However, pyruvate, which is found in red apples, cheese, and red wine, has not been thoroughly studied and its weight loss potential has not been scientifically established.

Alternative Medicine

Recommendations for medicinal plants for weight loss target five basic bodily mechanisms: managing or controlling appetite, stimulating thermogenesis and lipid metabolism, inhibiting pancreatic lipase activity, preventing adipogenesis, and promoting lipolysis.

A 2015 review of the available literature, gathered from books, journals, and a variety of electronic sources published in the period of 1991 to 2014, suggests that consumption of recommended medicinal plants in the one prescribed form, and at an optimized evidence-based dosage, could possibly be part of a safe and effective complementary treatment for obesity.

However, some currently available supplements and alternative medicine have insufficient evidence to support or oppose their use.

Product	Claim	Effectiveness	Side effects
Conjugated linoleic acid	Helps reduce obesity	Ineffective	
ECA Stack	weight loss; athletic performance	Modest short term weight loss; ineffective in long term	possible adverse effects on the mental, digestive, and nervous systems; heart palpitations

Side Effects

Some anti-obesity drugs can have severe, even, lethal side effects, fen-phen being a famous example. Fen-phen was reported through the FDA to cause abnormal echocardiograms, heart valve problems, and rare valvular diseases. One of, if not the first, to sound alarms was Sir Arthur MacNalty, Chief Medical Officer (United Kingdom). As early as the 1930s, he warned against the use of dinitrophenol as an anti-obesity medication and the injudicious and/or medically unsupervised use of thyroid hormone to achieve weight reduction. The side effects are often associated with the medication's mechanism of action. In general, stimulants carry a risk of high blood pressure, faster heart rate, palpitations, closed-angle glaucoma, drug addiction, restlessness, agitation, and insomnia.

Another drug, orlistat, blocks absorption of dietary fats, and as a result may cause oily spotting bowel movements (steatorrhea), oily stools, stomach pain, and flatulence. A similar medication designed for patients with Type 2 diabetes is Acarbose; which partially blocks absorption of carbohydrates in the small intestine, and produces similar side effects including stomach pain and flatulence.

Limitations of Current Knowledge

The limitation of - or knowledge gap concerning - drugs for obesity is that we do not fully understand the neural basis of appetite and how to modulate it. Appetite is clearly a very important instinct to promote survival.

Because the human body uses various chemicals and hormones to protect its stores of fat (a reaction probably useful to our ancestors when food was scarce in the past,) there has not yet been found a 'silver bullet', or a way to completely circumvent this natural habit of protecting excess food stores.

In order to circumvent the number of feedback mechanisms that prevent most monotherapies from producing sustained large amounts of weight loss, it has been hypothesized that combinations of drugs may be more effective by targeting multiple pathways and possibly inhibiting feedback pathways that work to cause a plateau in weight loss. This was evidenced by the success of the combination of phentermine and fenfluramine or dexfenfluramine, popularly referred to phen-fen, in producing significant weight loss but fenfluramine and dexfenfluramine were pulled from the market due to safety fears regarding a potential link to heart valve damage. The damage was found to be a result of activity of fenfluramine and dexfenfluramine at the 5-HT2B serotonin receptor in heart valves. Newer combinations of SSRIs and phentermine, known as phenpro, have been used with equal efficiency as fenphen with no known heart valve damage due to lack of activity at this particular serotonin receptor due to SSRIs. There has been a recent resurgence in combination therapy clinical development with the development of 3 combinations: Qsymia (topiramate + phentermine), Empatic (bupropion + zonisamide) and Contrave (bupropion + naltrexone).

Future Developments

Other classes of drugs in development include lipase inhibitors, similar to orlistat. Another lipase inhibitor, called GT 389-255, was being developed by Peptimmune (licensed from Genzyme). This was a novel combination of an inhibitor and a polymer designed to bind the undigested triglycerides therefore allowing increased fat expulsion without side effects such as oily stools that occur with orlistat. The development stalled as Phase 1 trials were conducted in 2004 and there was no further human clinical development afterward. In 2011, Peptimmune filed for Chapter 7 Liquidation.

Another potential long-term approach to anti-obesity medication is through the development of ribonucleic acid interference (RNAi). Animal studies have illustrated that the deletion of the RIP140 gene in mice by genetic knockdown results in the lack of fat accumulation, even when mice are fed a high fat diet. Similarly, another nuclear hormone receptor co-repressor, SMRT, has demonstrated an opposing effect in genetically engineered mice. Dr. Russell Nofsinger and Dr. Ronald Evans of the Salk Institute showed that disruption of the molecular interaction between

SMRT and their nuclear hormone receptor partners leads to increased adiposity and a decreased metabolic rate. These studies suggest that new drugs targeting the molecular interaction between nuclear hormone receptors and their regulatory cofactors could provide a useful new category of therapeutic targets to be developed in an effort to control obesity.

Another approach is to induce a sense of satiety by occupying space in the gastric and intestinal cavities. One clinical trial involves a hydrogel (Gelesis) made of indigestible, food-grade materials. Another pilot study uses pseudobezoars.

Other drugs in clinical trials as of October 2009 include Cetilistat and TM38837.

Anti-diabetic Medication

Drugs used in diabetes treat diabetes mellitus by lowering glucose levels in the blood. With the exceptions of insulin, exenatide, liraglutide and pramlintide, all are administered orally and are thus also called oral hypoglycemic agents or oral antihyperglycemic agents. There are different classes of anti-diabetic drugs, and their selection depends on the nature of the diabetes, age and situation of the person, as well as other factors.

Diabetes mellitus type 1 is a disease caused by the lack of insulin. Insulin must be used in Type I, which must be injected.

Diabetes mellitus type 2 is a disease of insulin resistance by cells. Type 2 diabetes mellitus is the most common type of diabetes. Treatments include (1) agents that increase the amount of insulin secreted by the pancreas, (2) agents that increase the sensitivity of target organs to insulin, and (3) agents that decrease the rate at which glucose is absorbed from the gastrointestinal tract.

Several groups of drugs, mostly given by mouth, are effective in Type II, often in combination. The therapeutic combination in Type II may include insulin, not necessarily because oral agents have failed completely, but in search of a desired combination of effects. The great advantage of injected insulin in Type II is that a well-educated patient can adjust the dose, or even take additional doses, when blood glucose levels measured by the patient, usually with a simple meter, as needed by the measured amount of sugar in the blood.

Insulin

Insulin is usually given subcutaneously, either by injections or by an insulin pump. Research of other routes of administration is underway. In acute-care settings, insulin may also be given intravenously. In general, there are three types of insulin, characterized by the rate which they are metabolized by the body. They are rapid acting insulins, intermediate acting insulins and long acting insulins.

Examples of rapid acting insulins include

- Regular insulin (Humulin R, Novolin R)
- Insulin lispro (Humalog)
- Insulin aspart (Novolog)
- Insulin glulisine (Apidra)

- Prompt insulin zinc (Semilente, Slightly slower acting)

Examples of intermediate acting insulins include

- Isophane insulin, neutral protamine Hagedorn (NPH) (Humulin N, Novolin N)

- Insulin zinc (Lente)

Examples of long acting insulins include

- Extended insulin zinc insulin (Ultralente)

- Insulin glargine (Lantus)

- Insulin detemir (Levemir)

Most anti-diabetic agents are contraindicated in pregnancy, in which insulin is preferred.

Sensitizers

Insulin sensitizers address the core problem in Type II diabetes—insulin resistance.

Biguanides

Biguanides reduce hepatic glucose output and increase uptake of glucose by the periphery, including skeletal muscle. Although it must be used with caution in patients with impaired liver or kidney function, metformin, a biguanide, has become the most commonly used agent for type 2 diabetes in children and teenagers. Among common diabetic drugs, metformin is the only widely used oral drug that does not cause weight gain.

Typical reduction in glycated hemoglobin (A1C) values for metformin is 1.5–2.0%

- Metformin (Glucophage) may be the best choice for patients who also have heart failure, but it should be temporarily discontinued before any radiographic procedure involving intravenous iodinated contrast, as patients are at an increased risk of lactic acidosis.

- Phenformin (DBI) was used from 1960s through 1980s, but was withdrawn due to lactic acidosis risk.

- Buformin also was withdrawn due to lactic acidosis risk.

Metformin is usually the first-line medication used for treatment of type 2 diabetes. In general, it is prescribed at initial diagnosis in conjunction with exercise and weight loss, as opposed to in the past, where it was prescribed after diet and exercise had failed. There is an immediate release as well as an extended-release formulation, typically reserved for patients experiencing GI side-effects. It is also available in combination with other oral diabetic medications.

Thiazolidinediones

Thiazolidinediones (TZDs), also known as "glitazones," bind to PPARγ, a type of nuclear regulatory protein involved in transcription of genes regulating glucose and fat metabolism. These PPARs act on peroxysome proliferator responsive elements (PPRE). The PPREs influence insulin-sensitive genes, which enhance production of mRNAs of insulin-dependent enzymes. The final result is better use of glucose by the cells.

Typical reductions in glycated hemoglobin (A1C) values are 1.5–2.0%. Some examples are:

- rosiglitazone (Avandia): the European Medicines Agency recommended in September 2010 that it be suspended from the EU market due to elevated cardiovascular risks.

- pioglitazone (Actos)

- troglitazone (Rezulin): used in 1990s, withdrawn due to hepatitis and liver damage risk

Multiple retrospective studies have resulted in a concern about rosiglitazone's safety, although it is established that the group, as a whole, has beneficial effects on diabetes. The greatest concern is an increase in the number of severe cardiac events in patients taking it. The ADOPT study showed that initial therapy with drugs of this type may prevent the progression of disease, as did the DREAM trial.

Concerns about the safety of rosiglitazone arose when a retrospective meta-analysis was published in the New England Journal of Medicine. There have been a significant number of publications since then, and a Food and Drug Administration panel voted, with some controversy, 20:3 that available studies "supported a signal of harm," but voted 22:1 to keep the drug on the market. The meta-analysis was not supported by an interim analysis of the trial designed to evaluate the issue, and several other reports have failed to conclude the controversy. This weak evidence for adverse effects has reduced the use of rosiglitazone, despite its important and sustained effects on glycemic control. Safety studies are continuing.

In contrast, at least one large prospective study, PROactive 05, has shown that pioglitazone may decrease the overall incidence of cardiac events in people with type 2 diabetes who have already had a heart attack.

Secretagogues

Secretagogues are drugs that increase insulin output from the pancreas.

Sulfonylureas

Sulfonylureas were the first widely used oral anti-hyperglycaemic medications. They are *insulin secretagogues*, triggering insulin release by inhibiting the K_{ATP} channel of the pancreatic beta cells. Eight types of these pills have been marketed in North America, but not all remain available. The "second-generation" drugs are now more commonly used. They are more effective than first-generation drugs and have fewer side-effects. All may cause weight gain.

Sulfonylureas bind strongly to plasma proteins. Sulfonylureas are useful only in Type II diabetes, as they work by stimulating endogenous release of insulin. They work best with patients over 40 years old who have had diabetes mellitus for under ten years. They cannot be used with type I diabetes, or diabetes of pregnancy. They can be safely used with metformin or -glitazones. The primary side-effect is hypoglycemia.

Typical reductions in glycated hemoglobin (A1C) values for second-generation sulfonylureas are 1.0–2.0%.

- First-generation agents

    o tolbutamide

    o acetohexamide

    o tolazamide

    o chlorpropamide

- Second-generation agents

    o glipizide

    o glyburide or glibenclamide

    o glimepiride

    o gliclazide

    o glycopyramide

    o gliquidone

Nonsulfonylurea Secretagogues

Meglitinides

Meglitinides help the pancreas produce insulin and are often called "short-acting secretagogues." They act on the same potassium channels as sulfonylureas, but at a different binding site. By closing the potassium channels of the pancreatic beta cells, they open the calcium channels, thereby enhancing insulin secretion.

They are taken with or shortly before meals to boost the insulin response to each meal. If a meal is skipped, the medication is also skipped.

Typical reductions in glycated hemoglobin (A1C) values are 0.5–1.0%.

- repaglinide

- nateglinide

Adverse reactions include weight gain and hypoglycemia.

Alpha-glucosidase Inhibitors

Alpha-glucosidase inhibitors are "diabetes pills" but not technically hypoglycemic agents because they do not have a direct effect on insulin secretion or sensitivity. These agents slow the digestion of starch in the small intestine, so that glucose from the starch of a meal enters the bloodstream more slowly, and can be matched more effectively by an impaired insulin response or sensitivity. These agents are effective by themselves only in the earliest stages of impaired glucose tolerance, but can be helpful in combination with other agents in type 2 diabetes.

Typical reductions in glycated hemoglobin (A1C) values are 0.5–1.0%.

- miglitol

- acarbose

- voglibose

These medications are rarely used in the United States because of the severity of their side-effects (flatulence and bloating). They are more commonly prescribed in Europe. They do have the potential to cause weight loss by lowering the amount of sugar metabolized.

Peptide Analogs

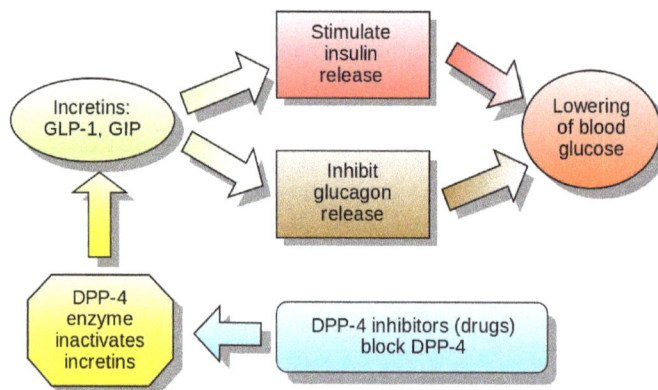

Overview of insulin secretion

Injectable Incretin Mimetics

Incretins are insulin secretagogues. The two main candidate molecules that fulfill criteria for being an incretin are glucagon-like peptide-1 (GLP-1) and gastric inhibitory peptide (glucose-dependent insulinotropic peptide, GIP). Both GLP-1 and GIP are rapidly inactivated by the enzyme dipeptidyl peptidase-4 (DPP-4).

Injectable Glucagon-like Peptide Analogs and Agonists

Glucagon-like peptide (GLP) agonists bind to a membrane GLP receptor. As a consequence, insulin release from the pancreatic beta cells is increased. Endogenous GLP has a half-life of only a few minutes, thus an analogue of GLP would not be practical.

- Exenatide (also Exendin-4, marketed as Byetta) is the first GLP-1 agonist approved for the treatment of type 2 diabetes. Exenatide is not an analogue of GLP but rather a GLP agonist. Exenatide has only 53% homology with GLP, which increases its resistance to degradation by DPP-4 and extends its half-life. Typical reductions in A1C values are 0.5–1.0%.

- Liraglutide, a once-daily human analogue (97% homology), has been developed by Novo Nordisk under the brand name Victoza. The product was approved by the European Medicines Agency (EMEA) on July 3, 2009, and by the U.S. Food and Drug Administration (FDA) on January 25, 2010.

- Taspoglutide is presently in Phase III clinical trials with Hoffman-La Roche.

- Lixisenatide (Lyxumia) Sanofi Aventis

These agents may also cause a decrease in gastric motility, responsible for the common side-effect of nausea, and is probably the mechanism by which weight loss occurs.

Gastric Inhibitory Peptide Analogs

Dipeptidyl Peptidase-4 Inhibitors

GLP-1 analogs resulted in weight loss and had more gastrointestinal side-effects, while in general DPP-4 inhibitors were weight-neutral and increased risk for infection and headache, but both classes appear to present an alternative to other antidiabetic drugs. However, weight gain and/or hypoglycaemia have been observed when DPP-4 inhibitors were used with sulfonylureas; effect on long-term health and morbidity rates are still unknown.

Dipeptidyl peptidase-4 (DPP-4) inhibitors increase blood concentration of the incretin GLP-1 by inhibiting its degradation by dipeptidyl peptidase-4.

Examples are:

- vildagliptin (Galvus) EU Approved 2008

- sitagliptin (Januvia) FDA approved Oct 2006

- saxagliptin (Onglyza) FDA Approved July 2009

- linagliptin (Tradjenta) FDA Approved May 2, 2011

- alogliptin

- septagliptin

- Teneligliptin

DPP-4 inhibitors lowered hemoglobin A1C values by 0.74%, comparable to other antidiabetic drugs.

A result in one RCT comprising 206 patients aged 65 or older (mean baseline HgbA1c of 7.8%) receiving either 50 or 100 mg/d of Sitagliptin was shown to reduce HbA1c by 0.7% (combined result of both doses). A combined result of 5 RCTs enlisting a total of 279 patients aged 65 or older (mean baseline HbA1c of 8%) receiving 5 mg/d of Saxagliptin was shown to reduce HbA1c by 0.73%. A combined result of 5 RCTs enlisting a total of 238 patients aged 65 or older (mean baseline HbA1c of 8.6%) receiving 100 mg/d of Vildagliptin was shown to reduce HbA1c by 1.2%. Another set of 6 combined RCTs involving Alogliptin (not yet approved, might be released in 2012) was shown to reduce HbA1c by 0.73% in 455 patients aged 65 or older who received 12.5 or 25 mg/d of the medication.

Injectable Amylin Analogues

Amylin agonist analogues slow gastric emptying and suppress glucagon. They have all the incretins actions except stimulation of insulin secretion. As of 2007, pramlintide is the only clinically available amylin analogue. Like insulin, it is administered by subcutaneous injection. The most frequent and severe adverse effect of pramlintide is nausea, which occurs mostly at the beginning of treatment and gradually reduces. Typical reductions in A1C values are 0.5–1.0%.

Glycosurics

SGLT-2 inhibitors block the re-uptake of glucose in the renal tubules, promoting loss of glucose in the urine. This causes both mild weight loss, and a mild reduction in blood sugar levels with little risk of hypoglycaemia.

Comparison

The following table compares some common anti-diabetic agents, generalizing classes, although there may be substantial variation in individual drugs of each class. When the table makes a comparison such as "lower risk" or "more convenient" the comparison is with the other drugs on the table.

Generic

Many anti-diabetes drugs are available as generics. These include:

- Sulfonylureas - glimepiride, glipizide, glyburide
- Biguanides - metformin
- Thiazolidinediones (Tzd) - pioglitazone, Actos generic
- Alpha-glucosidase inhibitors - Acarbose
- Meglitinides - nateglinide
- Combination of sulfonylureas plus metformin - known by generic names of the two drugs

No generics are available for dipeptidyl peptidase-4 inhibitors (Januvia, Onglyza) and other combinations.

Antibiotics

Antibiotics, also called antibacterials, are a type of antimicrobial drug used in the treatment and prevention of bacterial infections. They may either kill or inhibit the growth of bacteria. A limited number of antibiotics also possess antiprotozoal activity. Antibiotics are not effective against viruses such as the common cold or influenza, and their inappropriate use allows the emergence of resistant organisms. In 1928, Alexander Fleming identified penicillin, the first chemical compound with antibiotic properties. Fleming was working on a culture of disease-causing bacteria when he noticed the spores of a little green mold (*Penicillium chrysogenum*), in one of his culture plates. He observed that the presence of the mold killed or prevented the growth of the bacteria.

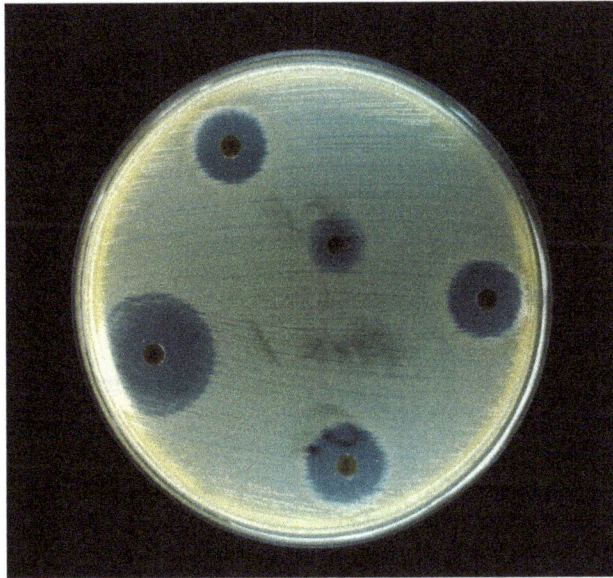

Testing the susceptibility of *Staphylococcus aureus* to antibiotics by the Kirby-Bauer disk diffusion method – antibiotics diffuse from antibiotic-containing disks and inhibit growth of *S. aureus*, resulting in a zone of inhibition.

Antibiotics revolutionized medicine in the 20th century, and have together with vaccination led to the near eradication of diseases such as tuberculosis in the developed world. Their effectiveness and easy access led to overuse, especially in livestock raising, prompting bacteria to develop resistance. This has led to widespread problems with antimicrobial and antibiotic resistance, so much as to prompt the World Health Organization to classify antimicrobial resistance as a "serious threat [that] is no longer a prediction for the future, it is happening right now in every region of the world and has the potential to affect anyone, of any age, in any country".

The era of antibacterial treatment began with the discovery of arsphenamine, first synthesized by Alfred Bertheim and Paul Ehrlich in 1907, and used to treat syphilis. The first systemically active antibacterial drug, prontosil was discovered in 1933 by Gerhard Domagk, for which he was awarded the 1939 Nobel Prize. All classes of antibiotics in use today were first discovered prior to the mid 1980s.

Sometimes the term antibiotic is used to refer to any substance used against microbes, synonymous with antimicrobial, leading to the widespread but incorrect belief that antibiotics can be used against viruses. Some sources distinguish between antibacterial and antibiotic; antibacterials are used in soaps and cleaners generally and antibiotics are used as medicine.

Medical Uses

Antibiotics are used to treat or prevent bacterial infections, and sometimes protozoan infections. (Metronidazole is effective against a number of parasitic diseases). When an infection is suspected of being responsible for an illness but the responsible pathogen has not been identified, an empiric therapy is adopted. This involves the administration of a broad-spectrum antibiotic based on the signs and symptoms presented and is initiated pending laboratory results that can take several days.

When the responsible pathogenic microorganism is already known or has been identified, definitive therapy can be started. This will usually involve the use of a narrow-spectrum antibiotic. The choice of antibiotic given will also be based on its cost. Identification is critically important as it can reduce the cost and toxicity of the antibiotic therapy and also reduce the possibility of the emergence of antimicrobial resistance. To avoid surgery antibiotics may be given for non-complicated acute appendicitis. Effective treatment has been evidenced.

Antibiotics may be given as a preventive measure (prophylactic) and this is usually limited to at-risk populations such as those with a weakened immune system (particularly in HIV cases to prevent pneumonia), those taking immunosuppressive drugs, cancer patients and those having surgery. Their use in surgical procedures is to help prevent infection of incisions made. They have an important role in dental antibiotic prophylaxis where their use may prevent bacteremia and consequent infective endocarditis. Antibiotics are also used to prevent infection in cases of neutropenia particularly cancer-related.

Administration

There are different routes of administration for antibiotic treatment. Antibiotics are usually taken by mouth. In more severe cases, particularly deep-seated systemic infections, antibiotics can be given intravenously or by injection. Where the site of infection is easily accessed antibiotics may be given topically in the form of eye drops onto the conjunctiva for conjunctivitis or ear drops for ear infections and acute cases of swimmer's ear. Topical use is also one of the treatment options for some skin conditions including acne and cellulitis. Advantages of topical application include achieving high and sustained concentration of antibiotic at the site of infection; reducing the potential for systemic absorption and toxicity, and total volumes of antibiotic required are reduced, thereby also reducing the risk of antibiotic misuse. Topical antibiotics applied over certain types of surgical wounds have been reported to reduce the risk of surgical site infections. However, there are certain general causes for concern with topical administration of antibiotics. Some systemic absorption of the antibiotic may occur; the quantity of antibiotic applied is difficult to accurately dose, and there is also the possibility of local hypersensitivity reactions or contact dermatitis occurring.

Side-effects

Antibiotics are screened for any negative effects before their approval for clinical use, and are usually considered safe and well tolerated. However, some antibiotics have been associated with a wide extent of adverse side effects ranging from mild to very severe depending on the type of antibiotic used, the microbes targeted, and the individual patient. Side effects may reflect the pharmacological or toxicological properties of the antibiotic or may involve hypersensitivity or allergic reactions. Adverse effects range from fever and nausea to major allergic reactions, including photodermatitis and anaphylaxis. Safety profiles of newer drugs are often not as well established as for those that have a long history of use.

Common side-effects include diarrhea, resulting from disruption of the species composition in the intestinal flora, resulting, for example, in overgrowth of pathogenic bacteria, such as *Clostridium difficile*. Antibacterials can also affect the vaginal flora, and may lead to overgrowth of yeast species of the genus *Candida* in the vulvo-vaginal area. Additional side-effects can result from interaction with other drugs, such as the possibility of tendon damage from the administration of a quinolone antibiotic with a systemic corticosteroid.

Health advocacy messages such as this one encourage patients to talk with their doctor about safety in using antibiotics.

Obesity

Exposure to antibiotics early in life is associated with increased body mass in humans and mouse models. Early life is a critical period for the establishment of the intestinal microbiota and for metabolic development. Mice exposed to subtherapeutic antibiotic treatment (STAT)– with either penicillin, vancomycin, or chlortetracycline had altered composition of the gut microbiota as well as its metabolic capabilities. One study has reported that mice given low-dose penicillin (1 µg/g body weight) around birth and throughout the weaning process had an increased body mass and fat mass, accelerated growth, and increased hepatic expression of genes involved in adipogenesis, compared to control mice. In addition, penicillin in combination with a high-fat diet increased fasting insulin levels in mice. However, it is unclear whether or not antibiotics cause obesity in humans. Studies have found a correlation between early exposure of antibiotics (<6 months) and increased body mass (at 10 and 20 months). Another study found that the type of antibiotic exposure was also significant with the highest risk of being overweight in those given macrolides compared to penicillin and cephalosporin. Therefore, there is correlation between antibiotic exposure in early life and obesity in humans, but whether or not there is a causal relationship remains unclear. Although there is a correlation between antibiotic use in early life and obesity, the effect of antibiotics on obesity in humans needs to be weighed against the beneficial effects of clinically indicated treatment with antibiotics in infancy.

Interactions

Birth Control Pills

The majority of studies indicate antibiotics do interfere with birth control pills, such as clinical studies that suggest the failure rate of contraceptive pills caused by antibiotics is very low (about 1%). In cases where antibiotics have been suggested to affect the efficiency of birth control pills, such as for the broad-spectrum antibiotic rifampicin, these cases may be due to an increase in the activities of hepatic liver enzymes' causing increased breakdown of the pill's active ingredients. Effects on the intestinal flora, which might result in reduced absorption of estrogens in the colon, have also been suggested, but such suggestions have been inconclusive and controversial. Clinicians have recommended that extra contraceptive measures be applied during therapies using antibiotics that are suspected to interact with oral contraceptives.

Alcohol

Interactions between alcohol and certain antibiotics may occur and may cause side-effects and decreased effectiveness of antibiotic therapy. While moderate alcohol consumption is unlikely to interfere with many common antibiotics, there are specific types of antibiotics with which alcohol consumption may cause serious side-effects. Therefore, potential risks of side-effects and effectiveness depend on the type of antibiotic administered.

Antibiotics such as metronidazole, tinidazole, cephamandole, latamoxef, cefoperazone, cefmenoxime, and furazolidone, cause a disulfiram-like chemical reaction with alcohol by inhibiting its breakdown by acetaldehyde dehydrogenase, which may result in vomiting, nausea, and shortness of breath. In addition, the efficacy of doxycycline and erythromycin succinate may be reduced by alcohol consumption. Other effects of alcohol on antibiotic activity include altered activity of the liver enzymes that break down the antibiotic compound.

Pharmacodynamics

The successful outcome of antimicrobial therapy with antibacterial compounds depends on several factors. These include host defense mechanisms, the location of infection, and the pharmacokinetic and pharmacodynamic properties of the antibacterial. A bactericidal activity of antibacterials may depend on the bacterial growth phase, and it often requires ongoing metabolic activity and division of bacterial cells. These findings are based on laboratory studies, and in clinical settings have also been shown to eliminate bacterial infection. Since the activity of antibacterials depends frequently on its concentration, *in vitro* characterization of antibacterial activity commonly includes the determination of the minimum inhibitory concentration and minimum bactericidal concentration of an antibacterial. To predict clinical outcome, the antimicrobial activity of an antibacterial is usually combined with its pharmacokinetic profile, and several pharmacological parameters are used as markers of drug efficacy.

Combination Therapy

In important infectious diseases, including tuberculosis, combination therapy (i.e., the concurrent application of two or more antibiotics) has been used to delay or prevent the emergence of resistance. In acute bacterial infections, antibiotics as part of combination therapy are prescribed for their synergistic effects to improve treatment outcome as the combined effect of both antibiotics is better than their individual effect. Methicillin-resistant Staphylococcus aureus infections may be treated with a combination therapy of fusidic acid and rifampin. Antibiotics used in combination may also be antagonistic and the combined effects of the two antibiotics may be less than if the individual antibiotic was given as part of a monotherapy. For example, Chloramphenicol and tetracyclines are antagonists to penicillins and aminoglycosides. However, this can vary depending on the species of bacteria. In general, combinations of a bacteriostatic antibiotic and bactericidal antibiotic are antagonistic.

Classes

Antibiotics are commonly classified based on their mechanism of action, chemical structure, or spectrum of activity. Most target bacterial functions or growth processes. Those that target the bacterial cell wall (penicillins and cephalosporins) or the cell membrane (polymyxins), or interfere with essential bacterial enzymes (rifamycins, lipiarmycins, quinolones, and sulfonamides) have bactericidal activities. Those that target protein synthesis (macrolides, lincosamides and tetracyclines) are usually bacteriostatic (with the exception of bactericidal aminoglycosides). Further categorization is based on their target specificity. "Narrow-spectrum" antibiotics target specific types of bacteria, such as gram-negative or gram-positive, whereas broad-spectrum antibiotics affect a wide range of bacteria. Following a 40-year break in discovering new classes of antibacterial compounds, four new classes of antibiotics have been brought into clinical use in the late 2000s and early 2010s: cyclic lipopeptides (such as daptomycin), glycylcyclines (such as tigecycline), oxazolidinones (such as linezolid), and lipiarmycins (such as fidaxomicin).

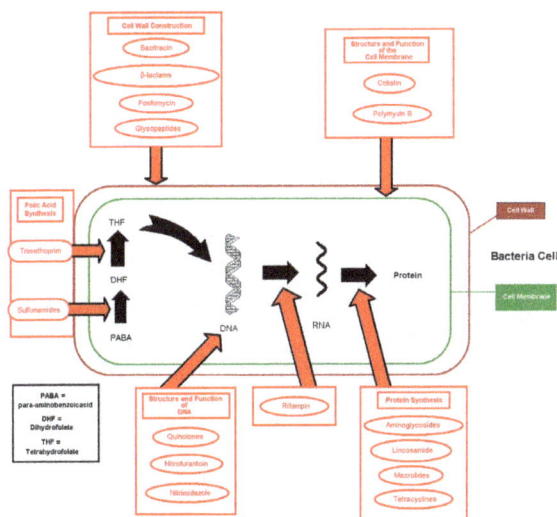

Molecular targets of antibiotics on the bacteria cell

Production

With advances in medicinal chemistry, most modern antibacterials are semisynthetic modifications of various natural compounds. These include, for example, the beta-lactam antibiotics, which include the penicillins (produced by fungi in the genus *Penicillium*), the cephalosporins, and the carbapenems. Compounds that are still isolated from living organisms are the aminoglycosides, whereas other antibacterials—for example, the sulfonamides, the quinolones, and the oxazolidinones—are produced solely by chemical synthesis. Many antibacterial compounds are relatively small molecules with a molecular weight of less than 1000 daltons.

Since the first pioneering efforts of Florey and Chain in 1939, the importance of antibiotics, including antibacterials, to medicine has led to intense research into producing antibacterials at large scales. Following screening of antibacterials against a wide range of bacteria, production of the active compounds is carried out using fermentation, usually in strongly aerobic conditions.

Resistance

The emergence of resistance of bacteria to antibiotics is a common phenomenon. Emergence of resistance often reflects evolutionary processes that take place during antibiotic therapy. The antibiotic treatment may select for bacterial strains with physiologically or genetically enhanced capacity to survive high doses of antibiotics. Under certain conditions, it may result in preferential growth of resistant bacteria, while growth of susceptible bacteria is inhibited by the drug. For example, antibacterial selection for strains having previously acquired antibacterial-resistance genes was demonstrated in 1943 by the Luria–Delbrück experiment. Antibiotics such as penicillin and erythromycin, which used to have a high efficacy against many bacterial species and strains, have become less effective, due to the increased resistance of many bacterial strains.

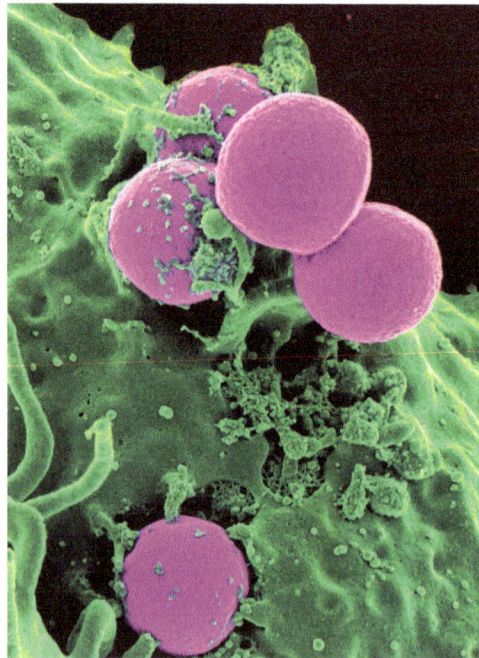

Scanning electron micrograph of a human neutrophil ingesting methicillin-resistant *Staphylococcus aureus* (MRSA)

Resistance may take the form of biodegredation of pharmaceuticals, such as sulfamethazine-degrading soil bacteria introduced to sulfamethazine through medicated pig feces. The survival of bacteria often results from an inheritable resistance, but the growth of resistance to antibacterials also occurs through horizontal gene transfer. Horizontal transfer is more likely to happen in locations of frequent antibiotic use.

Antibacterial resistance may impose a biological cost, thereby reducing fitness of resistant strains, which can limit the spread of antibacterial-resistant bacteria, for example, in the absence of antibacterial compounds. Additional mutations, however, may compensate for this fitness cost and can aid the survival of these bacteria.

Paleontological data show that both antibiotics and antibiotic resistance are ancient compounds and mechanisms. Useful antibiotic targets are those for which mutations negatively impact bacterial reproduction or viability.

Several molecular mechanisms of antibacterial resistance exist. Intrinsic antibacterial resistance may be part of the genetic makeup of bacterial strains. For example, an antibiotic target may be absent from the bacterial genome. Acquired resistance results from a mutation in the bacterial chromosome or the acquisition of extra-chromosomal DNA. Antibacterial-producing bacteria have evolved resistance mechanisms that have been shown to be similar to, and may have been transferred to, antibacterial-resistant strains. The spread of antibacterial resistance often occurs through vertical transmission of mutations during growth and by genetic recombination of DNA by horizontal genetic exchange. For instance, antibacterial resistance genes can be exchanged between different bacterial strains or species via plasmids that carry these resistance genes. Plasmids that carry several different resistance genes can confer resistance to multiple antibacterials. Cross-resistance to several antibacterials may also occur when a resistance mechanism encoded by a single gene conveys resistance to more than one antibacterial compound.

Antibacterial-resistant strains and species, sometimes referred to as "superbugs", now contribute to the emergence of diseases that were for a while well controlled. For example, emergent bacterial strains causing tuberculosis (TB) that are resistant to previously effective antibacterial treatments pose many therapeutic challenges. Every year, nearly half a million new cases of multidrug-resistant tuberculosis (MDR-TB) are estimated to occur worldwide. For example, NDM-1 is a newly identified enzyme conveying bacterial resistance to a broad range of beta-lactam antibacterials. The United Kingdom's Health Protection Agency has stated that "most isolates with NDM-1 enzyme are resistant to all standard intravenous antibiotics for treatment of severe infections." On May 26, 2016 an E coli bacteria "superbug" was identified in the United States resistant to colistin, "the last line of defence" antibiotic.

Misuse

Per the *The ICU Book* "The first rule of antibiotics is try not to use them, and the second rule is try not to use too many of them." Inappropriate antibiotic treatment and overuse of antibiotics have contributed to the emergence of antibiotic-resistant bacteria. Self prescription of antibiotics is an example of misuse. Many antibiotics are frequently prescribed to treat symptoms or diseases that do not respond to antibiotics or that are likely to resolve without treatment. Also, incorrect or suboptimal antibiotics are prescribed for certain bacterial infections. The overuse of antibiotics, like penicillin and erythromycin, has been associated with emerging antibiotic resistance since the 1950s. Widespread usage of antibiotics in hospitals has also been associated with increases in bacterial strains and species that no longer respond to treatment with the most common antibiotics.

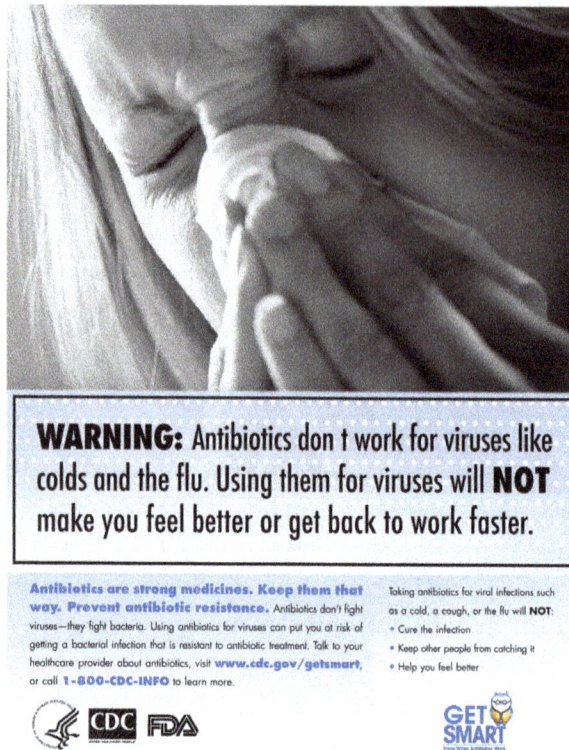

WARNING: Antibiotics don t work for viruses like colds and the flu. Using them for viruses will **NOT** make you feel better or get back to work faster.

Antibiotics are strong medicines. Keep them that way. Prevent antibiotic resistance. Antibiotics don't fight viruses—they fight bacteria. Using antibiotics for viruses can put you at risk of getting a bacterial infection that is resistant to antibiotic treatment. Talk to your healthcare provider about antibiotics, visit **www.cdc.gov/getsmart**, or call **1-800-CDC-INFO** to learn more.

Taking antibiotics for viral infections such as a cold, a cough, or the flu will **NOT**:
- Cure the infection
- Keep other people from catching it
- Help you feel better

CDC FDA   GET SMART

This poster from the US Centers for Disease Control and Prevention "Get Smart" campaign, intended for use in doctors' offices and other healthcare facilities, warns that antibiotics do not work for viral illnesses such as the common cold.

Common forms of antibiotic misuse include excessive use of prophylactic antibiotics in travelers and failure of medical professionals to prescribe the correct dosage of antibiotics on the basis of the patient's weight and history of prior use. Other forms of misuse include failure to take the entire prescribed course of the antibiotic, incorrect dosage and administration, or failure to rest for sufficient recovery. Inappropriate antibiotic treatment, for example, is their prescription to treat viral infections such as the common cold. One study on respiratory tract infections found "physicians were more likely to prescribe antibiotics to patients who appeared to expect them". Multifactorial interventions aimed at both physicians and patients can reduce inappropriate prescription of antibiotics.

Several organizations concerned with antimicrobial resistance are lobbying to eliminate the unnecessary use of antibiotics. The issues of misuse and overuse of antibiotics have been addressed by the formation of the US Interagency Task Force on Antimicrobial Resistance. This task force aims to actively address antimicrobial resistance, and is coordinated by the US Centers for Disease Control and Prevention, the Food and Drug Administration (FDA), and the National Institutes of Health (NIH), as well as other US agencies. An NGO campaign group is *Keep Antibiotics Working*. In France, an "Antibiotics are not automatic" government campaign started in 2002 and led to a marked reduction of unnecessary antibiotic prescriptions, especially in children.

The emergence of antibiotic resistance has prompted restrictions on their use in the UK in 1970 (Swann report 1969), and the EU has banned the use of antibiotics as growth-promotional agents since 2003. Moreover, several organizations (including the World Health Organization, the

National Academy of Sciences, and the U.S. Food and Drug Administration) have advocated restricting the amount of antibiotic use in food animal production. However, commonly there are delays in regulatory and legislative actions to limit the use of antibiotics, attributable partly to resistance against such regulation by industries using or selling antibiotics, and to the time required for research to test causal links between their use and resistance to them. Two federal bills (S.742 and H.R. 2562) aimed at phasing out nontherapeutic use of antibiotics in US food animals were proposed, but have not passed. These bills were endorsed by public health and medical organizations, including the American Holistic Nurses' Association, the American Medical Association, and the American Public Health Association (APHA).

There has been extensive use of antibiotics in animal husbandry. In the United States, the question of emergence of antibiotic-resistant bacterial strains due to use of antibiotics in livestock was raised by the US Food and Drug Administration (FDA) in 1977. In March 2012, the United States District Court for the Southern District of New York, ruling in an action brought by the Natural Resources Defense Council and others, ordered the FDA to revoke approvals for the use of antibiotics in livestock, which violated FDA regulations.

History

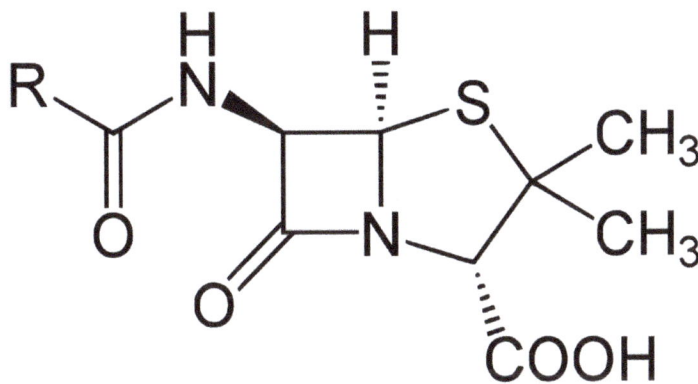

Penicillin, the first natural antibiotic discovered by Alexander Fleming in 1928

Before the early 20th century, treatments for infections were based primarily on medicinal folklore. Mixtures with antimicrobial properties that were used in treatments of infections were described over 2000 years ago. Many ancient cultures, including the ancient Egyptians and ancient Greeks, used specially selected mold and plant materials and extracts to treat infections. More recent observations made in the laboratory of antibiosis between microorganisms led to the discovery of natural antibacterials produced by microorganisms. Louis Pasteur observed, "if we could intervene in the antagonism observed between some bacteria, it would offer perhaps the greatest hopes for therapeutics". The term 'antibiosis', meaning "against life", was introduced by the French bacteriologist Jean Paul Vuillemin as a descriptive name of the phenomenon exhibited by these early antibacterial drugs. Antibiosis was first described in 1877 in bacteria when Louis Pasteur and Robert Koch observed that an airborne bacillus could inhibit the growth of *Bacillus anthracis*. These drugs were later renamed antibiotics by Selman Waksman, an American microbiologist, in 1942. Synthetic antibiotic chemotherapy as a science and development of antibacterials began in Germany with Paul Ehrlich in the late 1880s. Ehrlich noted certain dyes would color human, animal, or bacterial cells, whereas others did not. He then proposed the idea that it might be possible to create chemicals that would act as a selective drug that would bind to and kill bacteria without harming the human host. After screening hundreds of dyes against various organisms, in 1907, he discovered a medicinally useful drug, the first synthetic antibacterial salvarsan now called arsphenamine.

The effects of some types of mold on infection had been noticed many times over the course of history. In 1928, Alexander Fleming noticed the same effect in a Petri dish, where a number of disease-causing bacteria were killed by a fungus of the genus *Penicillium*. Fleming postulated that the effect is mediated by an antibacterial compound he named penicillin, and that its antibacterial properties could be exploited for chemotherapy. He initially characterized some of its biological properties, and attempted to use a crude preparation to treat some infections, but he was unable to pursue its further development without the aid of trained chemists.

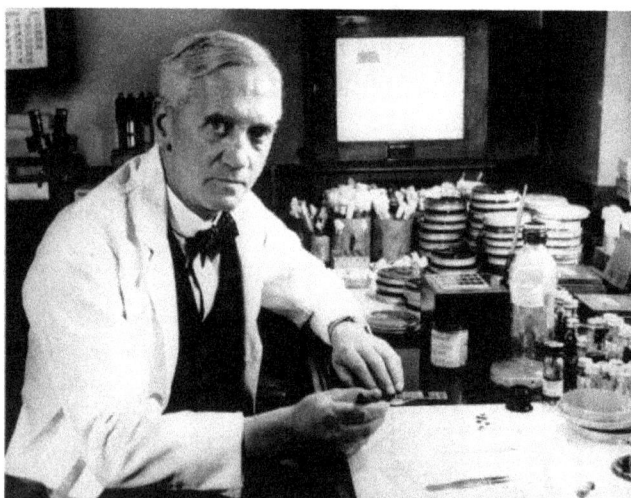

Alexander Fleming

The first sulfonamide and first commercially available antibacterial, Prontosil, was developed by a research team led by Gerhard Domagk in 1932 at the Bayer Laboratories of the IG Farben conglomerate in Germany. Domagk received the 1939 Nobel Prize for Medicine for his efforts. Prontosil had a relatively broad effect against Gram-positive cocci, but not against enterobacteria. Research was stimulated apace by its success. The discovery and development of this sulfonamide drug opened the era of antibacterials.

In 1939, coinciding with the start of World War II, Rene Dubos reported the discovery of the first naturally derived antibiotic, tyrothricin, a compound of 20% gramicidin and 80% tyrocidine, from *B. brevis*. It was one of the first commercially manufactured antibiotics universally and was very effective in treating wounds and ulcers during World War II. Gramicidin, however, could not be used systemically because of toxicity. Tyrocidine also proved too toxic for systemic usage. Research results obtained during that period were not shared between the Axis and the Allied powers during World War II and limited access during the Cold War.

Florey and Chain succeeded in purifying the first penicillin, penicillin G, in 1942, but it did not become widely available outside the Allied military before 1945. Later, Norman Heatley developed the back extraction technique for efficiently purifying penicillin in bulk. The chemical structure of penicillin was determined by Dorothy Crowfoot Hodgkin in 1945. Purified penicillin displayed potent antibacterial activity against a wide range of bacteria and had low toxicity in humans. Furthermore, its activity was not inhibited by biological constituents such as pus, unlike the synthetic sulfonamides. The discovery of such a powerful antibiotic was unprecedented, and the development of penicillin led to renewed interest in the search for antibiotic compounds with similar efficacy and safety. For their successful development of penicillin, which Fleming had accidentally discovered but could not develop himself, as a therapeutic drug, Ernst Chain and Howard Florey shared the 1945 Nobel Prize in Medicine with Fleming. Florey credited Dubos with pioneering the approach of deliberately and systematically searching for antibacterial compounds, which had led to the discovery of gramicidin and had revived Florey's research in penicillin.

Etymology

The term *antibiotic* was first used in 1942 by Selman Waksman and his collaborators in journal articles to describe any substance produced by a microorganism that is antagonistic to the growth of other microorganisms in high dilution. This definition excluded substances that kill bacteria but that are not produced by microorganisms (such as gastric juices and hydrogen peroxide). It also excluded synthetic antibacterial compounds such as the sulfonamides. In current usage, the term "antibiotic" is applied to any medication that kills bacteria or inhibits their growth, regardless of whether that medication is produced by a microorganism or not.

Research

Alternatives

The increase in bacterial strains that are resistant to conventional antibacterial therapies has prompted the development of bacterial disease treatment strategies that are alternatives to conventional antibacterials, including phage therapy.

Resistance-modifying Agents

One strategy to address bacterial drug resistance is the discovery and application of compounds that modify resistance to common antibacterials. Resistance modifying agents are capable of partly or completely suppressing bacterial resistance mechanisms. For example, some resistance-modifying agents may inhibit multidrug resistance mechanisms, such as drug efflux from the cell, thus increasing the susceptibility of bacteria to an antibacterial. Targets include:

- The efflux inhibitor Phe-Arg-β-naphthylamide.

- Beta-lactamase inhibitors, such as clavulanic acid and sulbactam

Metabolic stimuli such as sugar can help eradicate a certain type of antibiotic-tolerant bacteria by keeping their metabolism active.

Vaccines

Vaccines rely on immune modulation or augmentation. Vaccination either excites or reinforces the immune competence of a host to ward off infection, leading to the activation of macrophages, the production of antibodies, inflammation, and other classic immune reactions. Antibacterial vaccines have been responsible for a drastic reduction in global bacterial diseases. Vaccines made from attenuated whole cells or lysates have been replaced largely by less reactogenic, cell-free vaccines consisting of purified components, including capsular polysaccharides and their conjugates, to protein carriers, as well as inactivated toxins (toxoids) and proteins.

Phage Therapy

Phage therapy is another method for treating antibiotic-resistant strains of bacteria. Phage therapy infects pathogenic bacteria with their own viruses, bacteriophages. Bacteriophages, also known simply as phages, infect and can kill bacteria. Phages insert their DNA into the bacterium, where it is transcribed and used to make new phages, after which the cell will lyse, releasing new phage able to infect and destroy further bacteria of the same strain. The high specificity of phage protects "good" bacteria from destruction. When applicable, bacteriophage therapy defeats antibiotic resistant bacteria.

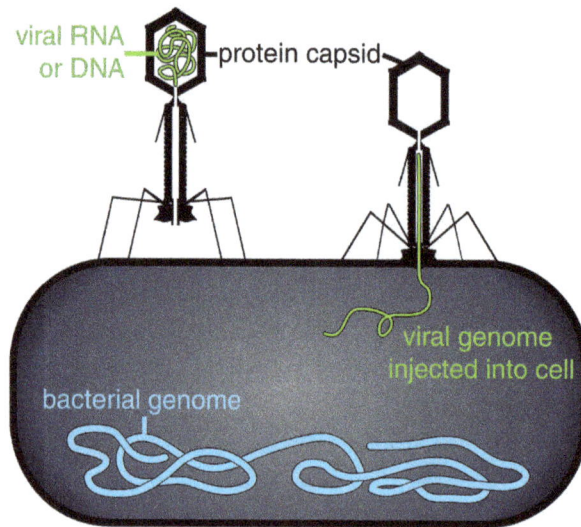

Phage injecting its genome into bacterial cell

Supplements

Some antioxidant dietary supplements contain polyphenols, such as grape seed extract, and demonstrate *in vitro* anti-bacterial properties.

Development of New Antibiotics

In April 2013, the Infectious Disease Society of America (IDSA) reported that the weak antibiotic pipeline does not match bacteria's increasing ability to develop resistance. Since 2009, only 2 new antibiotics were approved in the United States. The number of new antibiotics approved for marketing per year declines continuously. The report identified seven antibiotics against the Gram-negative bacilli (GNB) currently in phase 2 or phase 3 clinical trials. However, these drugs do not address the entire spectrum of resistance of GNB. Some of these antibiotics are combination of existent treatments:

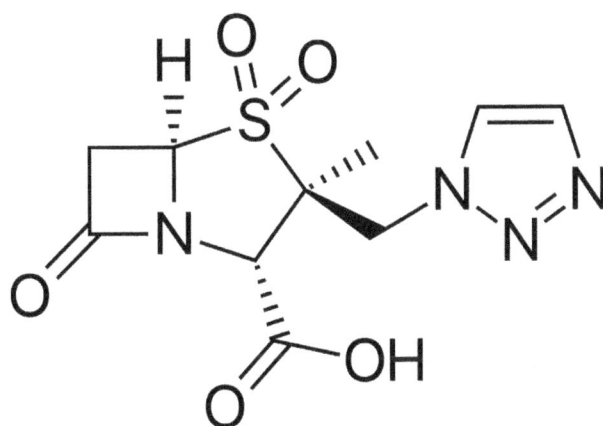

Tazobactam

- Ceftolozane/tazobactam (CXA-201; CXA-101/tazobactam): Antipseudomonal cephalosporin/β-lactamase inhibitor combination (cell wall synthesis inhibitor). FDA approved on 12/19/2014.

- Ceftazidime/avibactam (ceftazidime/NXL104): Antipseudomonal cephalosporin/β-lactamase inhibitor combination (cell wall synthesis inhibitor). In phase 3.

- Ceftaroline/avibactam (CPT-avibactam; ceftaroline/NXL104): Anti-MRSA cephalosporin/β-lactamase inhibitor combination (cell wall synthesis inhibitor)

- Imipenem/MK-7655: Carbapenem/ β-lactamase inhibitor combination (cell wall synthesis inhibitor). In phase 2.

- Plazomicin (ACHN-490): Aminoglycoside (protein synthesis inhibitor). In phase 2.

- Eravacycline (TP-434): Synthetic tetracycline derivative / protein synthesis inhibitor targeting the ribosome. Development by Tetraphase, Phase 2 trials complete.

- Brilacidin (PMX-30063): Peptide defense protein mimetic (cell membrane disruption). In phase 2.

Streptomyces research is expected to provide new antibiotics, including treatment against MRSA and infections resistant to commonly used medication. Efforts of John Innes Centre and universities in the UK, supported by BBSRC, resulted in the creation of spin-out companies, for example Novacta Biosystems, which has designed the type-b lantibiotic-based compound NVB302 (in phase 1) to treat *Clostridium difficile* infections. Possible improvements include clarification of clinical trial regulations by FDA. Furthermore, appropriate economic incentives could persuade pharmaceutical companies to invest in this endeavor. In the US, the Antibiotic Development to Advance Patient Treatment (ADAPT) Act was introduced with the aim of fast tracking the drug development of antibiotics to combat the growing threat of 'superbugs'. Under this Act, FDA can approve antibiotics and antifungals treating life-threatening infections based on smaller clinical trials. The CDC will monitor the use of antibiotics and the emerging resistance, and publish the data. The FDA antibiotics labeling process, 'Susceptibility Test Interpretive Criteria for Microbial Organisms' or 'breakpoints', will provide accurate data to healthcare professionals. According to

Allan Coukell, senior director for health programs at The Pew Charitable Trusts, "By allowing drug developers to rely on smaller datasets, and clarifying FDA's authority to tolerate a higher level of uncertainty for these drugs when making a risk/benefit calculation, ADAPT would make the clinical trials more feasible."

Antiviral Drug

Antiviral drugs are a class of medication used specifically for treating viral infections rather than bacterial ones. Most antivirals are used for specific viral infections, while a broad-spectrum antiviral is effective against a wide range of viruses. Unlike most antibiotics, antiviral drugs do not destroy their target pathogen; instead they inhibit their development.

Antiviral drugs are one class of antimicrobials, a larger group which also includes antibiotic (also termed antibacterial), antifungal and antiparasitic drugs, or antiviral drugs based on monoclonal antibodies. Most antivirals are considered relatively harmless to the host, and therefore can be used to treat infections. They should be distinguished from viricides, which are not medication but deactivate or destroy virus particles, either inside or outside the body. Natural antivirals are produced by some plants such as eucalyptus.

Medical Uses

Most of the antiviral drugs now available are designed to help deal with HIV, herpes viruses, the hepatitis B and C viruses, and influenza A and B viruses. Researchers are working to extend the range of antivirals to other families of pathogens.

Designing safe and effective antiviral drugs is difficult, because viruses use the host's cells to replicate. This makes it difficult to find targets for the drug that would interfere with the virus without also harming the host organism's cells. Moreover, the major difficulty in developing vaccines and anti-viral drugs is due to viral variation.

The emergence of antivirals is the product of a greatly expanded knowledge of the genetic and molecular function of organisms, allowing biomedical researchers to understand the structure and function of viruses, major advances in the techniques for finding new drugs, and the intense pressure placed on the medical profession to deal with the human immunodeficiency virus (HIV), the cause of the deadly acquired immunodeficiency syndrome (AIDS) pandemic.

The first experimental antivirals were developed in the 1960s, mostly to deal with herpes viruses, and were found using traditional trial-and-error drug discovery methods. Researchers grew cultures of cells and infected them with the target virus. They then introduced into the cultures chemicals which they thought might inhibit viral activity, and observed whether the level of virus in the cultures rose or fell. Chemicals that seemed to have an effect were selected for closer study.

This was a very time-consuming, hit-or-miss procedure, and in the absence of a good knowledge of how the target virus worked, it was not efficient in discovering effective antivirals which had few side effects. Only in the 1980s, when the full genetic sequences of viruses began to be unraveled, did researchers begin to learn how viruses worked in detail, and exactly what chemicals were needed to thwart their reproductive cycle.

Virus Life Cycle

Viruses consist of a genome and sometimes a few enzymes stored in a capsule made of protein (called a capsid), and sometimes covered with a lipid layer (sometimes called an 'envelope'). Viruses cannot reproduce on their own, and instead propagate by subjugating a host cell to produce copies of themselves, thus producing the next generation.

Researchers working on such "rational drug design" strategies for developing antivirals have tried to attack viruses at every stage of their life cycles. Some species of mushrooms have been found to contain multiple antiviral chemicals with similar synergistic effects. Viral life cycles vary in their precise details depending on the type of virus, but they all share a general pattern:

- Attachment to a host cell.

- Release of viral genes and possibly enzymes into the host cell.

- Replication of viral components using host-cell machinery.

- Assembly of viral components into complete viral particles.

- Release of viral particles to infect new host cells.

Limitations and Policy Implications

Several factors including cost, vaccination stigma, and acquired resistance limit the effectiveness of antiviral therapies. These issues are explored via a health policy perspective.

Research and Prices

Rising Costs

Cost is an important factor that limits access to antivirals therapies in the United States and internationally. The recommended treatment regimen for hepatitis C virus infection, for example, includes sofosbuvir-velpatasvir (Epclusa) and ledipasvir-sofosbuvir (Harrvoni). A twelve week supply of these drugs amount to $113,400 and $89,712, respectively. These drugs can be manufactured generically at a cost of $100 - $250 per 12 week treatment. Pharmaceutical companies attribute the majority of these costs to research and development expenses. On average, the research and development costs required to bring a new drug to market amount to $17.2 billion. However, critics point to monopolistic market conditions that allow manufacturers to increase prices without facing a reduction in sales, leading to higher profits at patient's expense. Intellectual property laws, anti-importation policies, and the slow pace of FDA review limit alternative options. Recently, private-public research partnerships have been established to promote expedited, cost-effective research.

Vaccinations and Stigma

Vaccines and Population Health

While most antivirals treat viral infection, vaccines are a preemptive first line of defense against pathogens. Vaccination involves the introduction (i.e. via injection) of a small amount of typically inactivated or attenuated antigenic material to stimulate an individual's immune system. The immune system responds by developing white blood cells to specifically combat the introduced pathogen, resulting in adaptive immunity. Vaccination in a population results in herd immunity and greatly improved population health, with significant reductions in viral infection and disease.

Vaccination Policy

Vaccination policy in the United States consists of public and private vaccination requirements. For instance, public schools require students to receive vaccinations (termed "vaccination schedule") for viruses such as diphtheria, pertussis, and tetanus (DTaP), measles, mumps, rubella (MMR), varicella (chickenpox), hepatitis B, rotavirus, polio, and more. Private institutions might require annual influenza vaccination. The Center for Disease Control and Prevention has estimated that routine immunization of newborns prevents about 42,000 deaths and 20 million cases of disease each year, saving about $13.6 billion.

Vaccination Controversy

Despite their successes, there is plenty of stigma surrounding vaccines that cause people to be incompletely vaccinated. These "gaps" in vaccination result in unnecessary infection, death, and costs. There are two major reasons for incomplete vaccination:

1. Vaccines, like other medical treatments, have a risk of causing serious complications in some individuals (i.e. severe allergic reactions). While these complications are less common than the risks faced when not vaccinated, negative media coverage can instill fear in a population. Other controversies involve the association of autism with vaccines, although the Center for Disease Control and Prevention, Institute of Medicine, and National Health Service regard this link as unfounded.

2. Low vaccine-preventable disease rates as a result of herd immunity also make vaccines seem unnecessary and leave many unvaccinated.

Although the American Academy of Pediatrics endorses universal immunization, they note that physicians should respect parents' refusal to vaccinate their children after sufficient advising and provided the child does not face a significant risk of infection. Parents can also cite religious reasons to avoid public school vaccination mandates, but this reduces herd immunity and increases risk of viral infection.

Public Policy

Use and Distribution

Guidelines regarding viral diagnoses and treatments change frequently and limit quality care. Even when physicians diagnose older patients with influenza, use of antiviral treatment can be low. Provider knowledge of antiviral therapies can improve patient care, especially in geriatric medicine. Furthermore, in local health departments (LHDs) with access to antivirals, guidelines may be unclear, causing delays in treatment. With time-sensitive therapies, delays could lead to lack of treatment. Overall, national guidelines regarding infection control and management standardize care and improve patient and health care worker safety. Guidelines such as those provided by the Centers for Disease Control and Prevention (CDC) during the 2009 flu pandemic caused by the H1N1 virus, recommend antiviral treatment regimens, clinical assessment algorithms for co-ordination of care, and antiviral chemoprophylaxis guidelines for exposed persons, among others. Roles of pharmacists and pharmacies have also expanded to meet the needs of public during public health emergencies.

Stockpiling

Public Health Emergency Preparedness initiatives are managed by the CDC via the Office of Public Health Preparedness and Response. Funds aim to support communities in preparing for public health emergencies, including pandemic influenza. Also managed by the CDC, the Strategic National Stockpile (SNS) consists of bulk quantities of medicines and supplies for use during such emergencies. Antiviral stockpiles prepare for shortages of antiviral medications in cases of public health emergencies. During the H1N1 pandemic in 2009-2010, guidelines for SNS use by local health departments was unclear, revealing gaps in antiviral planning. For example, local health departments that received antivirals from the SNS did not have transparent guidance on the use of the treatments. The gap made it difficult to create plans and policies for their use and future availabilities, causing delays in treatment.

Limitations of Vaccines

Vaccines bolster the body's immune system to better attack viruses in the "complete particle" stage, outside of the organism's cells. They traditionally consist of an attenuated (a live weakened) or inactivated (killed) version of the virus. These vaccines can, in very rare cases, harm the host by inadvertently infecting the host with a full-blown viral occupancy. Recently "subunit" vaccines have been devised that consist strictly of protein targets from the pathogen. They stimulate the immune system without doing serious harm to the host. In either case, when the real pathogen attacks the subject, the immune system responds to it quickly and blocks it.

Vaccines are very effective on stable viruses, but are of limited use in treating a patient who has already been infected. They are also difficult to successfully deploy against rapidly mutating viruses, such as influenza (the vaccine for which is updated every year) and HIV. Antiviral drugs are particularly useful in these cases.

Anti-viral Targeting

The general idea behind modern antiviral drug design is to identify viral proteins, or parts of proteins, that can be disabled. These "targets" should generally be as unlike any proteins or parts of proteins in humans as possible, to reduce the likelihood of side effects. The targets should also be common across many strains of a virus, or even among different species of virus in the same family, so a single drug will have broad effectiveness. For example, a researcher might target a critical enzyme synthesized by the virus, but not the patient, that is common across strains, and see what can be done to interfere with its operation.

Once targets are identified, candidate drugs can be selected, either from drugs already known to have appropriate effects, or by actually designing the candidate at the molecular level with a computer-aided design program.

The target proteins can be manufactured in the lab for testing with candidate treatments by inserting the gene that synthesizes the target protein into bacteria or other kinds of cells. The cells are then cultured for mass production of the protein, which can then be exposed to various treatment candidates and evaluated with "rapid screening" technologies.

Approaches by Life Cycle Stage

Before Cell Entry

One anti-viral strategy is to interfere with the ability of a virus to infiltrate a target cell. The virus must go through a sequence of steps to do this, beginning with binding to a specific "receptor" molecule on the surface of the host cell and ending with the virus "uncoating" inside the cell and releasing its contents. Viruses that have a lipid envelope must also fuse their envelope with the target cell, or with a vesicle that transports them into the cell, before they can uncoat.

This stage of viral replication can be inhibited in two ways:

1. Using agents which mimic the virus-associated protein (VAP) and bind to the cellular receptors. This may include VAP anti-idiotypic antibodies, natural ligands of the receptor and anti-receptor antibodies.

2. Using agents which mimic the cellular receptor and bind to the VAP. This includes anti-VAP antibodies, receptor anti-idiotypic antibodies, extraneous receptor and synthetic receptor mimics.

This strategy of designing drugs can be very expensive, and since the process of generating anti-idiotypic antibodies is partly trial and error, it can be a relatively slow process until an adequate molecule is produced.

Entry Inhibitor

A very early stage of viral infection is viral entry, when the virus attaches to and enters the host cell. A number of "entry-inhibiting" or "entry-blocking" drugs are being developed to fight HIV. HIV most heavily targets the immune system's white blood cells known as "helper T cells", and identifies these target cells through T-cell surface receptors designated "CD4" and "CCR5". Attempts to interfere with the binding of HIV with the CD4 receptor have failed to stop HIV from infecting helper T cells, but research continues on trying to interfere with the binding of HIV to the CCR5 receptor in hopes that it will be more effective.

HIV infects a cell through fusion with the cell membrane, which requires two different cellular molecular participants, CD4 and a chemokine receptor (differing depending on the cell type). Approaches to blocking this virus/cell fusion have shown some promise in preventing entry of the virus into a cell. At least one of theses entry inhibitors—a biomimetic peptide marketed under the brand name Fuzeon—has received FDA approval and has been in use for some time. Potentially, one of the benefits from the use of an effective entry-blocking or entry-inhibiting agent is that it potentially may not only prevent the spread of the virus within an infected individual but also the spread from an infected to an uninfected individual.

One possible advantage of the therapeutic approach of blocking viral entry (as opposed to the currently dominant approach of viral enzyme inhibition) is that it may prove more difficult for the virus to develop resistance to this therapy than for the virus to mutate or evolve its enzymatic protocols.

Uncoating Inhibitor

Inhibitors of uncoating have also been investigated.

Amantadine and rimantadine have been introduced to combat influenza. These agents act on penetration and uncoating.

Pleconaril works against rhinoviruses, which cause the common cold, by blocking a pocket on the surface of the virus that controls the uncoating process. This pocket is similar in most strains of rhinoviruses and enteroviruses, which can cause diarrhea, meningitis, conjunctivitis, and encephalitis.

Some scientists are making the case that a vaccine against rhinoviruses, the predominant cause of the common cold, is achievable. Vaccines that combine dozens of varieties of rhinovirus at once are effective in stimulating antiviral antibodies in mice and monkeys, researchers have reported in Nature Communications in 2016.

The quest for a vaccine against rhinoviruses may have seemed quixotic, because there are more than 100 varieties circulating around the world. But the immune system can handle the challenge.

Rhinoviruses are the most common cause of the common cold; other viruses such as respiratory syncytial virus, parainfluenza virus and adenoviruses can cause them too. Rhinoviruses also exacerbate asthma attacks. Although rhinoviruses come in many varieties, they do not drift to the same degree that influenza viruses do. A mixture of 50 inactivated rhinovirus types should be able to stimulate neutralizing antibodies against all of them to some degree.

During Viral Synthesis

A second approach is to target the processes that synthesize virus components after a virus invades a cell.

Reverse Transcription

One way of doing this is to develop nucleotide or nucleoside analogues that look like the building blocks of RNA or DNA, but deactivate the enzymes that synthesize the RNA or DNA once the analogue is incorporated. This approach is more commonly associated with the inhibition of reverse transcriptase (RNA to DNA) than with "normal" transcriptase (DNA to RNA).

The first successful antiviral, acyclovir, is a nucleoside analogue, and is effective against herpesvirus infections. The first antiviral drug to be approved for treating HIV, zidovudine (AZT), is also a nucleoside analogue.

An improved knowledge of the action of reverse transcriptase has led to better nucleoside analogues to treat HIV infections. One of these drugs, lamivudine, has been approved to treat hepatitis

B, which uses reverse transcriptase as part of its replication process. Researchers have gone further and developed inhibitors that do not look like nucleosides, but can still block reverse transcriptase.

Another target being considered for HIV antivirals include RNase H – which is a component of reverse transcriptase that splits the synthesized DNA from the original viral RNA.

On 10 August 2011 researchers at MIT announced the publication of a new method of inhibiting RNA, the process selectively affected infected cells. The team named the process "Double-stranded RNA Activated Caspase Oligomerizer" (DRACO). According to the lead researcher "In theory, [DRACO] should work against all viruses."

Integrase

Another target is integrase, which splices the synthesized DNA into the host cell genome.

Transcription

Once a virus genome becomes operational in a host cell, it then generates messenger RNA (mRNA) molecules that direct the synthesis of viral proteins. Production of mRNA is initiated by proteins known as transcription factors. Several antivirals are now being designed to block attachment of transcription factors to viral DNA.

Translation/Antisense

Genomics has not only helped find targets for many antivirals, it has provided the basis for an entirely new type of drug, based on "antisense" molecules. These are segments of DNA or RNA that are designed as complementary molecule to critical sections of viral genomes, and the binding of these antisense segments to these target sections blocks the operation of those genomes. A phosphorothioate antisense drug named fomivirsen has been introduced, used to treat opportunistic eye infections in AIDS patients caused by cytomegalovirus, and other antisense antivirals are in development. An antisense structural type that has proven especially valuable in research is morpholino antisense.

Morpholino oligos have been used to experimentally suppress many viral types:

- caliciviruses
- flaviviruses (including WNV)
- dengue[43]
- HCV[44]
- coronaviruses[45]

Translation/Ribozymes

Yet another antiviral technique inspired by genomics is a set of drugs based on ribozymes, which are enzymes that will cut apart viral RNA or DNA at selected sites. In their natural course, ribozymes are used as part of the viral manufacturing sequence, but these synthetic ribozymes are designed to cut RNA and DNA at sites that will disable them.

A ribozyme antiviral to deal with hepatitis C has been suggested, and ribozyme antivirals are being developed to deal with HIV. An interesting variation of this idea is the use of genetically modified cells that can produce custom-tailored ribozymes. This is part of a broader effort to create genetically modified cells that can be injected into a host to attack pathogens by generating specialized proteins that block viral replication at various phases of the viral life cycle.

Protein Processing and Targeting

Interference with post translational modifications or with targeting of viral proteins in the cell is also possible.

Protease Inhibitors

Some viruses include an enzyme known as a protease that cuts viral protein chains apart so they can be assembled into their final configuration. HIV includes a protease, and so considerable research has been performed to find "protease inhibitors" to attack HIV at that phase of its life cycle. Protease inhibitors became available in the 1990s and have proven effective, though they can have unusual side effects, for example causing fat to build up in unusual places. Improved protease inhibitors are now in development.

Protease inhibitors have also been seen in nature. A protease inhibitor was isolated from the Shiitake mushroom (*Lentinus edodes*). The presence of this may explain the Shiitake mushrooms noted antiviral activity *in vitro*.

Assembly

Rifampicin acts at the assembly phase.

Release Phase

The final stage in the life cycle of a virus is the release of completed viruses from the host cell, and this step has also been targeted by antiviral drug developers. Two drugs named zanamivir (Relenza) and oseltamivir (Tamiflu) that have been recently introduced to treat influenza prevent the release of viral particles by blocking a molecule named neuraminidase that is found on the surface of flu viruses, and also seems to be constant across a wide range of flu strains.

Immune System Stimulation

A second category of tactics for fighting viruses involves encouraging the body's immune system to attack them, rather than attacking them directly. Some antivirals of this sort do not focus on a specific pathogen, instead stimulating the immune system to attack a range of pathogens.

One of the best-known of this class of drugs are interferons, which inhibit viral synthesis in infected cells. One form of human interferon named "interferon alpha" is well-established as part of the standard treatment for hepatitis B and C, and other interferons are also being investigated as treatments for various diseases.

A more specific approach is to synthesize antibodies, protein molecules that can bind to a pathogen and mark it for attack by other elements of the immune system. Once researchers identify a particular target on the pathogen, they can synthesize quantities of identical "monoclonal" antibodies to link up that target. A monoclonal drug is now being sold to help fight respiratory syncytial virus in babies, and antibodies purified from infected individuals are also used as a treatment for hepatitis B.

Acquired Resistance

Antiviral resistance can be defined by a decreased susceptibility to a drug through either a minimally effective, or completely ineffective, treatment response to prevent associated illnesses from a particular virus. The issue inevitably remains a major obstacle to antiviral therapy as it has developed to almost all specific and effective antimicrobials, including antiviral agents.

The Centers for Disease Control and Prevention (CDC) inclusively recommends those six months and older to get a yearly vaccination to protect from influenza A viruses (H1N1) and (H3N2) and up to two influenza B viruses (depending on the vaccination). Comprehensive protection starts by ensuring vaccinations are current and complete. The three FDA-approved neuraminidase antiviral flu drugs available in the United States, recommended by the CDC, include: oseltamivir (Tamiflu®), zanamivir (Relenza®), and peramivir (Rapivab®).

A study published in 2009 in Nature Biotechnology emphasized the urgent need for augmentation of oseltamivir (Tamiflu®) stockpiles with additional antiviral drugs including zanamivir (Relenza®). This finding was based on a performance evaluation of these drugs supposing the 2009 H1N1 'Swine Flu' neuraminidase (NA) were to acquire the Tamiflu-resistance (His274Tyr) mutation which is currently widespread in seasonal H1N1 strains.

Origin of Antiviral Resistance

The genetic makeup of viruses is constantly changing and therefore may alter the virus resistant to the treatments currently available. Viruses can become resistant through spontaneous or intermittent mechanisms throughout the course of an antiviral treatment. Immunocompromised patients, more often than immunocompetent patients, hospitalized with pneumonia are at the highest risk of developing oseltamivir resistance during treatment. Subsequent to exposure to someone else with the flu, those who received oseltamivir for "post-exposure prophylaxis" are also at higher risk of resistance.

Detection of Antiviral Resistance

National and international surveillance is performed by the CDC to determine effectiveness of the current FDA-approved antiviral flu drugs. Public health officials use this information to make current recommendations about the use of flu antiviral medications. WHO further recommends in-depth epidemiological investigations to control potential transmission of the resistant virus and prevent future progression. As novel treatments and detection techniques to antiviral resistance are enhanced so can the establishment of strategies to combat the inevitable emergence of antiviral resistance.

Nonsteroidal Anti-inflammatory Drug

Nonsteroidal anti-inflammatory drugs (NSAIDs) are a drug class that groups together drugs that provide analgesic (pain-killing) and antipyretic (fever-reducing) effects, and, in higher doses, anti-inflammatory effects.

The term *nonsteroidal* distinguishes these drugs from steroids, which, among a broad range of other effects, have a similar eicosanoid-depressing, anti-inflammatory action. First used in 1960, the term served to distance new drugs from steroid-related iatrogenic tragedies.

The most prominent members of this group of drugs are, aspirin, ibuprofen and naproxen, all available over the counter in most countries. Paracetamol (acetaminophen) is generally not considered an NSAID because it has only little anti-inflammatory activity. It treats pain mainly by blocking COX-2 mostly in the central nervous system, but not much in the rest of the body.

Most NSAIDs inhibit the activity of cyclooxygenase-1 (COX-1) and cyclooxygenase-2 (COX-2), and thereby the synthesis of prostaglandins and thromboxanes. It is thought that inhibiting COX-2 leads to the anti-inflammatory, analgesic and antipyretic effects and that those NSAIDs also inhibiting COX-1, particularly aspirin, may cause gastrointestinal bleeding and ulcers.

Medical Uses

NSAIDs are usually used for the treatment of acute or chronic conditions where pain and inflammation are present.

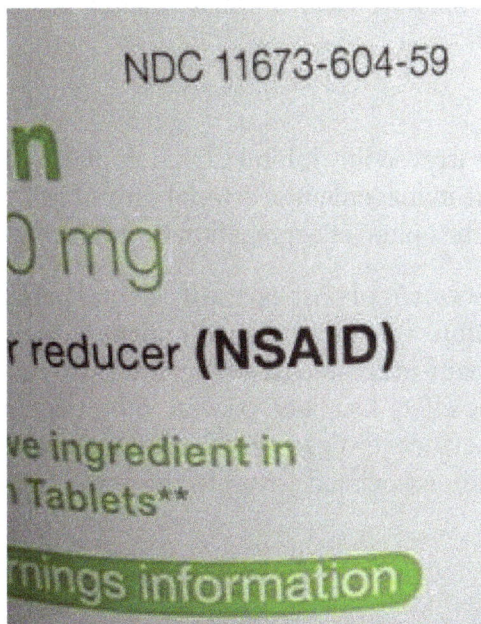

NSAID identification on label of generic ibuprofen, an OTC NSAID

NSAIDs are generally used for the symptomatic relief of the following conditions:

- Osteoarthritis
- Rheumatoid arthritis

- Mild-to-moderate pain due to inflammation and tissue injury

- Low back pain

- Inflammatory arthropathies (e.g., ankylosing spondylitis, psoriatic arthritis, reactive arthritis)

- Tennis elbow

- Headache

- Migraine

- Acute gout

- Dysmenorrhoea (menstrual pain)

- Metastatic bone pain

- Postoperative pain

- Muscle stiffness and pain due to Parkinson's disease

- Pyrexia (fever)

- Ileus

- Renal colic

- They are also given to neonate infants whose ductus arteriosus is not closed within 24 hours of birth

- Macular edema

Aspirin, the only NSAID able to irreversibly inhibit COX-1, is also indicated for inhibition of platelet aggregation. This is useful in the management of arterial thrombosis and prevention of adverse cardiovascular events. Aspirin inhibits platelet aggregation by inhibiting the action of thromboxane A_2.

NSAIDs are useful in the management of post-operative dental pain following invasive dental procedures such as dental extraction. When not contra-indicated they are favoured over the use of paracetamol alone due to the anti-inflammatory effect they provide. When used in combination with paracetamol the analgesic effect has been proven to be improved. A 2012 Cochrane review found that there is some weak evidence suggesting that taking pre-operative analgesia can reduce the length of post operative pain associated with placing orthodontic spacers under local anaesthetic.

Contraindications

NSAIDs may be used with caution by people with the following conditions:

- Irritable bowel syndrome

- Persons who are over age 50, and who have a family history of GI (gastrointestinal) problems

- Persons who have had past GI problems from NSAID use

NSAIDs should usually be avoided by people with the following conditions:

- Peptic ulcer or stomach bleeding

- Uncontrolled hypertension

- Kidney disease

- People that suffer with inflammatory bowel disease (Crohn's disease or ulcerative colitis)

- Past transient ischemic attack (excluding ibuprofen)

- Past stroke (excluding ibuprofen)

- Past myocardial infarction (excluding ibuprofen)

- Coronary artery disease (excluding ibuprofen)

- Undergoing coronary artery bypass surgery

- Taking ibuprofen for heart

- Congestive heart failure (excluding low-dose ibuprofen)

- In third trimester of pregnancy

- Persons who have undergone gastric bypass surgery

- Persons who have a history of allergic or allergic-type NSAID hypersensitivity reactions, e.g. aspirin-induced asthma

Adverse Effects

The widespread use of NSAIDs has meant that the adverse effects of these drugs have become increasingly common. Use of NSAIDs increases risk of having a range of gastrointestinal (GI) problems. When NSAIDs are used for pain management after surgery they cause increased risk of kidney problems.

An estimated 10–20% of NSAID patients experience dyspepsia. In the 1990s high doses of prescription NSAIDs were associated with serious upper gastrointestinal adverse events, including bleeding. Over the past decade, deaths associated with gastric bleeding have declined.

NSAIDs, like all drugs, may interact with other medications. For example, concurrent use of NSAIDs and quinolones may increase the risk of quinolones' adverse central nervous system effects, including seizure.

There is argument over the benefits and risks of NSAIDs for treating chronic musculoskeletal pain. Each drug has a benefit-risk profile and balancing the risk of no treatment with the competing potential risks of various therapies is the clinician's responsibility.

Combinational Risk

If a COX-2 inhibitor is taken, a traditional NSAID (prescription or over-the-counter) should not be taken at the same time. In addition, people on daily aspirin therapy (e.g., for reducing cardiovascular risk) must be careful if they also use other NSAIDs, as these may inhibit the cardioprotective effects of aspirin.

Rofecoxib (Vioxx) was shown to produce significantly fewer gastrointestinal adverse drug reactions (ADRs) compared with naproxen. This study, the VIGOR trial, raised the issue of the cardiovascular safety of the coxibs. A statistically significant increase in the incidence of myocardial infarctions was observed in patients on rofecoxib. Further data, from the APPROVe trial, showed a statistically significant relative risk of cardiovascular events of 1.97 versus placebo—which caused a worldwide withdrawal of rofecoxib in October 2004.

Use of methotrexate together with NSAIDS in rheumatoid arthritis is safe, if adequate monitoring is done.

Cardiovascular

NSAIDs aside from aspirin, both newer selective COX-2 inhibitors and traditional anti-inflammatories, increase the risk of myocardial infarction and stroke. They are not recommended in those who have had a previous heart attack as they increase the risk of death and/or recurrent MI. Evidence indicates that naproxen may be the least harmful out of these.

NSAIDs aside from (low-dose) aspirin are associated with a doubled risk of heart failure in people without a history of cardiac disease. In people with such a history, use of NSAIDs (aside from low-dose aspirin) was associated with a more than 10-fold increase in heart failure. If this link is proven causal, researchers estimate that NSAIDs would be responsible for up to 20 percent of hospital admissions for congestive heart failure. In people with heart failure, NSAIDs increase mortality risk (hazard ratio) by approximately 1.2–1.3 for naproxen and ibuprofen, 1.7 for rofecoxib and celecoxib, and 2.1 for diclofenac.

On 9 July 2015, the FDA toughened warnings of increased heart attack and stroke risk associated with nonsteroidal anti-inflammatory drugs (NSAID). Aspirin is an NSAID but is not affected by the new warnings.

Possible Erectile Dysfunction Risk

A 2005 Finnish study linked long term (over 3 months) use of NSAIDs with an increased risk of erectile dysfunction. This study was correlational only, and depended solely on self-reports (questionnaires).

A 2011 publication in the Journal of Urology received widespread publicity. According to this study, men who used NSAIDs regularly were at significantly increased risk of erectile dysfunction. A link between NSAID use and erectile dysfunction still existed after controlling for several conditions. However, the study was observational and not controlled, with low original participation rate, potential participation bias, and other uncontrolled factors. The authors warned against drawing any conclusion regarding cause.

Gastrointestinal

The main adverse drug reactions (ADRs) associated with NSAID use relate to direct and indirect irritation of the gastrointestinal (GI) tract. NSAIDs cause a dual assault on the GI tract: the acidic molecules directly irritate the gastric mucosa, and inhibition of COX-1 and COX-2 reduces the levels of protective prostaglandins. Inhibition of prostaglandin synthesis in the GI tract causes increased gastric acid secretion, diminished bicarbonate secretion, diminished mucus secretion and diminished trophic effects on epithelial mucosa.

Common gastrointestinal ADRs include:

- Nausea/vomiting

- Dyspepsia

- Gastric ulceration/bleeding

- Diarrhea

Clinical NSAID ulcers are related to the systemic effects of NSAID administration. Such damage occurs irrespective of the route of administration of the NSAID (e.g., oral, rectal, or parenteral) and can occur even in patients with achlorhydria.

Ulceration risk increases with therapy duration, and with higher doses. To minimise GI ADRs, it is prudent to use the lowest effective dose for the shortest period of time—a practice that studies show is often not followed. Recent studies show that over 50% of patients who take NSAIDs have sustained some mucosal damage to their small intestine.

There are also some differences in the propensity of individual agents to cause gastrointestinal ADRs. Indomethacin, ketoprofen and piroxicam appear to have the highest prevalence of gastric ADRs, while ibuprofen (lower doses) and diclofenac appear to have lower rates.

Certain NSAIDs, such as aspirin, have been marketed in enteric-coated formulations that manufacturers claim reduce the incidence of gastrointestinal ADRs. Similarly, some believe that rectal formulations may reduce gastrointestinal ADRs. However, consistent with the systemic mechanism of such ADRs, and in clinical practice, these formulations have not demonstrated a reduced risk of GI ulceration.

Commonly, gastric (but not necessarily intestinal) adverse effects can be reduced through suppressing acid production, by concomitant use of a proton pump inhibitor, e.g., omeprazole, esomeprazole; or the prostaglandin analogue misoprostol. Misoprostol is itself associated with a high incidence of gastrointestinal ADRs (diarrhea). While these techniques may be effective, they are expensive for maintenance therapy.

Inflammatory Bowel Disease

NSAIDs should be used with caution in individuals with inflammatory bowel disease (e.g., Crohn's disease or ulcerative colitis) due to their tendency to cause gastric bleeding and form ulceration in the gastric lining. Pain relievers such as paracetamol (also known as acetaminophen) or drugs containing codeine (which slows down bowel activity) are safer medications for pain relief in IBD.

Renal

NSAIDs are also associated with a fairly high incidence of renal adverse drug reactions (ADRs). The mechanism of these renal ADRs is due to changes in renal haemodynamics (kidney blood flow), ordinarily mediated by prostaglandins, which are affected by NSAIDs. Prostaglandins normally cause vasodilation of the afferent arterioles of the glomeruli. This helps maintain normal glomerular perfusion and glomerular filtration rate (GFR), an indicator of renal function. This is particularly important in renal failure where the kidney is trying to maintain renal perfusion pressure by elevated angiotensin II levels. At these elevated levels, angiotensin II also constricts the afferent arteriole into the glomerulus in addition to the efferent arteriole it normally constricts. Prostaglandins serve to dilate the afferent arteriole; by blocking this prostaglandin-mediated effect, particularly in renal failure, NSAIDs cause unopposed constriction of the afferent arteriole and decreased RPF (renal perfusion pressure).

Common ADRs associated with altered renal function include:

- Salt (Sodium) and fluid retention

- Hypertension (high blood pressure)

These agents may also cause renal impairment, especially in combination with other nephrotoxic agents. Renal failure is especially a risk if the patient is also concomitantly taking an ACE inhibitor (which removes angiotensin II's vasoconstriction of the efferent arteriole) and a diuretic (which drops plasma volume, and thereby RPF)—the so-called "triple whammy" effect.

In rarer instances NSAIDs may also cause more severe renal conditions:

- Interstitial nephritis

- Nephrotic syndrome

- Acute renal failure

- Acute tubular necrosis

- Renal papillary necrosis

NSAIDs in combination with excessive use of phenacetin and/or paracetamol (acetaminophen) may lead to analgesic nephropathy.

Photosensitivity

Photosensitivity is a commonly overlooked adverse effect of many of the NSAIDs. The 2-arylpropionic acids are the most likely to produce photosensitivity reactions, but other NSAIDs have also been implicated including piroxicam, diclofenac and benzydamine.

Benoxaprofen, since withdrawn due to its hepatotoxicity, was the most photoactive NSAID observed. The mechanism of photosensitivity, responsible for the high photoactivity of the 2-arylpropionic acids, is the ready decarboxylation of the carboxylic acid moiety. The specific absorbance characteristics of the different chromophoric 2-aryl substituents, affects the decarboxylation mechanism. While ibuprofen has weak absorption, it has been reported as a weak photosensitising agent.

During Pregnancy

NSAIDs are not recommended during pregnancy, particularly during the third trimester. While NSAIDs as a class are not direct teratogens, they may cause premature closure of the fetal ductus arteriosus and renal ADRs in the fetus. Additionally, they are linked with premature birth and miscarriage. Aspirin, however, is used together with heparin in pregnant women with antiphospholipid antibodies. Additionally, Indomethacin is used in pregnancy to treat polyhydramnios by reducing fetal urine production via inhibiting fetal renal blood flow.

In contrast, paracetamol (acetaminophen) is regarded as being safe and well-tolerated during pregnancy, but Leffers et al. released a study in 2010 indicating that there may be associated male infertility in the unborn. Doses should be taken as prescribed, due to risk of hepatotoxicity with overdoses.

In France, the country's health agency contraindicates the use of NSAIDs, including aspirin, after the sixth month of pregnancy.

Allergy/Allergy-like Hypersensitivity Reactions

A variety of allergic or allergic-like NSAID hypersensitivity reactions follow the ingestion of NSAIDs. These hypersensitivity reactions differ from the other adverse reactions listed here which are toxicity reactions, i.e. unwanted reactions that result from the pharmacological action of a drug, are dose-related, and can occur in any treated individual; hypersensitivity reactions are idiosyncratic reactions to a drug. Some NSAID hypersensitivity reactions are truly allergic in origin: 1) repetitive IgE-mediated urticarial skin eruptions, angioedema, and anaphylaxis following immediately to hours after ingesting one structural type of NSAID but not after ingesting structurally unrelated NSAIDs; and 2) Comparatively mild to moderately severe T cell-mediated delayed onset (usually more than 24 hour), skin reactions such as maculopapular rash, fixed drug eruptions, photosensitivity reactions, delayed urticaria, and contact dermatitis; or 3) far more severe and potentially life-threatening t-cell mediated delayed systemic reactions such as the DRESS syndrome, acute generalized exanthematous pustulosis, the Stevens–Johnson syndrome, and toxic epidermal necrolysis. Other NSAID hypersensitivity reactions are allergy-like symptoms but do not involve true allergic mechanisms; rather, they appear due to the ability of NSAIDs to alter the metabolism of arachidonic acid in favor of forming metabolites that promote allergic symptoms. Afflicted individuals may be abnormally sensitive to these provocative metabolites and/or overproduce them and typically are susceptible to a wide range of structurally dissimilar NSAIDs, particularly those that inhibit COX1. Symptoms, which develop immediately to hours after ingesting any of various NSAIDs that inhibit COX-1, are: 1) exacerbations of asthmatic and rhinitis symptoms in individuals with a history of asthma or rhinitis and 2) exacerbation or first-time development of wheals and/or angioedema in individuals with or without a history of chronic urticarial lesions or angioedema.

Other

Common adverse drug reactions (ADR), other than listed above, include: raised liver enzymes, headache, dizziness. Uncommon ADRs include: hyperkalaemia, confusion, bronchospasm, rash. Rapid and severe swelling of the face and/or body. Ibuprofen may also rarely cause irritable bowel syndrome symptoms. NSAIDs are also implicated in some cases of Stevens–Johnson syndrome.

Most NSAIDs penetrate poorly into the central nervous system (CNS). However, the COX enzymes are expressed constitutively in some areas of the CNS, meaning that even limited penetration may cause adverse effects such as somnolence and dizziness.

In very rare cases, ibuprofen can cause aseptic meningitis.

As with other drugs, allergies to NSAIDs might exist. While many allergies are specific to one NSAID, up to 1 in 5 people may have unpredictable cross-reactive allergic responses to other NSAIDs as well.

Drug Interactions

NSAIDs reduce renal blood flow and thereby decrease the efficacy of diuretics, and inhibit the elimination of lithium and methotrexate.

NSAIDs cause hypocoagulability, which may be serious when combined with other drugs that also decrease blood clotting, such as warfarin.

NSAIDs may aggravate hypertension (high blood pressure) and thereby antagonize the effect of antihypertensives, such as ACE Inhibitors.

NSAIDs may interfere and reduce efficiency of SSRI antidepressants.

Various widely used nonsteroidal anti-inflammatory drugs (NSAIDs) enhance endocannabinoid signaling by blocking the anandamide-degrading membrane enzyme fatty acid amide hydrolase (FAAH).

Mechanism of Action

Most NSAIDs act as nonselective inhibitors of the enzyme cyclooxygenase (COX), inhibiting both the cyclooxygenase-1 (COX-1) and cyclooxygenase-2 (COX-2) isoenzymes. This inhibition is competitively reversible (albeit at varying degrees of reversibility), as opposed to the mechanism of aspirin, which is irreversible inhibition. COX catalyzes the formation of prostaglandins and thromboxane from arachidonic acid (itself derived from the cellular phospholipid bilayer by phospholipase A_2). Prostaglandins act (among other things) as messenger molecules in the process of inflammation. This mechanism of action was elucidated by John Vane (1927–2004), who received a Nobel Prize for his work.

COX-1 is a constitutively expressed enzyme with a "house-keeping" role in regulating many normal physiological processes. One of these is in the stomach lining, where prostaglandins serve a protective role, preventing the stomach mucosa from being eroded by its own acid. COX-2 is an enzyme facultatively expressed in inflammation, and it is inhibition of COX-2 that produces the desirable effects of NSAIDs.

When nonselective COX-1/COX-2 inhibitors (such as aspirin, ibuprofen, and naproxen) lower stomach prostaglandin levels, ulcers of the stomach or duodenum internal bleeding can result.

NSAIDs have been studied in various assays to understand how they affect each of these enzymes. While the assays reveal differences, unfortunately different assays provide differing ratios.

The discovery of COX-2 led to research to development of selective COX-2 inhibiting drugs that do not cause gastric problems characteristic of older NSAIDs.

Paracetamol (acetaminophen) is not considered an NSAID because it has little anti-inflammatory activity. It treats pain mainly by blocking COX-2 mostly in the central nervous system, but not much in the rest of the body.

However, many aspects of the mechanism of action of NSAIDs remain unexplained, and for this reason further COX pathways are hypothesized. The COX-3 pathway was believed to fill some of this gap but recent findings make it appear unlikely that it plays any significant role in humans and alternative explanation models are proposed.

NSAIDs are also used in the acute pain caused by gout because they inhibit urate crystal phagocytosis besides inhibition of prostaglandin synthase.

Antipyretic Activity

NSAIDS have antipyretic activity and can be used to treat fever. Fever is caused by elevated levels of prostaglandin E2, which alters the firing rate of neurons within the hypothalamus that control thermoregulation. Antipyretics work by inhibiting the enzyme COX, which causes the general inhibition of prostanoid biosynthesis (PGE2) within the hypothalamus. PGE2 signals to the hypothalamus to increase the body's thermal set point. Ibuprofen has been shown more effective as an antipyretic than paracetamol (acetaminophen). Arachidonic acid is the precursor substrate for cyclooxygenase leading to the production of prostaglandins F, D & E.

Classification

NSAIDs can be classified based on their chemical structure or mechanism of action. Older NSAIDs were known long before their mechanism of action was elucidated and were for this reason classified by chemical structure or origin. Newer substances are more often classified by mechanism of action.

Salicylates

- Aspirin (acetylsalicylic acid)

- Diflunisal (Dolobid)

- Salicylic acid and other salicylates

- Salsalate (Disalcid)

Propionic Acid Derivatives

- Ibuprofen
- Dexibuprofen
- Naproxen
- Fenoprofen
- Ketoprofen
- Dexketoprofen
- Flurbiprofen
- Oxaprozin
- Loxoprofen

Acetic Acid Derivatives

- Indomethacin
- Tolmetin
- Sulindac
- Etodolac
- Ketorolac
- Diclofenac
- Aceclofenac
- Nabumetone (drug itself is non-acidic but the active, principal metabolite has a carboxylic acid group)

Enolic Acid (Oxicam) Derivatives

- Piroxicam
- Meloxicam
- Tenoxicam
- Droxicam
- Lornoxicam
- Isoxicam (withdrawn from market 1985)
- Phenylbutazone (Bute)

Anthranilic Acid Derivatives (Fenamates)

The following NSAIDs are derived from fenamic acid. which is a derivative of anthranilic acid, which in turn is a nitrogen isostere of salicylic acid, which is the active metabolite of aspirin.

- Mefenamic acid

- Meclofenamic acid

- Flufenamic acid

- Tolfenamic acid

Selective COX-2 Inhibitors (Coxibs)

- Celecoxib (FDA alert)

- Rofecoxib (withdrawn from market)

- Valdecoxib (withdrawn from market)

- Parecoxib FDA withdrawn, licensed in the EU

- Lumiracoxib TGA cancelled registration

- Etoricoxib not FDA approved, licensed in the EU

- Firocoxib used in dogs and horses

Sulfonanilides

- Nimesulide (systemic preparations are banned by several countries for the potential risk of hepatotoxicity)

Others

- Clonixin

- Licofelone acts by inhibiting LOX (lipooxygenase) & COX and hence known as 5-LOX/COX inhibitor

- H-harpagide in Figwort or Devil's Claw

Chirality

Most NSAIDs are chiral molecules (diclofenac is a notable exception). However, the majority are prepared in a racemic mixture. Typically, only a single enantiomer is pharmacologically active. For some drugs (typically profens), an isomerase enzyme *in vivo* converts the inactive enantiomer into the active form, although its activity varies widely in individuals. This phenomenon is likely responsible for the poor correlation between NSAID efficacy and plasma concentration observed in older studies, when specific analysis of the active enantiomer was not performed.

Ibuprofen and ketoprofen are now available in single, active enantiomer preparations (dexibuprofen and dexketoprofen), which purport to offer quicker onset and an improved side-effect profile. Naproxen has always been marketed as the single active enantiomer.

Main Practical Differences

NSAIDs within a group tend to have similar characteristics and tolerability. There is little difference in clinical efficacy among the NSAIDs when used at equivalent doses. Rather, differences among compounds usually relate to dosing regimens (related to the compound's elimination half-life), route of administration, and tolerability profile.

Regarding adverse effects, selective COX-2 inhibitors have lower risk of gastrointestinal bleeding, but a substantially more increased risk of myocardial infarction than the increased risk from non-selective inhibitors. Some data also supports that the partially selective nabumetone is less likely to cause gastrointestinal events. The nonselective naproxen appears risk-neutral with regard to cardiovascular events.

A consumer report noted that ibuprofen, naproxen, and salsalate are less expensive than other NSAIDs, and essentially as effective and safe when used appropriately to treat osteoarthritis and pain.

Pharmacokinetics

Most nonsteroidal anti-inflammatory drugs are weak acids, with a pKa of 3–5. They are absorbed well from the stomach and intestinal mucosa. They are highly protein-bound in plasma (typically >95%), usually to albumin, so that their volume of distribution typically approximates to plasma volume. Most NSAIDs are metabolised in the liver by oxidation and conjugation to inactive metabolites that typically are excreted in the urine, though some drugs are partially excreted in bile. Metabolism may be abnormal in certain disease states, and accumulation may occur even with normal dosage.

Ibuprofen and diclofenac have short half-lives (2–3 hours). Some NSAIDs (typically oxicams) have very long half-lives (e.g. 20–60 hours).

History

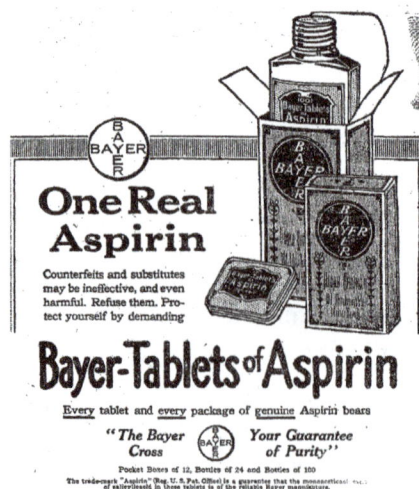

One of the first advertisements for Bayer Aspirin, published in *The New York Times* in 1917

From the era of Greek medicine to the mid-19th century, the discovery of medicinal agents was classed as an empirical art; folklore and mythological guidance were combined in deploying the vegetable and mineral products that made up the expansive pharmacopoeia of the time. Myrtle leaves were in use by 1500 BCE. Hippocrates (460–377 BCE) first reported using willow bark and in 30 BCE Celsus described the signs of inflammation and also used willow bark to mitigate them. On 25 April 1763, Edward Stone wrote to the Royal Society describing his observations on the use of willow bark-based medicines in febrile patients. The active ingredient of willow bark, a glycoside called salicin, was first isolated by Johann Andreas Buchner in 1827. By 1829, French chemist Henri Leroux had improved the extraction process to obtain about 30g of purified salicin from 1.5 kg of bark.

By hydrolysis, salicin releases glucose and salicylic alcohol which can be converted into salicylic acid, both in vivo and through chemical methods. The acid is more effective than salicin and, in addition to its fever-reducing properties, is anti-inflammatory and analgesic. In 1869, Hermann Kolbe synthesised salicylate, although it was too acidic for the gastric mucosa. The reaction used to synthesise aromatic acid from a phenol in the presence of CO_2 is known as the Kolbe-Schmitt reaction.

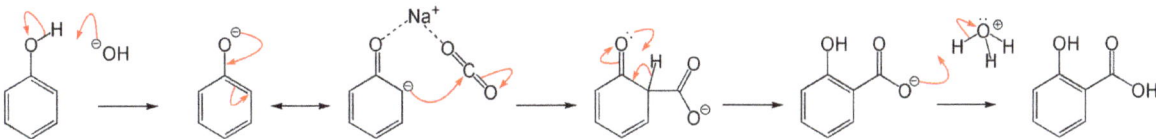

By 1897 the German chemist Felix Hoffmann and the Bayer company prompted a new age of pharmacology by converting salicylic acid into acetylsalicylic acid—named aspirin by Heinrich Dreser. Other NSAIDs were developed from the 1950s forward. In 2001, NSAIDs accounted for 70,000,000 prescriptions and 30 billion over-the-counter doses sold annually in the United States.

Research

While studies have been conducted to see if various NSAIDs can improve behavior in transgenic mouse models of Alzheimer's disease and observational studies in humans have shown promise, there is no good evidence from randomized clinical trials that NSAIDs can treat or prevent Alzheimer's in humans; clinical trials of NSAIDs for treatment of Alzheimer's have found more harm than benefit. Non-Steroidal Anti-Inflammatory Drugs (NSAIDs) coordinate with Metal ions affecting the cellular function

Veterinary Use

Research supports the use of NSAIDs for the control of pain associated with veterinary procedures such as dehorning and castration of calves. The best effect is obtained by combining a short-term local anesthetic such as lidocaine with an NSAID acting as a longer term analgesic. However, as different species have varying reactions to different medications in the NSAID family, little of the existing research data can be extrapolated to animal species other than those specifically studied, and the relevant government agency in one area sometimes prohibits uses approved in other jurisdictions.

For example, ketoprofen's effects have been studied in horses more than in ruminants but, due to controversy over its use in racehorses, veterinarians who treat livestock in the United States more commonly prescribe flunixin meglumine, which, while labeled for use in such animals, is not indicated for post-operative pain.

In the United States, meloxicam is approved for use only in canines, whereas (due to concerns about liver damage) it carries warnings against its use in cats except for one-time use during surgery. In spite of these warnings, meloxicam is frequently prescribed "off-label" for non-canine animals including cats and livestock species. In other countries, for example The European Union (EU), there is a label claim for use in cats.

Generic Drug

A generic drug is a pharmaceutical drug that is equivalent to a brand-name product in dosage, strength, route of administration, quality, performance, and intended use. The term may also refer to any drug marketed under its chemical name without advertising, or to the chemical makeup of a drug rather than the brand name under which the drug is sold.

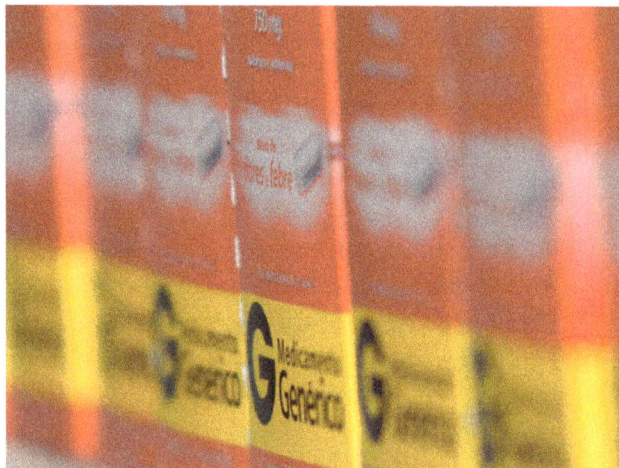

In some countries, such as Brazil (photo) and France, more than 20% of all drug sales are generic.

Although they may not be associated with a particular company, generic drugs are usually subject to government regulations in the countries where they are dispensed. They are labeled with the name of the manufacturer and a generic nonproprietary name such as the United States Adopted Name or international nonproprietary name of the drug. A generic drug must contain the same active ingredients as the original brand-name formulation. The U.S. Food and Drug Administration (FDA) requires that generics be identical to, or within an acceptable bioequivalent range of, their brand-name counterparts with respect to pharmacokinetic and pharmacodynamic properties. (The FDA's use of the word "identical" is a legal interpretation, not literal.)

Biopharmaceuticals such as monoclonal antibodies differ biologically from small molecule drugs. Generic versions of these drugs, known as biosimilars, are typically regulated under an extended set of rules.

In most cases, generic products become available after the patent protections afforded to a drug's original developer expire. Once generic drugs enter the market, competition often leads to substantially lower prices for both the original brand-name product and its generic equivalents. In most countries, patents give 20 years of protection. However, many countries and regions, such as the European Union and the United States, may grant up to five years of additional protection ("patent term restoration") if manufacturers meet specific goals, such as conducting clinical trials for pediatric patients. Manufacturers, wholesalers, insurers, and drugstores can each increase prices at various stages of production and distribution.

In 2014, according to an analysis by the Generic Pharmaceutical Association, generic drugs accounted for 88% of the 4.3 billion prescriptions filled in the United States.

Nomenclature

Generic drug names are constructed using standardized affixes that distinguish drugs between and within classes and suggest their action.

Economics

When a pharmaceutical company first markets a drug, it is usually under a patent that, until it expires, the company can use to exclude competitors by suing them for patent infringement. Pharmaceutical companies that develop new drugs generally only invest in drug candidates with strong patent protection as a strategy to recoup their costs to develop the drug (include the costs of the drug candidates that fail) and to make a profit. The average cost to a brand-name company of discovering, testing, and obtaining regulatory approval for a new drug, with a new chemical entity, was estimated to be as much as $800 million in 2003 and $2.6 billion in 2014. Drug companies that bring new products have several product line extension strategies they use to extend their exclusivity, some of which are seen as gaming the system and referred to by critics as "evergreening", but at some point there is no patent protection available. For as long as a drug patent lasts, a brand-name company enjoys a period of market exclusivity, or monopoly, in which the company is able to set the price of the drug at a level that maximizes profit. This profit often greatly exceeds the development and production costs of the drug, allowing the company to offset the cost of research and development of other drugs that are not profitable or do not pass clinical trials.

Large pharmaceutical companies often spend millions of dollars protecting their patents from generic competition. Apart from litigation, they may reformulate a drug or license a subsidiary (or another company) to sell generics under the original patent. Generics sold under license from the patent holder are known as authorized generics.

Generic drugs are usually sold for significantly lower prices than their branded equivalents and at lower profit margins. One reason for this is that competition increases among producers when a drug is no longer protected by patents. Generic companies incur fewer costs in creating generic drugs—only the cost of manufacturing, without the costs of drug discovery and drug development—and are therefore able to maintain profitability at a lower price. The prices are often low enough for users in less-prosperous countries to afford them. For example, Thailand has imported millions of doses of a generic version of the blood-thinning drug Plavix (used to help prevent heart attacks) from India, the leading manufacturer of generic drugs, at a cost of 3 US cents per dose.

Generic drug companies may also receive the benefit of the previous marketing efforts of the brand-name company, including advertising, presentations by drug representatives, and distribution of free samples. Many drugs introduced by generic manufacturers have already been on the market for a decade or more and may already be well known to patients and providers, although often under their branded name.

In the United Kingdom, generic drug pricing is controlled by the government's reimbursement rate. The price paid by pharmacists and doctors is determined mainly by the number of license holders, the sales value of the original brand, and the ease of manufacture. A typical price decay graph will show a "scalloped" curve, which usually starts at the brand-name price on the day of generic launch and then falls as competition intensifies. After some years, the graph typically flattens out at approximately 20% of the original brand price. In about 20% of cases, the price "bounces": Some license holders withdraw from the market when the selling price dips below their cost of goods, and the price then rises for a while until the license holders re-enter the market with new stock.

In In 2012, 84% of prescriptions in the US were filled with generic drugs, and in 2014, the use of generic drugs in the United States led to $254 billion in health care savings.

Regulation

Most nations require generic drug manufacturers to prove that their formulations are bioequivalent to their brand-name counterparts.

Bioequivalence does not mean generic drugs must be exactly the same as the brand-name product ("pharmaceutical equivalent"). Chemical differences may exist; a different salt or ester may be used, for instance. However, the therapeutic effect of the drug must be the same ("pharmaceutical alternative"). Most small molecule drugs are accepted as bioequivalent if their pharmacokinetic parameters of AUC (area under concentration) and Cmax (maximum concentration) are within a 90% confidence interval of 80–125%; most approved generics are well within this limit. For more complex products—such as inhalers, patch delivery systems, liposomal preparations, or biosimilar drugs—demonstrating pharmacodynamic or clinical equivalence is more challenging.

United States

Enacted in 1984, the Drug Price Competition and Patent Term Restoration Act, informally known as the Hatch-Waxman Act, standardized procedures for recognition of generic drugs. In 2007, the FDA launched the Generic Initiative for Value and Efficiency (GIVE): an effort to modernize and streamline the generic drug approval process, and to increase the number and variety of generic products available.

Before a company can market a generic drug, it needs to file an Abbreviated New Drug Application (ANDA) with the Food and Drug Administration, seeking to demonstrate therapeutic equivalence to a previously approved "reference-listed drug" and proving that it can manufacture the drug safely and consistently. For an ANDA to be approved, the FDA requires the bioequivalence of a generic drug to be between 80% and 125% of the innovator product. (This range is part of a statistical calculation, and does not mean that generic drugs are allowed to differ from their brand-name counterparts by up to 25 percent.) The FDA evaluated 2,070 studies conducted between 1996 and 2007 that compared the absorption of brand-name and generic drugs into a person's body. The average difference in absorption between the generic and the brand-name drug was 3.5 percent, comparable to the difference between two batches of a brand-name drug. Generic versions of biologic drugs, or biosimilars, require clinical trials for immunogenicity in addition to tests establishing bioequivalency. These products cannot be entirely identical because of batch-to-batch variability and their biological nature, and they are subject to extra rules.

When an application is approved, the FDA adds the generic drug to its Approved Drug Products with Therapeutic Equivalence Evaluations list and annotates the list to show equivalence between the reference-listed drug and the generic. The FDA also recognizes drugs that use the same ingredients with different bioavailability, and divides them into therapeutic equivalence groups. For example, as of 2006, diltiazem hydrochloride had four equivalence groups, all using the same active ingredient, but considered equivalent only within each group.

In order to start selling a drug promptly after the patent on innovator drug expires, a generic company has to file its ANDA well before the patent expires. This puts the generic company at risk of being sued for patent infringement, since the act of filing the ANDA is considered "constructive infringement" of the patent. In order to incentivize generic companies to take that risk the Hatch-Waxman act granted a 180-day administrative exclusivity period to generic drug manufacturers who are the first to file an ANDA.

When faced with patent litigation from the drug innovator, generic companies will often counter-sue, challenging the validity of the patent. Like any litigation between private parties, the innovator and generic companies may choose to settle the litigation. Some of these settlement agreements have been stuck down by courts when they took the form of reverse payment patent settlement agreements, in which the generic company basically accepts a payment to drop the litigation, delaying the introduction of the generic product and frustrating the purpose of the Hatch-Waxman Act.

Innovator companies sometimes try to maintain some of the revenue from their drug after patents expire by allowing another company to sell an authorized generic; a 2011 FTC report found that consumers benefitted from lower costs when an authorized generic was introduced during the 180 exclusivity period, as it created competition.

Innovator companies may also present arguments to the FDA that the ANDA should not be accepted by filing a "citizen petition" with the FDA. Citizen petitions are part of the basic law governing everything the FDA does - at any time, any "interested person" can request that the FDA "issue, amend, or revoke a regulation or order," or "take or refrain from taking any other form of administrative action." Originally there was no deadline by which the FDA had to respond to citizen petitions filed to protest ANDAs, leading to significant delays in approving generics. In 2007 the law was amended to include a new section, Section 505(q), in the part of the federal code created by the Hatch-Waxman Act; this section said that the FDA could not delay approving an ANDA due to concerns raised in a citizen petition unless the delay was "necessary to protect public health"; it also mandated that the FDA needed to respond to a petition within 180 days - this was shorted to 150 days in a 2011 amendment. In 2014 the FDA issued guidance to industry about submitting citizen petitions and how it would consider them.

Acceptance

A series of scandals around the approval of generic drugs in the late 1980s shook public confidence in generic drugs; there were several instances in which companies obtained bioequivalence data fraudulently, by using the branded drug in their tests instead of their own product, and a congressional investigation found corruption at the FDA, where employees were accepting bribes to approve some generic companies' applications and delaying or denying others.

Some generic drugs are viewed with suspicion by doctors. For example, warfarin (Coumadin) has a narrow therapeutic window and requires frequent blood tests to make sure patients do not have a subtherapeutic or a toxic level. A study performed in Ontario showed that replacing Coumadin with generic warfarin was safe, but many physicians are not comfortable with their patients taking branded generic equivalents. In some countries (for example, Australia) where a drug is prescribed under more than one brand name, doctors may choose not to allow pharmacists to substitute a brand different from the one prescribed unless the consumer requests it.

Recalls

In 2007, North Carolina Public Radio's *The People's Pharmacy* began reporting on consumers' complaints that generic versions of bupropion (Wellbutrin) were yielding unexpected effects. Subsequently, Impax Laboratories's 300 mg extended-release tablets, marketed by Teva Pharmaceutical Industries, were withdrawn from the US market after the FDA determined in 2012 that they were not bioequivalent.

Litigation

Two women, each claiming to have suffered severe medical complications from a generic version of metoclopramide, lost their Supreme Court appeal on June 23, 2011. In a 5-4 ruling in PLIVA, Inc. v. Mensing, in which the court held that generic companies cannot be held liable for information, or the lack of information, on the originator's label.

India

The Indian government began encouraging more drug manufacturing by Indian companies in the early 1960s, and with the Patents Act in 1970. The Patents Act removed composition patents for foods and drugs, and though it kept process patents, these were shortened to a period of five to seven years. The resulting lack of patent protection created a niche in both the Indian and global markets that Indian companies filled by reverse-engineering new processes for manufacturing low-cost drugs. Mumbai, India headquartered Sun Pharmaceutical's consolidated revenues for the 12 months ending March 2015 are US$4.5 billion.

China

Generic drug production is a large part of the pharmaceutical industry in China. Western observers have said that China lacks administrative protection for patents. However, entry to the World Trade Organization has brought a stronger patent system.

References

- Finkel, Richard; Cubeddu, Luigi; Clark, Michelle (2009). Lippencott's Illustrated Reviews: Pharmacology 4th Edition. Lippencott Williams & Wilkins. pp. 1–4. ISBN 978-0-7817-7155-9.

- H. F. J. Horstmanshoff, Marten Stol, Cornelis Tilburg (2004), Magic and Rationality in Ancient Near Eastern and Graeco-Roman Medicine, p. 99, Brill Publishers, ISBN 90-04-13666-5.

- Kenneth G. Zysk, Asceticism and Healing in Ancient India: Medicine in the Buddhist Monastery, Oxford University Press, rev. ed. (1998) ISBN 0-19-505956-5.

- Miller, AA; Miller, PF (editor) (2011). Emerging Trends in Antibacterial Discovery: Answering the Call to Arms. Caister Academic Press. ISBN 978-1-904455-89-9.

- World Health Organization (2003). Introduction to drug utilization research (PDF). Geneva: World Health Organization. p. 33. ISBN 924156234X.

- Kolata, Gina (2007). Rethinking thin: The new science of weight loss – and the myths and realities of dieting. Picador. ISBN 0-312-42785-9.

- Chemical Analysis of Antibiotic Residues in Food. (PDF). John Wiley & Sons, Inc. 2012. pp. 1–60. ISBN 9781449614591.

- "Antimicrobial resistance: global report on surveillance" (PDF). The World Health Organization. April 2014. ISBN 978 92 4 156474 8. Retrieved 13 June 2016.

- Gualerzi, Claudio O.; Brandi, Letizia; Fabbretti, Attilio; Pon, Cynthia L. (2013-12-04). Antibiotics: Targets, Mechanisms and Resistance. John Wiley & Sons. p. 1. ISBN 9783527333059.

- Dyer, Betsey Dexter (2003). "Chapter 9, Pathogens". A Field Guide To Bacteria. Cornell University Press. ISBN 978-0-8014-8854-2.

Pharmacokinetics and Pharmacodynamics

Pharmacokinetics is a branch of pharmacology; it is the study of how an organism is affected by drugs. It includes the effects of dosage and the adverse reactions to drugs. The aspects explained in the section are clearance, biological half-life, bioavailability, adverse drug reaction, ADME, drug metabolism and others. The chapter serves as a source to understand the major categories related to pharmacokinetics and pharmacodynamics.

Pharmacokinetics

Pharmacokinetics, sometimes abbreviated as PK, is a branch of pharmacology dedicated to determining the fate of substances administered to a living organism. The substances of interest include any chemical xenobiotic such as: pharmaceutical drugs, pesticides, food additives, cosmetic ingredients, etc. It attempts to analyze chemical metabolism and to discover the fate of a chemical from the moment that it is administered up to the point at which it is completely eliminated from the body. Pharmacokinetics is the study of how an organism affects a drug, whereas pharmacodynamics is the study of how the drug affects the organism. Both together influence dosing, benefit, and adverse effects, as seen in PK/PD models.

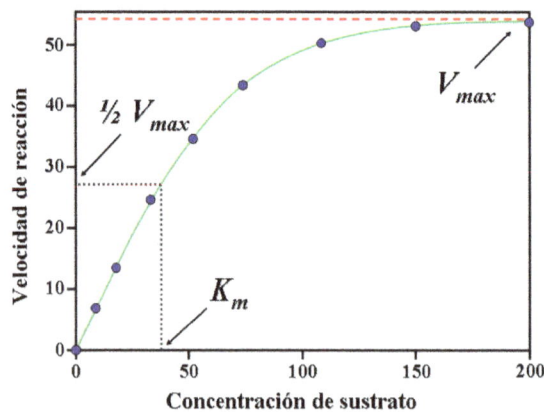

Graph that demonstrates the Michaelis-Menten kinetics model for the relationship between an enzyme and a substrate: one of the parameters studies in pharmacokinetics, where the substrate is a pharmaceutical drug.

Pharmacokinetics describes how the body affects a specific xenobiotic/chemical after administration through the mechanisms of absorption and distribution, as well as the metabolic changes of the substance in the body (e.g. by metabolic enzymes such as cytochrome P450 or glucuronosyltransferase enzymes), and the effects and routes of excretion of the metabolites of the drug. Pharmacokinetic properties of chemicals are affected by the route of administration and the dose of administered drug. These may affect the absorption rate.

Models have been developed to simplify conceptualization of the many processes that take place in the interaction between an organism and a chemical substance. One of these, the multi-compartmental model, gives the best approximation to reality; however, the complexity involved means that *monocompartmental models* and above all *two compartmental models* are the most-frequently used. The various compartments that the model is divided into are commonly referred to as the ADME scheme (also referred to as LADME if liberation is included as a separate step from absorption):

- Liberation - the process of release of a drug from the pharmaceutical formulation.

- Absorption - the process of a substance entering the blood circulation.

- Distribution - the dispersion or dissemination of substances throughout the fluids and tissues of the body.

- Metabolism (or biotransformation, or inactivation) – the recognition by the organism that a foreign substance is present and the irreversible transformation of parent compounds into daughter metabolites.

- Excretion - the removal of the substances from the body. In rare cases, some drugs irreversibly accumulate in body tissue.

The two phases of metabolism and excretion can also be grouped together under the title elimination. The study of these distinct phases involves the use and manipulation of basic concepts in order to understand the process dynamics. For this reason in order to fully comprehend the *kinetics* of a drug it is necessary to have detailed knowledge of a number of factors such as: the properties of the substances that act as excipients, the characteristics of the appropriate biological membranes and the way that substances can cross them, or the characteristics of the enzyme reactions that inactivate the drug.

All these concepts can be represented through mathematical formulas that have a corresponding graphical representation. The use of these models allows an understanding of the characteristics of a molecule, as well as how a particular drug will behave given information regarding some of its basic characteristics such as its acid dissociation constant (pKa), bioavailability and solubility, absorption capacity and distribution in the organism.

The model outputs for a drug can be used in industry (for example, in calculating bioequivalence when designing generic drugs) or in the clinical application of pharmacokinetic concepts. Clinical pharmacokinetics provides many performance guidelines for effective and efficient use of drugs for human-health professionals and in veterinary medicine.

Metrics

The following are the most commonly measured pharmacokinetic metrics:

Characteristic	Description	Example value	Symbol	Formula
Dose	Amount of drug administered.	500 mg	D	Design parameter

Dosing interval	Time between drug dose administrations.	24 h	τ	Design parameter
C_{max}	The peak plasma concentration of a drug after administration.	60.9 mg/L	C_{max}	Direct measurement
t_{max}	Time to reach C_{max}.	3.9 h	t_{max}	Direct measurement
C_{min}	The lowest (trough) concentration that a drug reaches before the next dose is administered.	27.7 mg/L	$C_{min,ss}$	Direct measurement
Volume of distribution	The apparent volume in which a drug is distributed (i.e., the parameter relating drug concentration to drug amount in the body).	6.0 L	V_d	$= \dfrac{D}{C_0}$
Concentration	Amount of drug in a given volume of plasma.	83.3 mg/L	C_0, C_{ss}	$= \dfrac{D}{V_d}$
Elimination half-life	The time required for the concentration of the drug to reach half of its original value.	12 h	$t_{\frac{1}{2}}$	$= \dfrac{\ln(2)}{k_e}$
Elimination rate constant	The rate at which a drug is removed from the body.	0.0578 h^{-1}	k_e	$= \dfrac{\ln(2)}{t_{\frac{1}{2}}} = \dfrac{CL}{V_d}$
Infusion rate	Rate of infusion required to balance elimination.	50 mg/h	k_{in}	$= C_{ss} \cdot CL$
Area under the curve	The integral of the concentration-time curve (after a single dose or in steady state).	1,320 mg/L·h	$AUC_{0-\infty}$	$= \int_0^\infty C dt$
			$AUC_{T,ss}$	$= \int_t^{t+\tau} C dt$
Clearance	The volume of plasma cleared of the drug per unit time.	0.38 L/h	CL	$= V_d \cdot k_e = \dfrac{D}{AUC}$
Bioavailability	The systemically available fraction of a drug.	0.8	f	$= \dfrac{AUC_{po} \cdot D_{iv}}{AUC_{iv} \cdot D_{po}}$
Fluctuation	Peak trough fluctuation within one dosing interval at steady state	41.8 %	%PTF	$= \dfrac{C_{max,ss} - C_{min,ss}}{C_{av,ss}} \cdot 100$ where $C_{av,ss} = \dfrac{1}{\tau} AUC_{\delta,ss}$

In pharmacokinetics, *steady state* refers to the situation where the overall intake of a drug is fairly in dynamic equilibrium with its elimination. In practice, it is generally considered that steady state is reached when a time of 4 to 5 times the half-life for a drug after regular dosing is started.

The following graph depicts a typical time course of drug plasma concentration and illustrates main pharmacokinetic metrics:

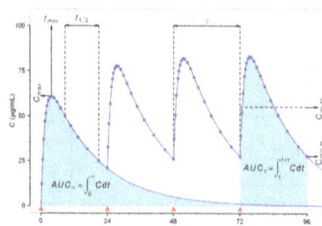

The time course of drug plasma concentrations over 96 hours following oral administrations every 24 hours. Note that the AUC in steady state equals AUC_∞ after the first dose.

Pharmacokinetic Models

Pharmacokinetic modelling is performed by noncompartmental or compartmental methods. Noncompartmental methods estimate the exposure to a drug by estimating the area under the curve of a concentration-time graph. Compartmental methods estimate the concentration-time graph using kinetic models. Noncompartmental methods are often more versatile in that they do not assume any specific compartmental model and produce accurate results also acceptable for bioequivalence studies. The final outcome of the transformations that a drug undergoes in an organism and the rules that determine this fate depend on a number of interrelated factors. A number of functional models have been developed in order to simplify the study of pharmacokinetics. These models are based on a consideration of an organism as a number of related compartments. The simplest idea is to think of an organism as only one homogenous compartment. This *monocompartimental model* presupposes that blood plasma concentrations of the drug are a true reflection of the drug's concentration in other fluids or tissues and that the elimination of the drug is directly proportional to the drug's concentration in the organism (first order kinetics).

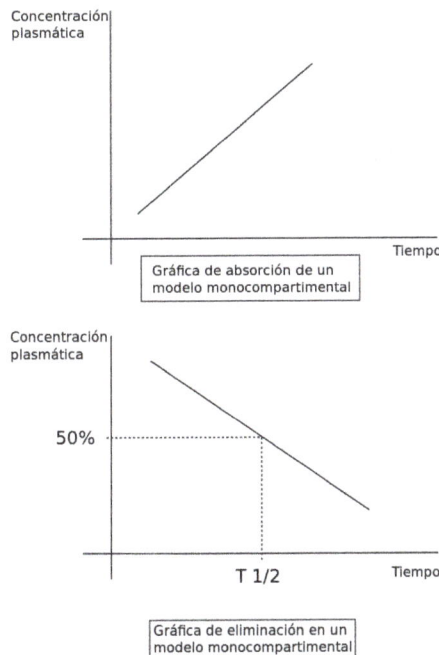

Graph representing the monocompartmental action model.

However, these models do not always truly reflect the real situation within an organism. For example, not all body tissues have the same blood supply, so the distribution of the drug will be slower in these tissues than in others with a better blood supply. In addition, there are some tissues (such as the brain tissue) that present a real barrier to the distribution of drugs, that can be breached with greater or lesser ease depending on the drug's characteristics. If these relative conditions for the different tissue types are considered along with the rate of elimination, the organism can be considered to be acting like two compartments: one that we can call the *central compartment* that has a more rapid distribution, comprising organs and systems with a well-developed blood supply; and a *peripheral compartment* made up of organs with a lower blood flow. Other tissues, such as the brain, can occupy a variable position depending on a drug's ability to cross the barrier that separates the organ from the blood supply.

This *two compartment model* will vary depending on which compartment elimination occurs in. The most common situation is that elimination occurs in the central compartment as the liver and kidneys are organs with a good blood supply. However, in some situations it may be that elimination occurs in the peripheral compartment or even in both. This can mean that there are three possible variations in the two compartment model, which still do not cover all possibilities.

This model may not be applicable in situations where some of the enzymes responsible for metabolizing the drug become saturated, or where an active elimination mechanism is present that is independent of the drug's plasma concentration. In the real world each tissue will have its own distribution characteristics and none of them will be strictly linear. If we label the drug's volume of distribution within the organism Vd_F and its volume of distribution in a tissue Vd_T the former will be described by an equation that takes into account all the tissues that act in different ways, that is:

$$Vd_F = Vd_{T1} + Vd_{T2} + Vd_{T3} + \ldots + Vd_{Tn}$$

This represents the *multi-compartment model* with a number of curves that express complicated equations in order to obtain an overall curve. A number of computer programs have been developed to plot these equations. However complicated and precise this model may be, it still does not truly represent reality despite the effort involved in obtaining various distribution values for a drug. This is because the concept of distribution volume is a relative concept that is not a true reflection of reality. The choice of model therefore comes down to deciding which one offers the lowest margin of error for the drug involved.

Noncompartmental Analysis

Noncompartmental PK analysis is highly dependent on estimation of total drug exposure. Total drug exposure is most often estimated by area under the curve (AUC) methods, with the trapezoidal rule (numerical integration) the most common method. Due to the dependence on the length of 'x' in the trapezoidal rule, the area estimation is highly dependent on the blood/plasma sampling schedule. That is, the closer time points are, the closer the trapezoids reflect the actual shape of the concentration-time curve.

Compartmental Analysis

Compartmental PK analysis uses kinetic models to describe and predict the concentration-time curve. PK compartmental models are often similar to kinetic models used in other scientific disciplines such as chemical kinetics and thermodynamics. The advantage of compartmental over some noncompartmental analyses is the ability to predict the concentration at any time. The disadvantage is the difficulty in developing and validating the proper model. Compartment-free modelling based on curve stripping does not suffer this limitation. The simplest PK compartmental model is the one-compartmental PK model with IV bolus administration and first-order elimination. The most complex PK models (called PBPK models) rely on the use of physiological information to ease development and validation.

Single-compartment Model

Linear pharmacokinetics is so-called because the graph of the relationship between the various factors involved (dose, blood plasma concentrations, elimination, etc.) gives a straight line or an approximation to one. For drugs to be effective they need to be able to move rapidly from blood plasma to other body fluids and tissues.

The change in concentration over time can be expressed as $C = C_{initial} * e^{-kelt}$

Multi-compartmental Models

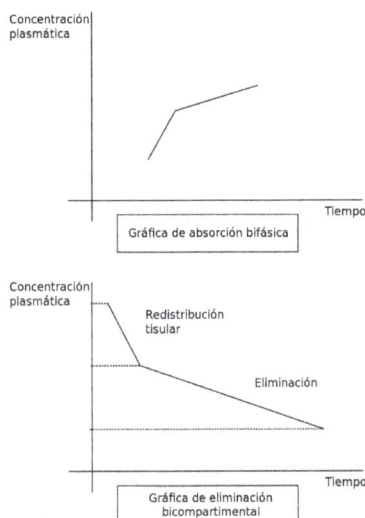

Graphs for absorption and elimination for a non-linear pharmacokinetic model.

The graph for the non-linear relationship between the various factors is represented by a curve, the relationships between the factors can then be found by calculating the dimensions of different areas under the curve. The models used in '*non linear pharmacokinetics*' are largely based on Michaelis-Menten kinetics. A reaction's factors of non linearity include the following:

- Multiphasic absorption : Drugs injected intravenously are removed from the plasma through two primary mechanisms: (1) Distribution to body tissues and (2) metabolism + excretion of the drugs. The resulting decrease of the drug's plasma concentration follows a biphasic pattern (see figure).

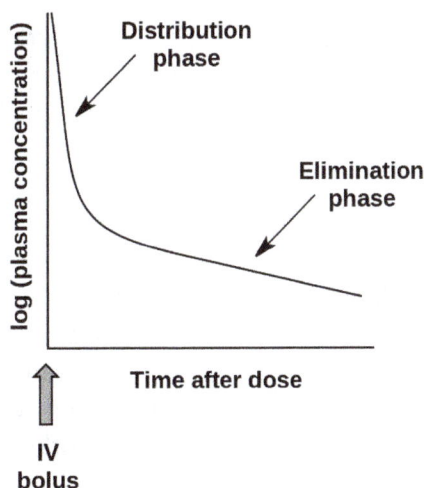

Plasma drug concentration vs time after an IV dose

o Alpha phase: An initial phase of rapid decrease in plasma concentration. The decrease is primarily attributed to drug distribution from the central compartment (circulation) into the peripheral compartments (body tissues). This phase ends when a pseudo-equilibrium of drug concentration is established between the central and peripheral compartments.

o Beta phase: A phase of gradual decrease in plasma concentration after the alpha phase. The decrease is primarily attributed to drug metabolism and excretion.

o Additional phases (gamma, delta, etc.) are sometimes seen.

- A drug's characteristics make a clear distinction between tissues with high and low blood flow.

- Enzymatic saturation: When the dose of a drug whose elimination depends on biotransformation is increased above a certain threshold the enzymes responsible for its metabolism become saturated. The drug's plasma concentration will then increase disproportionately and its elimination will no longer be constant.

- Induction or enzymatic inhibition: Some drugs have the capacity to inhibit or stimulate their own metabolism, in negative or positive feedback reactions. As occurs with fluvoxamine, fluoxetine and phenytoin. As larger doses of these pharmaceuticals are administered the plasma concentrations of the unmetabolized drug increases and the elimination half-life increases. It is therefore necessary to adjust the dose or other treatment parameters when a high dosage is required.

- The kidneys can also establish active elimination mechanisms for some drugs, independent of plasma concentrations.

It can therefore be seen that non-linearity can occur because of reasons that affect the entire pharmacokinetic sequence: absorption, distribution, metabolism and elimination.

Variable Volume in Time Models

Variable volume pharmacokinetic models can be a drug centered models that assign a volume of drug distribution to be where the drug is at that time. Another possibility occurs when the body volume is changing in time, which would occur, for example, during dialysis when the volume in which a drug can be distributed is itself changing in time.

Bioavailability

At a practical level, a drug's bioavailability can be defined as the proportion of the drug that reaches its site of action. From this perspective the intravenous administration of a drug provides the greatest possible bioavailability, and this method is considered to yield a bioavailability of 1 (or 100%). Bioavailability of other delivery methods is compared with that of intravenous injection («absolute bioavailability») or to a standard value related to other delivery methods in a particular study («relative bioavailability»).

$$B_A = \frac{[ABC]_P . D_{IV}}{[ABC]_{IV} . D_P}$$

$$B_R = \frac{[ABC]_A . dose_B}{[ABC]_B . dose_A}$$

Once a drug's bioavailability has been established it is possible to calculate the changes that need to be made to its dosage in order to reach the required blood plasma levels. Bioavailability is therefore a mathematical factor for each individual drug that influences the administered dose. It is possible to calculate the amount of a drug in the blood plasma that has a real potential to bring about its effect using the formula: $De = B.Da$; where De is the effective dose, B bioavailability and Da the administered dose.

Therefore, if a drug has a bioavailability of 0.8 (or 80%) and it is administered in a dose of 100 mg, the equation will demonstrate the following:

De = 0.8 x 100 mg = 80 mg

That is the 100 mg administered represents a blood plasma concentration of 80 mg that has the capacity to have a pharmaceutical effect.

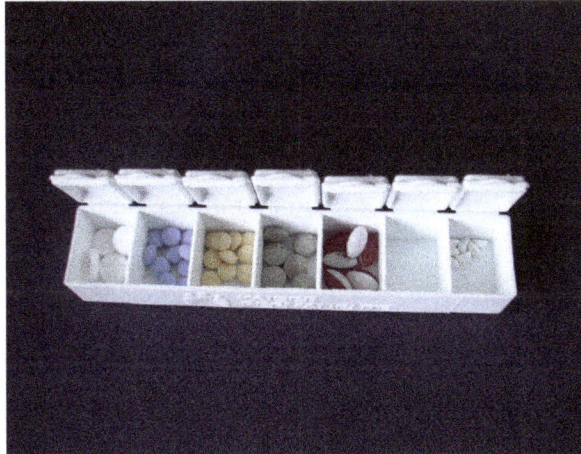

Different forms of tablets, which will have different pharmacokinetic behaviours after their administration.

This concept depends on a series of factors inherent to each drug, such as:

- Pharmaceutical form

- Chemical form

- Route of administration

- Stability

- Metabolism

These concepts, which are discussed in detail in their respective titled articles, can be mathematically quantified and integrated to obtain an overall mathematical equation:

$$De = Q.Da.B$$

where Q is the drug's purity.

$$Va = \frac{Da.B.Q}{\tau}$$

where Va is the drug's rate of administration and τ is the rate at which the absorbed drug reaches the circulatory system.

Finally, using the Henderson-Hasselbalch equation, and knowing the drug's pKa (pH at which there is an equilibrium between its ionized and non ionized molecules), it is possible to calculate the non ionized concentration of the drug and therefore the concentration that will be subject to absorption:

$$pH = pKa + log\frac{B}{A}$$

When two drugs have the same bioavailability, they are said to be biological equivalents or bioequivalents. This concept of bioequivalence is important because it is currently used as a yardstick in the authorization of generic drugs in many countries .

LADME

A number of phases occur once the drug enters into contact with the organism, these are described using the acronym LADME:

- Liberation of the active substance from the delivery system,

- Absorption of the active substance by the organism,

- Distribution through the blood plasma and different body tissues,

- Metabolism that is, inactivation of the xenobiotic substance, and finally

- Excretion or elimination of the substance or the products of its metabolism.

Some textbooks combine the first two phases as the drug is often administered in an active form, which means that there is no liberation phase. Others include a phase that combines distribution, metabolism and excretion into a «disposition phase». Other authors include the drug's toxicological aspect in what is known as *ADME-Tox* or *ADMET*.

Each of the phases is subject to physico-chemical interactions between a drug and an organism, which can be expressed mathematically. Pharmacokinetics is therefore based on mathematical equations that allow the prediction of a drug's behavior and which place great emphasis on the relationships between drug plasma concentrations and the time elapsed since the drug's administration.

Analysis

Bioanalytical Methods

Bioanalytical methods are necessary to construct a concentration-time profile. Chemical techniques are employed to measure the concentration of drugs in biological matrix, most often plasma. Proper bioanalytical methods should be selective and sensitive. For example, microscale thermophoresis can be used to quantify how the biological matrix/liquid affects the affinity of a drug to its target.

Mass Spectrometry

Pharmacokinetics is often studied using mass spectrometry because of the complex nature of the matrix (often plasma or urine) and the need for high sensitivity to observe concentrations after a low dose and a long time period. The most common instrumentation used in this application is LC-MS with a triple quadrupole mass spectrometer. Tandem mass spectrometry is usually employed for added specificity. Standard curves and internal standards are used for quantitation of usually a single pharmaceutical in the samples. The samples represent different time points as a pharmaceutical is administered and then metabolized or cleared from the body. Blank samples taken before administration are important in determining background and ensuring data integrity with such complex sample matrices. Much attention is paid to the linearity of the standard curve; however it is common to use curve fitting with more complex functions such as quadratics since the response of most mass spectrometers is less than linear across large concentration ranges.

There is currently considerable interest in the use of very high sensitivity mass spectrometry for microdosing studies, which are seen as a promising alternative to animal experimentation.

Population Pharmacokinetics

Population pharmacokinetics is the study of the sources and correlates of variability in drug concentrations among individuals who are the target patient population receiving clinically relevant doses of a drug of interest. Certain patient demographic, pathophysiological, and therapeutical features, such as body weight, excretory and metabolic functions, and the presence of other therapies, can regularly alter dose-concentration relationships. For example, steady-state concentrations of drugs eliminated mostly by the kidney are usually greater in patients suffering from renal failure than they are in patients with normal renal function receiving the same drug dosage. Population pharmacokinetics seeks to identify the measurable pathophysiologic factors that cause changes in the dose-concentration relationship and the extent of these changes so that, if such changes are associated with clinically significant shifts in the therapeutic index, dosage can be appropriately modified. An advantage of population pharmacokinetic modelling is its ability to analyse sparse data sets (sometimes only one concentration measurement per patient is available).

Software packages used in population pharmacokinetics modelling include NONMEM, which was developed at the UCSF and newer packages which incorporate GUIs like Monolix as well as graphical model building tools; Phoenix NLME.

Clinical Pharmacokinetics

Clinical pharmacokinetics (arising from the clinical use of population pharmacokinetics) is the direct application to a therapeutic situation of knowledge regarding a drug's pharmacokinetics and the characteristics of a population that a patient belongs to (or can be ascribed to).

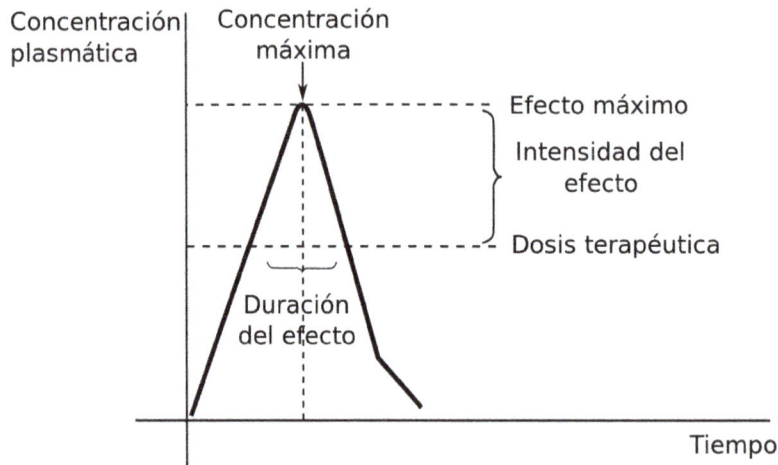

Basic graph for evaluating the therapeutic implications of pharmacokinetics.

An example is the relaunch of the use of ciclosporin as an immunosuppressor to facilitate organ transplant. The drug's therapeutic properties were initially demonstrated, but it was almost never used after it was found to cause nephrotoxicity in a number of patients. However, it was then realized that it was possible to individualize a patient's dose of ciclosporin by analysing the patients plasmatic concentrations (pharmacokinetic monitoring). This practice has allowed this drug to be used again and has facilitated a great number of organ transplants.

Clinical monitoring is usually carried out by determination of plasma concentrations as this data is usually the easiest to obtain and the most reliable. The main reasons for determining a drug's plasma concentration include:

- Narrow therapeutic range (difference between toxic and therapeutic concentrations)

- High toxicity

- High risk to life.

Drugs where pharmacokinetic monitoring is recommended include:

Medication for which monitoring is recommended.			
• Antiepileptic medication + Phenytoin + Carbamazepine + Valproic acid + Lamotrigine + Ethosuximide + Phenobarbital + Primidone	• Cardioactive medication + Digoxin + Lidocaine	• Immunosuppressor medication + Ciclosporin + Tacrolimus + Sirolimus + Everolimus + Mycophenolate	• Antibiotic medication + Gentamicin + Tobramycin + Amikacin + Vancomycin

Bronchodilator medication + Theophylline	• Cytostatic medication + Methotrexate + 5-Fluorouracil + Irinotecan	* Antiviral (HIV) medication + Efavirenz + Tenofovir + Ritonavir	• Coagulation factors + Factor VIII, + Factor IX, + Factor VIIa, + Factor XI

Ecotoxicology

Ecotoxicology is the branch of science that deals with the nature, effects, and interactions of substances that are harmful to the environment.

Liberation (Pharmacology)

Liberation is the first step in the process by which medication enters the body and liberates the active ingredient that has been administered. The pharmaceutical drug must separate from the vehicle or the excipient that it was mixed with during manufacture. Some authors split the process of liberation into three steps: disintegration, disaggregation and dissolution. A limiting factor in the adsorption of pharmaceutical drugs is the degree to which they are ionized, as cell membranes are relatively impermeable to ionized molecules. Many health professionals advise patients to chew the tablets or pills they take in order to facilitate the liberation process, particularly disaggregation.

The characteristics of a medication's excipient play a fundamental role in creating a suitable environment for the correct absorption of a drug. This can mean that the same dose of a drug in different forms can have different bioequivalence, as they yield different plasma concentrations and therefore have different therapeutic effects.

Dissolution

In a typical situation a pill taken orally will pass through the oesophagus and into the stomach. As the stomach has an aqueous environment it is the first place where the pill can dissolve. The rate of dissolution is a key element in controlling the duration of a drug's effect. For this reason, different forms of the same medication can have the same active ingredients but different dissolution rates. If a drug is administered in a form that is not rapidly dissolved the drug will be adsorbed more gradually over time and its action will have a longer duration. A consequence of this is that patients will comply more closely to a prescribed course of treatment, as the medication does not have to be taken so frequently. In addition, a slow release system will maintain drug concentrations within a therapeutically acceptable range for longer than quicker releasing delivery systems as these result in more pronounced peaks in plasma concentration.

The dissolution rate is described by the Noyes–Whitney equation:

$$\frac{dW}{dt} = \frac{DA(C_s - C)}{L}$$

Where:

- $\dfrac{dW}{dt}$ is the dissolution rate.

- A is the solid's surface area.

- C is the concentration of the solid in the bulk dissolution medium.

- is the concentration of the solid in the diffusion layer surrounding the solid.

- D is the diffusion coefficient.

- L is the thickness of the diffusion layer.

As the solution is already in a dissolved state it does not have to go through a dissolution stage before absorption begins.

Ionization

Cell membranes present a greater barrier to the movement of ionized molecules than non-ionized liposoluble substances. This is particularly important for substances that are weakly amphoteric. The stomach's acidic pH and the subsequent alkalization in the intestine modifies the degree of ionization of acids and weak bases depending on a substance's pKa. The pKa is the pH at which a substance is present at an equilibrium between ionized and non-ionized molecules. The Henderson–Hasselbalch equation is used to calculate pKa.

Absorption (Pharmacokinetics)

In pharmacology (and more specifically pharmacokinetics), absorption is the movement of a drug into the bloodstream.

Absorption involves several phases. First, the drug needs to be introduced via some route of administration (oral, topical-dermal, *etc.*) and in a specific dosage form such as a tablet, capsule, solution and so on.

In other situations, such as intravenous therapy, intramuscular injection, enteral nutrition and others, absorption is even more straightforward and there is less variability in absorption and bioavailability is often near 100%. It is considered that intravascular administration (e.g. IV) does not involve absorption, and there is no loss of drug. The fastest route of absorption is inhalation, and not as mistakenly considered the intravenous administration.

Absorption is a primary focus in drug development and medicinal chemistry, since the drug must be absorbed before any medicinal effects can take place. Moreover, the drug's pharmacokinetic profile can be easily and significantly changed by adjusting factors that affect absorption.

Dissolution

In the most common situation, a tablet is ingested and passes through the esophagus to the stomach.

The rate of dissolution is a key target for controlling the duration of a drug's effect, and as such, several dosage forms that contain the same active ingredient may be available, differing only in the rate of dissolution. If a drug is supplied in a form that is not readily dissolved, the drug may be released more gradually over time with a longer duration of action. Having a longer duration of action may improve compliance since the medication will not have to be taken as often. Additionally, slow-release dosage forms may maintain concentrations within an acceptable therapeutic range over a long period of time, as opposed is quick-release dosage forms which may result in sharper peaks and troughs in serum concentrations.

The rate of dissolution is described by the Noyes–Whitney equation as shown below:

$$\frac{dW}{dt} = \frac{DA(C_s - C)}{L}$$

Where:

- $\frac{dW}{dt}$ is the rate of dissolution.
- A is the surface area of the solid.
- C is the concentration of the solid in the bulk dissolution medium.
- C_s is the concentration of the solid in the diffusion layer surrounding the solid.
- D is the diffusion coefficient.
- L is the diffusion layer thickness.

As can be inferred by the Noyes-Whitney equation, the rate of dissolution may be modified primarily by altering the surface area of the solid. The surface area may be adjusted by altering the particle size (e.g. micronization). For many drugs, reducing the particle size leads to a reduction in the dose that is required to achieve the same therapeutic effect. The reduction of particle size increases the specific surface area and the dissolution rate, and it does not affect solubility.

The rate of dissolution may also be altered by choosing a suitable polymorph of a compound. Different polymorphs exhibit different solubility and dissolution rate characteristics. Specifically, crystalline forms dissolve slower than amorphous forms, since crystalline forms require more energy to leave lattice during dissolution. The most stable crystalline polymorph has the lowest dissolution rate. Dissolution is also different for anhydrous and hydrous forms of a drug. Anhydrous often dissolve faster than hydrated; however, anhydrous forms sometimes exhibit lower solubility.

Chemical modification by esterification is also used to control solubility. For example, stearate and estolate esters of a drug have decreased solubility in gastric fluid. Later, esterases in the GIT wall and blood hydrolze these esters to release the parent drug.

Also, coatings on a tablet or a pellet may act as a barrier to reduce the rate of dissolution. Coating may also be used to modify where dissolution takes place. For example, enteric coatings may be applied to a drug, so that the coating only dissolves in the basic environment of the intestines. This will prevent release of the drug before reaching the intestines.

Since solutions are already dissolved, they do not need to undergo dissolution before being absorbed. Lipid-soluble drugs are less absorbed than water-soluble drugs, especially when they are enteral.

Ionization

The gastrointestinal tract is lined with epithelial cells. Drugs must pass or permeate through these cells in order to be absorbed into the circulatory system. One particular cellular barrier that may prevent absorption of a given drug is the cell membrane. Cell membranes are essentially lipid bilayers which form a semipermeable membrane. Pure lipid bilayers are generally permeable only to small, uncharged solutes. Hence, whether or not a molecule is ionized will affect its absorption, since ionic molecules are charged. Solubility favors charged species, and permeability favors neutral species. Some molecules have special exchange proteins and channels to facilitate movement from the lumen into the circulation.

Ions cannot passively diffuse through the gastrointestinal tract because the epithelial cell membrane is made up of a phospholipid bilayer. The bilayer is made up of two layers of phospholipids in which the charged hydrophilic heads face outwards and the non-charged hydrophobic fatty acid chains are in the middle of the layer. The uncharged fatty acid chains repel ionized, charged molecules. Which mean the ionized molecules cannot pass through the intestinal membrane and be absorbed.

The Henderson-Hasselbalch equation offers a way to determine the proportion of a substance that is ionized at a given pH. In the stomach, drugs that are weak acids (such as aspirin) will be present mainly in their non-ionic form, and weak bases will be in their ionic form. Since non-ionic species diffuse more readily through cell membranes, weak acids will have a higher absorption in the highly acidic stomach.

However, the reverse is true in the basic environment of the intestines-- weak bases (such as caffeine) will diffuse more readily since they will be non-ionic.

This aspect of absorption has been targeted by medicinal chemistry. For example, a suitable analog may be chosen so that the drug is more likely to be in a non-ionic form. Also, prodrugs of a compound may be developed by medicinal chemists-- these chemical variants may be more readily absorbed and then metabolized by the body into the active compound. However, changing the structure of a molecule is less predictable than altering dissolution properties, since changes in chemical structure may affect the pharmacodynamic properties of a drug.

Other Factors

Other facts that affect absorption include, but are not limited to, bioactivity, resonance, the inductive effect, isosterism, bio-isosterism, and consideration.

Distribution (Pharmacology)

Distribution in pharmacology is a branch of pharmacokinetics which describes the reversible transfer of a drug from one location to another within the body.

Once a drug enters into systemic circulation by absorption or direct administration, it must be distributed into interstitial and intracellular fluids. Each organ or tissue can receive different doses of the drug and the drug can remain in the different organs or tissues for a varying amount of time. The distribution of a drug between tissues is dependent on vascular permeability, regional blood flow, cardiac output and perfusion rate of the tissue and the ability of the drug to bind tissue and plasma proteins and its lipid solubility. pH partition plays a major role as well. The drug is easily distributed in highly perfused organs such as the liver, heart and kidney. It is distributed in small quantities through less perfused tissues like muscle, fat and peripheral organs. The drug can be moved from the plasma to the tissue until the equilibrium is established (for unbound drug present in plasma).

The concept of compartmentalization of an organism must be considered when discussing a drug's distribution. This concept is used in pharmacokinetic modelling.

Factors that Affect Distribution

There are many factors that affect a drug's distribution throughout an organism, but Pascuzzo considers that the most important ones are the following: an organism's physical volume, the removal rate and the degree to which a drug binds with plasma proteins and / or tissues.

Physical Volume of an Organism

This concept is related to multi-compartmentalization. Any drugs within an organism will act as a solute and the organism's tissues will act as solvents. The differing specificities of different tissues will give rise to different concentrations of the drug within each group. Therefore, the chemical characteristics of a drug will determine its distribution within an organism. For example, a liposoluble drug will tend to accumulate in body fat and water-soluble drugs will tend to accumulate in extracellular fluids. The volume of distribution (V_D) of a drug is a property that quantifies the extent of its distribution. It can be defined as the theoretical volume that a drug would have to occupy (if it were uniformly distributed), to provide the same concentration as it currently is in blood plasma. It can be determined from the following formula: $Vd = \dfrac{Ab}{Cp}$ Where: Ab is total amount of the drug in the body and Cp is the drug's plasma concentration.

As the value for Ab is equivalent to the dose of the drug that has been administered the formula shows us that there is an inversely proportional relationship between Vd and Cp. That is, that the greater Cp is the lower Vd will be and vice versa. It therefore follows that the factors that increase Cp will decrease Vd. This gives an indication of the importance of knowledge relating to the drug's plasma concentration and the factors that modify it.

If this formula is applied to the concepts relating to bioavailability, we can calculate the amount of drug to administer in order to obtain a required concentration of the drug in the organism ('*loading dose*):

$$Dc = \frac{Vd.Cp}{Da.B}$$

This concept is of clinical interest as it is sometimes necessary to reach a certain concentration of a drug that is known to be optimal in order for it to have the required effects on the organism (as occurs if a patient is to be scanned).

Removal Rate

A drug's removal rate will be determined by the proportion of the drug that is removed from circulation by each organ once the drug has been delivered to the organ by the circulating blood supply. This new concept builds on earlier ideas and it depends on a number of distinct factors:

- The drugs characteristics, including its pKa.

- Redistribution through an organism's tissues: Some drugs are distributed rapidly in some tissues until they reach equilibrium with the plasma concentration. However, other tissues with a slower rate of distribution will continue to absorb the drug from the plasma over a longer period. This will mean that the drug concentration in the first tissue will be greater than the plasma concentration and the drug will move from the tissue back into the plasma. This phenomenon will continue until the drug has reached equilibrium over the whole organism. The most sensitive tissue will therefore experience two different drug concentrations: an initial higher concentration and a later lower concentration as a consequence of tissue redistribution.

- Concentration differential between tissues.

- Exchange surface.

- Presence of natural barriers. These are obstacles to a drug's diffusion similar to those encountered during its absorption. The most interesting are:

  o Capillary bed permeability, which varies between tissues.

  o Blood-brain barrier: this is located between the blood plasma in the cerebral blood vessels and the brain's extracellular space. The presence of this barrier makes it hard for a drug to reach the brain.

  o Placental barrier: this prevents high concentrations of a potentially toxic drug from reaching the foetus.

Plasma Protein Binding

Some drugs have the capacity to bind with certain types of proteins that are carried in blood plasma. This is important as only drugs that are present in the plasma in their free form can be transported to the tissues. Drugs that are bound to plasma proteins therefore act as a reservoir of the drug within the organism and this binding reduces the drug's final concentration in the tissues. The binding between a drug and plasma protein is rarely specific and is usually labile and reversible. The binding generally involves ionic bonds, hydrogen bonds, Van der Waals forces and, less often, covalent bonds. This means that the bond between a drug and a protein can be broken and the drug can be replaced by another substance (or another drug) and that, regardless of this, the protein binding is subject to saturation. An equilibrium also exists between the free drug in the blood plasma and that bound to proteins, meaning that the proportion of the drug bound to plasma proteins will be stable, independent of its total concentration in the plasma.

In vitro studies carried out under optimum conditions have shown that the equilibrium between a drug's plasmatic concentration and its tissue concentration is only significantly altered at binding rates to plasma proteins of greater than 90%. Above these levels the drug is "sequestered", which decreases it presence in tissues by up to 50%. This is important when considering pharmacological interactions: the tissue concentration of a drug with a plasma protein binding rate of less than 90% is not going to significantly increase if that drug is displaced from its union with a protein by another substance. On the other hand, at binding rates of greater than 95% small changes can cause important modifications in a drug's tissue concentration. This will, in turn, increase the risk of the drug having a toxic effect on tissues.

Perhaps the most important plasma proteins are the albumins as they are present in relatively high concentrations and they readily bind to other substances. Other important proteins include the glycoproteins, the lipoproteins and to a lesser degree the globulins.

It is therefore easy to see that clinical conditions that modify the levels of plasma proteins (for example, hypoalbuminemias brought on by renal dysfunction) may affect the effect and toxicity of a drug that has a binding rate with plasma proteins of above 90%.

Redistribution

Highly lipid-soluble drugs given by intravenous or inhalation routes are initially distributed to organs with high blood flow. Later, less vascular but more bulky tissues (such as muscle and fat) take up the drug—plasma concentration falls and the drug is withdrawn from these sites. If the site of action of the drug was in one of the highly perfused organs, redistribution results in termination of the drug action. The greater the lipid solubility of the drug, the faster its redistribution will be. For example, the anaesthetic action of thiopentone is terminated in a few minutes due to redistribution. However, when the same drug is given repeatedly or continuously over long periods, the low-perfusion and high-capacity sites are progressively filled up and the drug becomes longer-acting.

It is reversible process of moving drug of sites of highly perfused to systemic circulation,FMAS

Clearance (Pharmacology)

In pharmacology, the clearance is a pharmacokinetic measurement of the volume of plasma from which a substance is completely removed per unit time; the usual units are mL/min. The quantity reflects the rate of drug elimination divided by plasma concentration.

The total body clearance will be equal to the renal clearance + hepatic clearance + lung clearance. Although for many drugs the clearance is simply considered as the renal excretion ability, that is, the rate at which waste substances are cleared from the blood by the kidney. In these cases clearance is almost synonymous with renal clearance or renal plasma clearance. Each substance has a specific clearance that depends on its filtration characteristics. Clearance is a function of glomerular filtration, secretion from the peritubular capillaries to the nephron, and re-absorption from the nephron back to the peritubular capillaries. Clearance is variable in zero-order kinetics because a constant amount of the drug is eliminated per unit time, but it is constant in first-order kinetics, because the amount of drug eliminated per unit time changes with the concentration of drug in the blood. The concept of clearance was described by Thomas Addis, a graduate of the University of Edinburgh Medical School.

It can refer to the amount of drug removed from the whole body per unit time, or in some cases the inter-compartmental clearances can be discussed referring to redistribution between body compartments such as plasma, muscle, fat.

Definition

When referring to the function of the kidney, clearance is considered to be the *amount of liquid filtered out of the blood that gets processed by the kidneys* or *the amount of blood cleaned per time* because it has the units of a volumetric flow rate [volume / time]. However, it does not refer to a real value; "the kidney does not completely remove a substance from the total renal plasma flow." From a mass transfer perspective and physiologically, volumetric blood flow (to the dialysis machine and/or kidney) is only one of several factors that determine blood concentration and removal of a substance from the body. Other factors include the mass transfer coefficient, dialysate flow and dialysate recirculation flow for hemodialysis, and the glomerular filtration rate and the tubular reabsorption rate, for the kidney. A physiologic interpretation of clearance (at steady-state) is that clearance is *a ratio of the mass generation and blood (or plasma) concentration.*

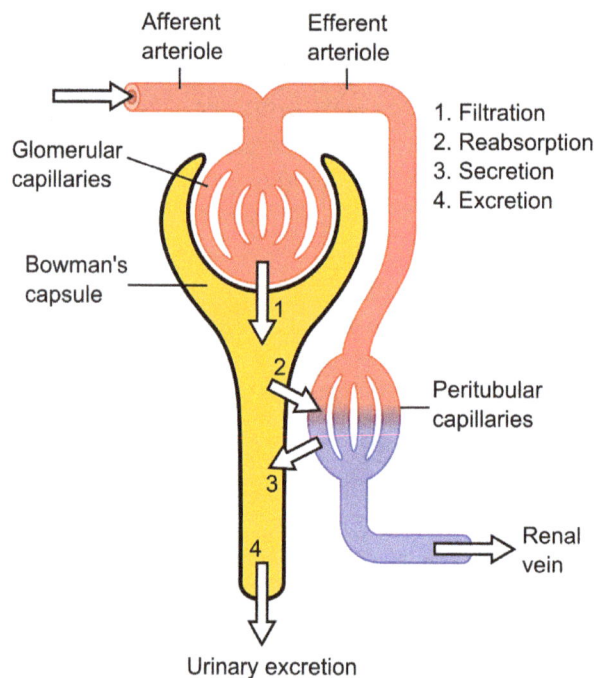

Excretion = Filtration − Reabsorption + Secretion
Diagram showing the basic physiologic mechanisms of the kidney

Its definition follows from the differential equation that describes exponential decay and is used to model kidney function and hemodialysis machine function:

$$V\frac{dC}{dt} = -K \cdot C + \dot{m} \qquad (1)$$

Where:

- $\dot{m}$ is the mass generation rate of the substance - assumed to be a constant, i.e. not a function of time (equal to zero for foreign substances/drugs) [mmol/min] or [mol/s]

- t is dialysis time or time since injection of the substance/drug [min] or [s]

- V is the volume of distribution or total body water [L] or [m³]

- K is the clearance [mL/min] or [m³/s]

- C is the concentration [mmol/L] or [mol/m³] (in the United States often [mg/mL])

From the above definitions it follows that $\dfrac{dC}{dt}$ is the first derivative of concentration with respect to time, i.e. the change in concentration with time.
It is derived from a mass balance.

Clearance of a substance is sometimes expressed as the inverse of the time constant that describes its removal rate from the body divided by its volume of distribution (or total body water).

In steady-state, it is defined as the mass generation rate of a substance (which equals the mass removal rate) divided by its concentration in the blood.

Effect of Plasma Protein Binding

For substances that exhibit substantial plasma protein binding, clearance is generally defined as the total concentration (free + protein-bound) and not the free concentration.

Most plasma substances have primarily their free concentrations regulated, which thus remains the same, so extensive protein binding increases total plasma concentration (free + protein-bound). This decreases clearance compared to what would have been the case if the substance did not bind to protein. However, the mass removal rate is the same, because it depends only on concentration of free substance, and is independent on plasma protein binding, even with the fact that plasma proteins increase in concentration in the distal renal glomerulus as plasma is filtered into Bowman's capsule, because the relative increases in concentrations of substance-protein and non-occupied protein are equal and therefore give no net binding or dissociation of substances from plasma proteins, thus giving a constant plasma concentration of free substance throughout the glomerulus, which also would have been the case without any plasma protein binding.

In other sites than the kidneys, however, where clearance is made by membrane transport proteins rather than filtration, extensive plasma protein binding may increase clearance by keeping concentration of free substance fairly constant throughout the capillary bed, inhibiting a decrease in clearance caused by decreased concentration of free substance through the capillary.

Derivation of Equation

Equation 1 is derived from a mass balance:

$$\Delta m_{body} = (-\dot{m}_{out} + \dot{m}_{in} + \dot{m}_{gen.})\Delta t \qquad (2)$$

where:

- Δt is a period of time
- Δm_{body} the change in mass of the toxin in the body during
- $\dot{m}_{in}$ is the toxin intake rate
- $\dot{m}_{out}$ is the toxin removal rate
- $\dot{m}_{gen.}$ is the toxin generation rate

In words, the above equation states:

The change in the mass of a toxin within the body ($\ddot{A}m$) during some time $\ddot{A}t$ is equal to the toxin intake plus the toxin generation minus the toxin removal.

Since

$$m_{body} = C \cdot V \qquad (3)$$

and

$$\dot{m}_{out} = K \cdot C \qquad (4)$$

Equation A1 can be rewritten as:

$$\Delta(C \cdot V) = (-K \cdot C + \dot{m}_{in} + \dot{m}_{gen.})\Delta t \qquad (5)$$

If one lumps the *in* and *gen.* terms together, i.e. $\dot{m} = \dot{m}_{in} + \dot{m}_{gen.}$ and divides by Δt the result is a difference equation:

$$\frac{\Delta(C \cdot V)}{\Delta t} = -K \cdot C + \dot{m} \qquad (6)$$

If one applies the limit $\Delta t \to 0$ one obtains a differential equation:

$$\frac{d(C \cdot V)}{dt} = -K \cdot C + \dot{m} \qquad (7)$$

Using the Product Rule this can be rewritten as:

$$C\frac{dV}{dt} + V\frac{dC}{dt} = -K \cdot C + \dot{m} \qquad (8)$$

If one assumes that the volume change is not significant, i.e. $C\frac{dV}{dt} = 0$, the result is Equation 1:

$$V\frac{dC}{dt} = -K \cdot C + \dot{m} \qquad (1)$$

Solution to the Differential Equation

The general solution of the above differential equation (*1*) is:

$$C = \frac{\dot{m}}{K} + \left(C_o - \frac{\dot{m}}{K}\right)e^{-\frac{K \cdot t}{V}} \qquad (9)$$

Where:

- C_o is the concentration at the beginning of dialysis *or* the initial concentration of the substance/drug (after it has distributed) [mmol/L] or [mol/m³]

- e is the base of the natural logarithm

Steady-state Solution

The solution to the above differential equation (9) at time infinity (steady state) is:

$$C_\infty = \frac{\dot{m}}{K} \quad (10a)$$

The above equation (*10a*) can be rewritten as:

$$K = \frac{\dot{m}}{C_\infty} \quad (10b)$$

The above equation (*10b*) makes clear the relationship between mass removal and *clearance*. It states that (with a constant mass generation) the concentration and clearance vary inversely with one another. If applied to creatinine (i.e. creatinine clearance), it follows from the equation that if the serum creatinine doubles the clearance halves and that if the serum creatinine quadruples the clearance is quartered.

Measurement of Renal Clearance

Renal clearance can be measured with a timed collection of urine and an analysis of its composition with the aid of the following equation (which follows directly from the derivation of (*10b*)):

$$K = \frac{C_U \cdot Q}{C_B} \quad (11)$$

Where:

- K is the clearance [mL/min]

- C_U is the urine concentration [mmol/L] (in the USA often [mg/mL])

- Q is the urine flow (volume/time) [mL/min] (often [mL/24 h])

- C_B is the plasma concentration [mmol/L] (in the USA often [mg/mL])

When the substance "C" is creatinine, an endogenous chemical that is excreted only by filtration, the calculated clearance is equivalent to the glomerular filtration rate. Inulin clearance is also used to estimate glomerular filtration rate.

Note - the above equation (*11*) is valid *only* for the steady-state condition. If the substance being cleared is *not* at a constant plasma concentration (i.e. *not* at steady-state) K must be obtained from the (full) solution of the differential equation (9).

Bioavailability

In pharmacology, bioavailability (*BA*) is a subcategory of absorption and is the fraction of an administered dose of unchanged drug that reaches the systemic circulation, one of the principal pharmacokinetic properties of drugs. By definition, when a medication is administered intravenously, its bioavailability is 100%. However, when a medication is administered via other routes (such as orally), its bioavailability generally decreases (due to incomplete absorption and first-pass metabolism) or may vary from patient to patient. Bioavailability is one of the essential tools in pharmacokinetics, as bioavailability must be considered when calculating dosages for non-intravenous routes of administration.

For dietary supplements, herbs and other nutrients in which the route of administration is nearly always oral, bioavailability generally designates simply the quantity or fraction of the ingested dose that is absorbed.

Bioavailability is defined slightly differently for drugs as opposed to dietary supplements primarily due to the method of administration and Food and Drug Administration regulations.

Bioaccessibility is a concept related to bioavailability in the context of biodegradation and environmental pollution. A molecule (often a persistent organic pollutant) is said to be bioaccessible when "[it] is available to cross an organism's cellular membrane from the environment, if the organism has access to the chemical."

Definitions

In Pharmacology

In pharmacology, bioavailability is a measurement of the rate and extent to which a drug reaches at the site of action. It is denoted by the letter f (or, if expressed in percent, by F).

In Nutritional Sciences

In nutritional sciences, which covers the intake of nutrients and non-drug dietary ingredients, the concept of bioavailability lacks the well-defined standards associated with the pharmaceutical industry. The pharmacological definition cannot apply to these substances because utilization and absorption is a function of the nutritional status and physiological state of the subject, resulting in even greater differences from individual to individual (inter-individual variation). Therefore, bioavailability for dietary supplements can be defined as the proportion of the administered substance capable of being absorbed and available for use or storage.

In both pharmacology and nutrition sciences, bioavailability is measured by calculating the area under curve (AUC) of the drug concentration time profile.

In Environmental Sciences or Science

Bioavailability is commonly a limiting factor in the production of crops (due to solubility limitation or adsorption of plant nutrients to soil colloids) and in the removal of toxic substances from the food chain by microorganisms (due to sorption to or partitioning of otherwise degradable substances into inaccessible phases in the environment). A noteworthy example for agriculture is plant phosphorus deficiency induced by precipitation with iron and aluminum phosphates at low soil pH and precipitation with calcium phosphates at high soil pH. Toxic materials in soil, such as lead from paint may be rendered unavailable to animals ingesting contaminated soil by supplying phosphorus fertilizers in excess. Organic pollutants such as solvents or pesticides may be rendered unavailable to microorganisms and thus persist in the environment when they are adsorbed to soil minerals or partition into hydrophobic organic matter.

Absolute Bioavailability

Absolute bioavailability compares the bioavailability of the active drug in systemic circulation following non-intravenous administration (i.e., after oral, ocular, rectal, transdermal, subcutaneous, or sublingual administration), with the bioavailability of the same drug following intravenous administration. It is the fraction of the drug absorbed through non-intravenous administration compared with the corresponding intravenous administration of the same drug. The comparison must be dose normalized (e.g., account for different doses or varying weights of the subjects); consequently, the amount absorbed is corrected by dividing the corresponding dose administered.

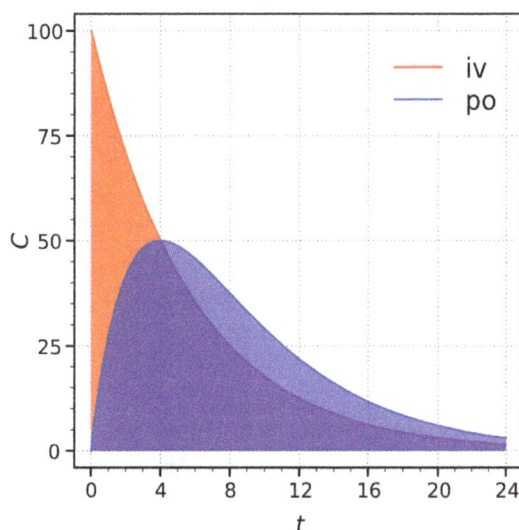

Absolute bioavailability is a ratio of areas under the curves. IV, intravenous; PO, oral route. C is plasma concentration (arbitrary units)

In pharmacology, in order to determine absolute bioavailability of a drug, a pharmacokinetic study must be done to obtain a *plasma drug concentration vs time* plot for the drug after both intravenous (iv) and extravascular (non-intravenous, i.e., oral) administration. The absolute bioavailability is the dose-corrected area under curve (*AUC*) non-intravenous divided by *AUC* intravenous. For example, the formula for calculating *F* for a drug administered by the oral route (po) is given below. (*D* is dose)

$$F_{abs} = 100 \cdot \frac{AUC_{po} \cdot D_{iv}}{AUC_{iv} \cdot D_{po}}$$

Therefore, a drug given by the intravenous route will have an absolute bioavailability of 100% (*f* = 1), whereas drugs given by other routes usually have an absolute bioavailability of less than one. If we compare the two different dosage forms having same active ingredients and compare the two drug bioavailability is called comparative bioavailability.

Although knowing the true extent of systemic absorption (referred to as absolute bioavailability) is clearly useful, in practice it is not determined as frequently as one may think. The reason for this is that its assessment requires an intravenous reference, that is, a route of administration that guarantees that all of the administered drug reaches the systemic circulation. Such studies come at considerable cost, not least of which is the necessity to conduct preclinical toxicity tests to ensure adequate safety, as well as there being potential problems due to solubility limitations. These limitations may be overcome, however, by administering a very low dose (typically a few micrograms) of an isotopically labelled drug concomitantly with a therapeutic non-labelled oral dose. Providing the isotopically-labelled intravenous dose is sufficiently low so as not to perturb the systemic drug concentrations achieved from the absorbed oral dose, then the intravenous and oral pharmacokinetics can be deconvoluted by virtue of their different isotopic constitution and thereby determine the oral and intravenous pharmacokinetics from the same dose administration. This technique eliminates pharmacokinetic issues on non-equivalent clearance as well as enabling the intravenous dose to be administered with a minimum of toxicology and formulation. The technique was first applied using stable-isotopes such as ^{13}C and mass-spectrometry to distinguish the isotopes by mass difference. More recently, ^{14}C labelled drugs are administered intravenously and accelerator mass spectrometry (AMS) used to measure the isotopically labelled drug along with mass spectrometry for the unlabelled drug.

There is no regulatory requirement to define the intravenous pharmacokinetics or absolute bioavailability however regulatory authorities do sometimes ask for absolute bioavailability information of the extravascular route in cases in which the bioavailability is apparently low or variable and there is a proven relationship between the pharmacodynamics and the pharmacokinetics at therapeutic doses. In all such cases, to conduct an absolute bioavailability study requires that the drug be given intravenously.

Intravenous administration of a developmental drug can provide valuable information on the fundamental pharmacokinetic parameters of volume of distribution (V) and clearance (CL).

Relative Bioavailability and Bioequivalence

In pharmacology, relative bioavailability measures the bioavailability (estimated as the AUC) of a formulation (A) of a certain drug when compared with another formulation (B) of the same drug, usually an established standard, or through administration via a different route. When the standard consists of intravenously administered drug, this is known as absolute bioavailability.

$$F_{rel} = 100 \cdot \frac{AUC_A \cdot D_B}{AUC_B \cdot D_A}$$

Relative bioavailability is one of the measures used to assess bioequivalence (*BE*) between two drug products. For FDA approval, a generic manufacturer must demonstrate that the 90% confidence interval for the ratio of the mean responses (usually of AUC and the maximum concentration, C_{max}) of its product to that of the "brand name drug" is within the limits of 80% to 125%.

Where AUC refers to the concentration of the drug in the blood over time $t = 0$ to $t = \infty$, C_{max} refers to the maximum concentration of the drug in the blood. When T_{max} is given, it refers to the time it takes for a drug to reach C_{max}.

While the mechanisms by which a formulation affects bioavailability and bioequivalence have been extensively studied in drugs, formulation factors that influence bioavailability and bioequivalence in nutritional supplements are largely unknown. As a result, in nutritional sciences, relative bioavailability or bioequivalence is the most common measure of bioavailability, comparing the bioavailability of one formulation of the same dietary ingredient to another.

Factors Influencing Bioavailability

The absolute bioavailability of a drug, when administered by an extravascular route, is usually less than one (i.e., $F < 100\%$). Various physiological factors reduce the availability of drugs prior to their entry into the systemic circulation. Whether a drug is taken with or without food will also affect absorption, other drugs taken concurrently may alter absorption and first-pass metabolism, intestinal motility alters the dissolution of the drug and may affect the degree of chemical degradation of the drug by intestinal microflora. Disease states affecting liver metabolism or gastrointestinal function will also have an effect.

Other factors may include, but are not limited to:

- Physical properties of the drug (hydrophobicity, pKa, solubility)

- The drug formulation (immediate release, excipients used, manufacturing methods, modified release – delayed release, extended release, sustained release, etc.)

- Whether the formulation is administered in a fed or fasted state

- Gastric emptying rate

- Circadian differences

- Interactions with other drugs/foods:

    o Interactions with other drugs (e.g., antacids, alcohol, nicotine)

    o Interactions with other foods (e.g., grapefruit juice, pomello, cranberry juice, brassica vegetables)

- Transporters: Substrate of efflux transporters (e.g. P-glycoprotein)

- Health of the gastrointestinal tract

- Enzyme induction/inhibition by other drugs/foods:

    o Enzyme induction (increased rate of metabolism), e.g., Phenytoin induces CYP1A2, CYP2C9, CYP2C19, and CYP3A4

    o Enzyme inhibition (decreased rate of metabolism), e.g., grapefruit juice inhibits CYP3A → higher nifedipine concentrations

- Individual variation in metabolic differences

- o Age: In general, drugs are metabolized more slowly in fetal, neonatal, and geriatric populations

- o Phenotypic differences, enterohepatic circulation, diet, gender

- Disease state

- o E.g., hepatic insufficiency, poor renal function

Each of these factors may vary from patient to patient (inter-individual variation), and indeed in the same patient over time (intra-individual variation). In clinical trials, inter-individual variation is a critical measurement used to assess the bioavailability differences from patient to patient in order to ensure predictable dosing.

Bioavailability of Drugs Versus Dietary Supplements

In comparison to drugs, there are significant differences in dietary supplements that impact the evaluation of their bioavailability. These differences include the following: the fact that nutritional supplements provide benefits that are variable and often qualitative in nature; the measurement of nutrient absorption lacks the precision; nutritional supplements are consumed for prevention and well-being; nutritional supplements do not exhibit characteristic dose-response curves; and dosing intervals of nutritional supplements, therefore, are not critical in contrast to drug therapy.

In addition, the lack of defined methodology and regulations surrounding the consumption of dietary supplements hinders the application of bioavailability measures in comparison to drugs. In clinical trials with dietary supplements, bioavailability primarily focuses on statistical descriptions of mean or average AUC differences between treatment groups, while often failing to compare or discuss their standard deviations or inter-individual variation. This failure leaves open the question of whether or not an individual in a group is likely to experience the benefits described by the mean-difference comparisons. Further, even if this issue were discussed, it would be difficult to communicate meaning of these inter-subject variances to consumers and/or their physicians.

Nutritional Science: Reliable and Universal Bioavailability

One way to resolve this problem is to define "reliable bioavailability" as positive bioavailability results (an absorption meeting a predefined criterion) that include 84% of the trial subjects and "universal bioavailability" as those that include 98% of the trial subjects. This reliable-universal framework would improve communications with physicians and consumers such that, if it were included on products labels for example, make educated choices as to the benefits of a formulation for them directly. In addition, the reliable-universal framework is similar to the construction of confidence intervals, which statisticians have long offered as one potential solution for dealing with small samples, violations of statistical assumptions or large standard deviations.

Biological Half-life

The biological half-life or terminal half-life of a substance is the time it takes for a substance (for example a metabolite, drug, signalling molecule, radioactive nuclide, or other substance) to lose half of its pharmacologic, physiologic, or radiologic activity, according to the Medical Subject Headings (MeSH) definition. Typically, this refers to the body's cleansing through the function of kidneys and liver in addition to excretion functions to eliminate a substance from the body. In a medical context, half-life may also describe the time it takes for the blood plasma concentration of a substance to halve (*plasma half-life*) its steady-state. The relationship between the biological and plasma half-lives of a substance can be complex depending on the substance in question, due to factors including accumulation in tissues (protein binding), active metabolites, and receptor interactions.

Biological half-life is an important pharmacokinetic parameter and is usually denoted by the abbreviation $t_{\frac{1}{2}}$.

While a radioactive isotope decays perfectly according to first order kinetics where the rate constant is fixed, the elimination of a substance from a living organism follows more complex chemical kinetics.

Examples

Water

The biological half-life of water in a human is about 7 to 14 days. It can be altered by behavior. Drinking large amounts of alcohol will reduce the biological half-life of water in the body. This has been used to decontaminate humans who are internally contaminated with tritiated water (tritium). The basis of this decontamination method (used at Harwell) is to increase the rate at which the water in the body is replaced with new water.

Alcohol

The removal of ethanol (drinking alcohol) through oxidation by alcohol dehydrogenase in the liver from the human body is limited. Hence the removal of a large concentration of alcohol from blood may follow zero-order kinetics. Also the rate-limiting steps for one substance may be in common with other substances. For instance, the blood alcohol concentration can be used to modify the biochemistry of methanol and ethylene glycol. In this way the oxidation of methanol to the toxic formaldehyde and formic acid in the human body can be prevented by giving an appropriate amount of ethanol to a person who has ingested methanol. Note that methanol is very toxic and causes blindness and death. A person who has ingested ethylene glycol can be treated in the same way. Half life is also relative to the subjective metabolic rate of the individual in question.

Common Prescription Medications

Substance	Biological half-life
Adenosine	<10 seconds
Norepinephrine	2 minutes
Oxaliplatin	14 minutes
Salbutamol	1.6 hours
Zaleplon	1–2 hours
Morphine	2–3 hours

Methotrexate	3–10 hours (lower doses), 8–15 hours (higher doses)
Phenytoin	12–42 hours
Methadone	15 hours to 3 days, in rare cases up to 8 days
Buprenorphine	16–72 hours
Clonazepam	18–50 hours
Diazepam	20–100 hours (active metabolite, nordazepam 1.5–8.3 days)
Flurazepam	0.8–4.2 days (active metabolite, desflurazepam 1.75–10.4 days)
Donepezil	70 hours (approx.)
Fluoxetine	4–6 days (active lipophilic metabolite 4–16 days)
Dutasteride	5 weeks
Amiodarone	25–110 days
Bedaquiline	5.5 months

Metals

The biological half-life of caesium in humans is between one and four months. This can be shortened by feeding the person prussian blue. The prussian blue in the digestive system acts as a solid ion exchanger which absorbs the caesium while releasing potassium ions.

For some substances, it is important to think of the human or animal body as being made up of several parts, each with their own affinity for the substance, and each part with a different biological half-life (physiologically-based pharmacokinetic modelling). Attempts to remove a substance from the whole organism may have the effect of increasing the burden present in one part of the organism. For instance, if a person who is contaminated with lead is given EDTA in a chelation therapy, then while the rate at which lead is lost from the body will be increased, the lead within the body tends to relocate into the brain where it can do the most harm.

- Polonium in the body has a biological half-life of about 30 to 50 days.

- Caesium in the body has a biological half-life of about one to four months.

- Mercury (as methylmercury) in the body has a half-life of about 65 days.

- Lead in the blood has a half life of 28–36 days.

- Lead in bone has a biological half-life of about ten years.

- Cadmium in bone has a biological half-life of about 30 years.

- Plutonium in bone has a biological half-life of about 100 years.

- Plutonium in the liver has a biological half-life of about 40 years.

Peripheral Half-life

Some substances may have different half-lives in different parts of the body. For example, oxytocin has a half-life of typically about three minutes in the blood when given intravenously. Peripherally administered (e.g. intravenous) peptides like oxytocin cross the blood-brain-barrier very poorly, although very small amounts (< 1%) do appear to enter the central nervous system in humans when given via this route. In contrast to peripheral administration, when administered intranasally via a nasal spray, oxytocin reliably crosses the blood–brain barrier and exhibits psychoactive effects in humans. In addition, also unlike the case of peripheral administration, intranasal oxytocin has a central duration of at least 2.25 hours and as long as 4 hours. In likely relation to this fact, endogenous oxytocin concentrations in the brain have been found to be as much as 1000-fold higher than peripheral levels.

Rate Equations

First-order Elimination

There are circumstances where the half-life varies with the concentration of the drug. Thus the half-life, under these circumstances, is proportional to the initial concentration of the drug A_0 and inversely proportional to the zero-order rate constant k_o where:

$$t_{\frac{1}{2}} = \frac{0.5 A_0}{k_0}$$

This process is usually a logarithmic process - that is, a constant proportion of the agent is eliminated per unit time. Thus the fall in plasma concentration after the administration of a single dose is described by the following equation:

$$C_t = C_0 e^{-kt}$$

- C_t is concentration after time t

- C_o is the initial concentration (t=0)

- k is the elimination rate constant

The relationship between the elimination rate constant and half-life is given by the following equation:

$$k = \frac{\ln 2}{t_{\frac{1}{2}}}$$

Half-life is determined by clearance (CL) and volume of distribution (V_D) and the relationship is described by the following equation:

$$t_{\frac{1}{2}} = \frac{\ln 2 \cdot V_D}{CL}$$

In clinical practice, this means that it takes 4 to 5 times the half-life for a drug's serum concentration to reach steady state after regular dosing is started, stopped, or the dose changed. So, for example, digoxin has a half-life (or $t_{1/2}$) of 24–36 h; this means that a change in the dose will take the best part of a week to take full effect. For this reason, drugs with a long half-life (e.g., amiodarone, elimination $t_{1/2}$ of about 58 days) are usually started with a loading dose to achieve their desired clinical effect more quickly.

Toxicokinetics

Toxicokinetics (often abbreviated as 'TK') is the description of what rate a chemical will enter the body and what happens to it once it is in the body.

Relation to Pharmacokinetics

It is an application of pharmacokinetics to determine the relationship between the systemic exposure of a compound in experimental animals and its toxicity. It is used primarily for establishing relationships between exposures in toxicology experiments in animals and the corresponding exposures in humans. However, it can also be used in environmental risk assessments in order to determine the potential effects of releasing chemicals into the environment. In order to quantify toxic effects toxicokinetics can be combined with toxicodynamics. Such toxicokinetic-toxicodynamic (TKTD) models are used in ecotoxicology.

Similarly, physiological toxicokinetic models are physiological pharmacokinetic models developed to describe and predict the behavior of a toxicant in an animal body; for example, what parts (compartments) of the body a chemical may tend to enter (e.g. fat, liver, spleen, etc.), and whether or not the chemical is expected to be metabolized or excreted and at what rate.

Processes

Four potential processes exist for a chemical interacting with an animal: absorption, distribution, metabolism and excretion (ADME). Absorption describes the entrance of the chemical into the body, and can occur through the air, water, food, or soil. Once a chemical is inside a body, it can be distributed to other areas of the body through diffusion or other biological processes. At this point, the chemical may undergo metabolism and be biotransformed into other chemicals (metabolites). These metabolites can be less or more toxic than the parent compound. After this potential biotransformation occurs, the metabolites may leave the body, be transformed into other compounds, or continue to be stored in the body compartments.

A well designed toxicokinetic study may involve several different strategies and depends on the scientific question to be answered. Controlled acute and repeated toxicokinetic animal studies are useful to identify a chemical's biological persistence, tissue and whole body half-life, and its potential to bioaccumulate. Toxicokinetic profiles can change with increasing exposure duration or dose. Real world environmental exposures generally occur as low level mixtures, such as from air, water, food, or tobacco products. Mixture effects may differ from individual chemical toxicokinetic profiles because of chemical interactions, synergistic, or competitive processes. For other reasons, it is equally important to characterize the toxicokinetics of individual chemicals constituents found in mixtures as information on behavior or fate of the individual chemical can help explain environmental, human, and wildlife biomonitoring studies.

Adverse Drug Reaction

An adverse drug reaction (ADR) is an injury caused by taking a medication. ADRs may occur following a single dose or prolonged administration of a drug or result from the combination of two or more drugs. The meaning of this expression differs from the meaning of "side effect", as this last expression might also imply that the effects can be beneficial. The study of ADRs is the concern of the field known as *pharmacovigilance*. An adverse drug event (ADE) refers to any injury occurring at the time a drug is used, whether or not it is identified as a cause of the injury. An ADR is a special type of ADE in which a causative relationship can be shown.

Classification

ADRs may be classified by e.g. cause and severity.

Cause

- Type A: Augmented pharmacologic effects - dose dependent and predictable

  Type A reactions, which constitute approximately 80% of adverse drug reactions, are usually a consequence of the drug's primary pharmacological effect (e.g. bleeding when using the anticoagulant warfarin) or a low therapeutic index of the drug (e.g. nausea from digoxin), and they are therefore predictable. They are dose-related and usually mild, although they may be serious or even fatal (e.g. intracranial bleeding from warfarin). Such reactions are usually due to inappropriate dosage, especially when drug elimination is impaired. The term 'side effects' is often applied to minor type A reactions.

- Type B: Idiosyncratic

Types A and B were proposed in the 1970s, and the other types were proposed subsequently when the first two proved insufficient to classify ADRs.

Severity

The American Food and Drug Administration defines a serious adverse event as one when the patient outcome is one of the following:

- Death
- Life-threatening
- Hospitalization (initial or prolonged)
- Disability - significant, persistent, or permanent change, impairment, damage or disruption in the patient's body function/structure, physical activities or quality of life.
- Congenital anomaly
- Requires intervention to prevent permanent impairment or damage

Severity is a point on an arbitrary scale of intensity of the adverse event in question. The terms "severe" and "serious" when applied to adverse events are technically very different. They are easily confused but can not be used interchangeably, requiring care in usage.

A headache is severe, if it causes intense pain. There are scales like "visual analog scale" that help clinicians assess the severity. On the other hand, a headache is not usually serious (but may be in case of subarachnoid haemorrhage, subdural bleed, even a migraine may temporally fit criteria), unless it also satisfies the criteria for seriousness listed above.

Location

Adverse effects may be local, i.e. limited to a certain location, or systemic, where a medication has caused adverse effects throughout the systemic circulation.

For instance, some ocular antihypertensives cause systemic effects, although they are administered locally as eye drops, since a fraction escapes to the systemic circulation.

Mechanisms

Adverse drug reaction leading to hepatitis (drug-induced hepatitis) with granulomata. Other causes were excluded with extensive investigations. Liver biopsy. H&E stain.

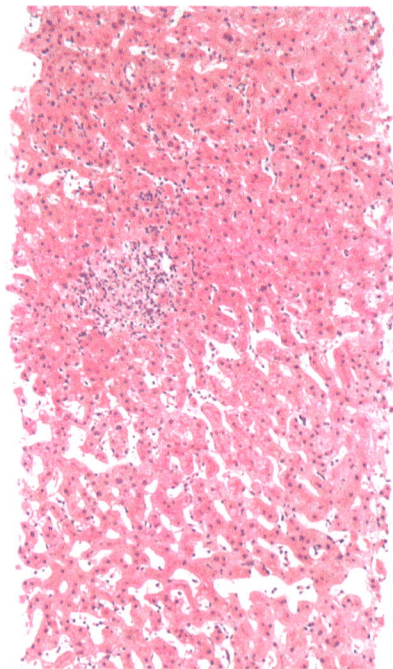

As research better explains the biochemistry of drug use, fewer ADRs are Type B and more are Type A. Common mechanisms are:

- Abnormal pharmacokinetics due to
    - genetic factors
    - comorbid disease states

- Synergistic effects between either

  o   a drug and a disease

  o   two drugs

Abnormal Pharmacokinetics

Comorbid Disease States

Various diseases, especially those that cause renal or hepatic insufficiency, may alter drug metabolism. Resources are available that report changes in a drug's metabolism due to disease states.

Genetic Factors

Abnormal drug metabolism may be due to inherited factors of either Phase I oxidation or Phase II conjugation. Pharmacogenomics is the study of the inherited basis for abnormal drug reactions.

Phase I Reactions

Inheriting abnormal alleles of cytochrome P450 can alter drug metabolism. Tables are available to check for drug interactions due to P450 interactions.

Inheriting abnormal butyrylcholinesterase (pseudocholinesterase) may affect metabolism of drugs such as succinylcholine

Phase II Reactions

Inheriting abnormal N-acetyltransferase which conjugated some drugs to facilitate excretion may affect the metabolism of drugs such as isoniazid, hydralazine, and procainamide.

Inheriting abnormal thiopurine S-methyltransferase may affect the metabolism of the thiopurine drugs mercaptopurine and azathioprine.

Interactions with Other Drugs

The risk of drug interactions is increased with polypharmacy.

Protein Binding

These interactions are usually transient and mild until a new steady state is achieved. These are mainly for drugs without much first-pass liver metabolism. The principal plasma proteins for drug binding are:

1. albumin

2. α1-acid glycoprotein

3. lipoproteins

Some drug interactions with warfarin are due to changes in protein binding.

Cytochrome P450

Patients have abnormal metabolism by cytochrome P450 due to either inheriting abnormal alleles or due to drug interactions. Tables are available to check for drug interactions due to P450 interactions.

Synergistic Effects

An example of synergism is two drugs that both prolong the QT interval.

Assessing Causality

Causality assessment is used to determine the likelihood that a drug caused a suspected ADR. There are a number of different methods used to judge causation, including the Naranjo algorithm, the Venulet algorithm and the WHO causality term assessment criteria. Each have pros and cons associated with their use and most require some level of expert judgement to apply. An ADR should not be labeled as 'certain' unless the ADR abates with a challenge-dechallenge-rechallenge protocol (stopping and starting the agent in question). The chronology of the onset of the suspected ADR is important, as another substance or factor may be implicated as a cause; co-prescribed medications and underlying psychiatric conditions may be factors in the ADR.

Assigning causality to a specific agent often proves difficult, unless the event is found during a clinical study or large databases are used. Both methods have difficulties and can be fraught with error. Even in clinical studies some ADRs may be missed as large numbers of test individuals are required to find that adverse drug reaction. Psychiatric ADRs are often missed as they are grouped together in the questionnaires used to assess the population.

Monitoring Bodies

Many countries have official bodies that monitor drug safety and reactions. On an international level, the WHO runs the Uppsala Monitoring Centre, and the European Union runs the European Medicines Agency (EMEA). In the United States, the Food and Drug Administration (FDA) is responsible for monitoring post-marketing studies. In Canada, the Marketed Health Products Directorate of Health Canada is responsible for the surveillance of marketed health products. In Australia, the Therapeutic Goods Administration (TGA) conducts postmarket monitoring of therapeutic products.

Epidemiology

A study by the Agency for Healthcare Research and Quality (AHRQ) found that in 2011, sedatives and hypnotics were a leading source for adverse drug events seen in the hospital setting. Approximately 2.8% of all ADEs present on admission and 4.4% of ADEs that originated during a hospital stay were caused by a sedative or hypnotic drug. A second study by AHRQ found that in 2011, the most common specifically identified causes of adverse drug events that originated during hospital stays in the U.S. were steroids, antibiotics, opiates and narcotics, and anticoagulants. Patients treated in urban teaching hospitals had higher rates of ADEs involving antibiotics and opiates/narcotics compared to those treated in urban nonteaching hospitals. Those treated in private, not-for-profit hospitals had higher rates of most ADE causes compared to patients treated in public or private, for-profit hospitals.

In the U.S., females had a higher rate of ADEs involving opiates and narcotics than males in 2011, while male patients had a higher rate of anticoagulant ADEs. Nearly 8 in 1,000 adults aged 65 years or older experienced one of the four most common ADEs (steroids, antibiotics, opiates and narcotics, and anticoagulants) during hospitalization. A study showed that 48% of patients had an adverse drug reaction to at least one drug, and pharmacist involvement help to pick up adverse drug reactions.

ADME

ADME is an abbreviation in pharmacokinetics and pharmacology for "absorption, distribution, metabolism, and excretion," and describes the disposition of a pharmaceutical compound within an organism. The four criteria all influence the drug levels and kinetics of drug exposure to the tissues and hence influence the performance and pharmacological activity of the compound as a drug.

Components

Absorption/Administration

For a compound to reach a tissue, it usually must be taken into the bloodstream - often via mucous surfaces like the digestive tract (intestinal absorption) - before being taken up by the target cells. Factors such as poor compound solubility, gastric emptying time, intestinal transit time, chemical instability in the stomach, and inability to permeate the intestinal wall can all reduce the extent to which a drug is absorbed after oral administration. Absorption critically determines the compound's bioavailability. Drugs that absorb poorly when taken orally must be administered in some less desirable way, like intravenously or by inhalation (e.g. zanamivir). Routes of administration is an important consideration

Distribution

The compound needs to be carried to its effector site, most often via the bloodstream. From there, the compound may distribute into muscle and organs, usually to differing extents. After entry into the systemic circulation, either by intravascular injection or by absorption from any of the various extracellular sites, the drug is subjected to numerous distribution processes that tend to lower its plasma concentration.

Distribution is defined as the reversible transfer of a drug between one compartment to another. Some factors affecting drug distribution include regional blood flow rates, molecular size, polarity and binding to serum proteins, forming a complex. Distribution can be a serious problem at some natural barriers like the blood–brain barrier.

Metabolism

Compounds begin to break down as soon as they enter the body. The majority of small-molecule drug metabolism is carried out in the liver by redox enzymes, termed cytochrome P450 enzymes.

As metabolism occurs, the initial (parent) compound is converted to new compounds called metabolites. When metabolites are pharmacologically inert, metabolism deactivates the administered dose of parent drug and this usually reduces the effects on the body. Metabolites may also be pharmacologically active, sometimes more so than the parent drug.

Excretion

Compounds and their metabolites need to be removed from the body via excretion, usually through the kidneys (urine) or in the feces. Unless excretion is complete, accumulation of foreign substances can adversely affect normal metabolism.

There are three main sites where drug excretion occurs. The kidney is the most important site and it is where products are excreted through urine. Biliary excretion or fecal excretion is the process that initiates in the liver and passes through to the gut until the products are finally excreted along with waste products or feces. The last main method of excretion is through the lungs (e.g. anesthetic gases).

Excretion of drugs by the kidney involves 3 main mechanisms:

- Glomerular filtration of unbound drug.

- Active secretion of (free & protein-bound) drug by transporters (e.g. anions such as urate, penicillin, glucuronide, sulfate conjugates) or cations such as choline, histamine.

- Filtrate 100-fold concentrated in tubules for a favorable concentration gradient so that it may be secreted by passive diffusion and passed out through the urine.

Toxicity

Sometimes, the potential or real toxicity of the compound is taken into account (ADME-Tox or ADMET).

Computational chemists try to predict the ADME-Tox qualities of compounds through methods like QSPR or QSAR.

The route of administration critically influences ADME.

Drug Metabolism

Drug metabolism is the metabolic breakdown of drugs by living organisms, usually through specialized enzymatic systems. More generally, xenobiotic metabolism is the set of metabolic pathways that modify the chemical structure of xenobiotics, which are compounds foreign to an organism's normal biochemistry, such any drug or poison. These pathways are a form of biotransformation present in all major groups of organisms, and are considered to be of ancient origin. These reactions often act to detoxify poisonous compounds (although in some cases the intermediates in xenobiotic metabolism can themselves cause toxic effects). The study of drug metabolism is called pharmacokinetics.

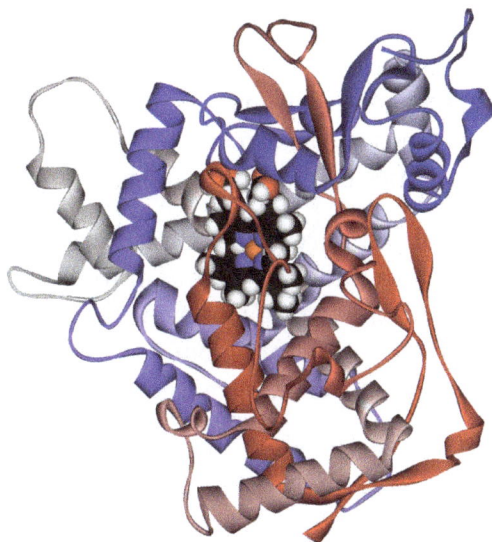

Cytochrome P450 oxidases are important enzymes in xenobiotic metabolism.

The metabolism of pharmaceutical drugs is an important aspect of pharmacology and medicine. For example, the rate of metabolism determines the duration and intensity of a drug's pharmacologic action. Drug metabolism also affects multidrug resistance in infectious diseases and in chemotherapy for cancer, and the actions of some drugs as substrates or inhibitors of enzymes involved in xenobiotic metabolism are a common reason for hazardous drug interactions. These pathways are also important in environmental science, with the xenobiotic metabolism of microorganisms determining whether a pollutant will be broken down during bioremediation, or persist in the environment. The enzymes of xenobiotic metabolism, particularly the glutathione S-transferases are also important in agriculture, since they may produce resistance to pesticides and herbicides.

Drug metabolism is divided into three phases. In phase I, enzymes such as cytochrome P450 oxidases introduce reactive or polar groups into xenobiotics. These modified compounds are then conjugated to polar compounds in phase II reactions. These reactions are catalysed by transferase enzymes such as glutathione S-transferases. Finally, in phase III, the conjugated xenobiotics may be further processed, before being recognised by efflux transporters and pumped out of cells. Drug metabolism often converts lipophilic compounds into hydrophilic products that are more readily excreted.

Permeability Barriers and Detoxification

The exact compounds an organism is exposed to will be largely unpredictable, and may differ widely over time; these are major characteristics of xenobiotic toxic stress. The major challenge faced by xenobiotic detoxification systems is that they must be able to remove the almost-limitless number of xenobiotic compounds from the complex mixture of chemicals involved in normal metabolism. The solution that has evolved to address this problem is an elegant combination of physical barriers and low-specificity enzymatic systems.

All organisms use cell membranes as hydrophobic permeability barriers to control access to their internal environment. Polar compounds cannot diffuse across these cell membranes, and the up-take of useful molecules is mediated through transport proteins that specifically select substrates from the extracellular mixture. This selective uptake means that most hydrophilic molecules can-not enter cells, since they are not recognised by any specific transporters. In contrast, the diffusion of hydrophobic compounds across these barriers cannot be controlled, and organisms, therefore, cannot exclude lipid-soluble xenobiotics using membrane barriers.

However, the existence of a permeability barrier means that organisms were able to evolve detox-ification systems that exploit the hydrophobicity common to membrane-permeable xenobiotics. These systems therefore solve the specificity problem by possessing such broad substrate specific-ities that they metabolise almost any non-polar compound. Useful metabolites are excluded since they are polar, and in general contain one or more charged groups.

The detoxification of the reactive by-products of normal metabolism cannot be achieved by the systems outlined above, because these species are derived from normal cellular constituents and usually share their polar characteristics. However, since these compounds are few in number, spe-cific enzymes can recognize and remove them. Examples of these specific detoxification systems are the glyoxalase system, which removes the reactive aldehyde methylglyoxal, and the various antioxidant systems that eliminate reactive oxygen species.

Phases of Detoxification

The metabolism of xenobiotics is often divided into three phases:- modification, conjugation, and excretion. These reactions act in concert to detoxify xenobiotics and remove them from cells.

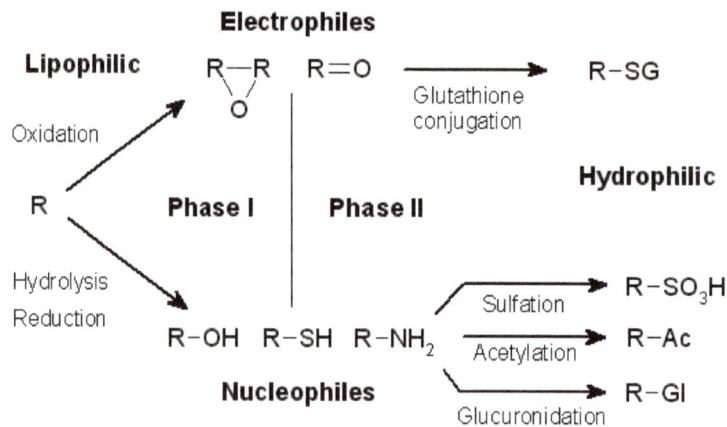

Phases I and II of the metabolism of a lipophilic xenobiotic.

Phase I – Modification

In phase I, a variety of enzymes act to introduce reactive and polar groups into their substrates. One of the most common modifications is hydroxylation catalysed by the cytochrome P-450-de-pendent mixed-function oxidase system. These enzyme complexes act to incorporate an atom of oxygen into nonactivated hydrocarbons, which can result in either the introduction of hydroxyl groups or N-, O- and S-dealkylation of substrates. The reaction mechanism of the P-450 oxidases proceeds through the reduction of cytochrome-bound oxygen and the generation of a highly-reactive oxyferryl species, according to the following scheme:

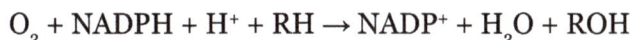

$$O_2 + NADPH + H^+ + RH \rightarrow NADP^+ + H_2O + ROH$$

Phase I reactions (also termed nonsynthetic reactions) may occur by oxidation, reduction, hydrolysis, cyclization, decyclization, and addition of oxygen or removal of hydrogen, carried out by mixed function oxidases, often in the liver. These oxidative reactions typically involve a cytochrome P450 monooxygenase (often abbreviated CYP), NADPH and oxygen. The classes of pharmaceutical drugs that utilize this method for their metabolism include phenothiazines, paracetamol, and steroids. If the metabolites of phase I reactions are sufficiently polar, they may be readily excreted at this point. However, many phase I products are not eliminated rapidly and undergo a subsequent reaction in which an endogenous substrate combines with the newly incorporated functional group to form a highly polar conjugate.

A common Phase I oxidation involves conversion of a C-H bond to a C-OH. This reaction sometimes converts a pharmacologically inactive compound (a prodrug) to a pharmacologically active one. By the same token, Phase I can turn a nontoxic molecule into a poisonous one (toxification). Simple hydrolysis in the stomach is normally an innocuous reaction, however there are exceptions. For example, phase I metabolism converts acetonitrile to $HOCH_2CN$, which rapidly dissociates into formaldehyde and hydrogen cyanide, both of which are toxic.

Phase I metabolism of drug candidates can be simulated in the laboratory using non-enzyme catalysts. This example of a biomimetic reaction tends to give products that often contains the Phase I metabolites. As an example, the major metabolite of the pharmaceutical trimebutine, desmethyltrimebutine (nor-trimebutine), can be efficiently produced by in vitro oxidation of the commercially available drug. Hydroxylation of an N-methyl group leads to expulsion of a molecule of formaldehyde, while oxidation of the O-methyl groups takes place to a lesser extent.

Oxidation

- Cytochrome P450 monooxygenase system
- Flavin-containing monooxygenase system
- Alcohol dehydrogenase and aldehyde dehydrogenase
- Monoamine oxidase
- Co-oxidation by peroxidases

Reduction

- NADPH-cytochrome P450 reductase

Cytochrome P450 reductase, also known as NADPH:ferrihemoprotein oxidoreductase, NADPH:hemoprotein oxidoreductase, NADPH:P450 oxidoreductase, P450 reductase, POR, CPR, CYPOR, is a membrane-bound enzyme required for electron transfer to cytochrome P450 in the microsome of the eukaryotic cell from a FAD- and FMN-containing enzyme NADPH:cytochrome P450 reductase The general scheme of electron flow in the POR/P450 system is:

$$NADPH \rightarrow FAD \rightarrow FMN \rightarrow P450 \rightarrow O_2$$

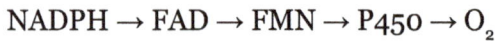

- Reduced (ferrous) cytochrome P450

During reduction reactions, a chemical can enter *futile cycling*, in which it gains a free-radical electron, then promptly loses it to oxygen (to form a superoxide anion).

Hydrolysis

- Esterases and amidase

- Epoxide hydrolase

Phase II – Conjugation

In subsequent phase II reactions, these activated xenobiotic metabolites are conjugated with charged species such as glutathione (GSH), sulfate, glycine, or glucuronic acid. Sites on drugs where conjugation reactions occur include carboxyl (-COOH), hydroxyl (-OH), amino (NH_2), and sulfhydryl (-SH) groups. Products of conjugation reactions have increased molecular weight and tend to be less active than their substrates, unlike Phase I reactions which often produce active metabolites. The addition of large anionic groups (such as GSH) detoxifies reactive electrophiles and produces more polar metabolites that cannot diffuse across membranes, and may, therefore, be actively transported.

These reactions are catalysed by a large group of broad-specificity transferases, which in combination can metabolise almost any hydrophobic compound that contains nucleophilic or electrophilic groups. One of the most important classes of this group is that of the glutathione S-transferases (GSTs).

Mechanism	Involved enzyme	Co-factor	Location
methylation	methyltransferase	S-adenosyl-L-methionine	liver, kidney, lung, CNS
sulphation	sulfotransferases	3'-phosphoadenosine-5'-phosphosulfate	liver, kidney, intestine
acetylation	• N-acetyltransferases • bile acid-CoA:amino acid N-acyltransferases	acetyl coenzyme A	liver, lung, spleen, gastric mucosa, RBCs, lymphocytes
glucuronidation	UDP-glucuronosyltransferases	UDP-glucuronic acid	liver, kidney, intestine, lung, skin, prostate, brain
glutathione conjugation	glutathione S-transferases	glutathione	liver, kidney
glycine conjugation	acetyl Co-enzyme As	glycine	liver, kidney

Phase III – Further Modification and Excretion

After phase II reactions, the xenobiotic conjugates may be further metabolised. A common example is the processing of glutathione conjugates to acetylcysteine (mercapturic acid) conjugates. Here, the γ-glutamate and glycine residues in the glutathione molecule are removed by Gamma-glu-tamyl transpeptidase and dipeptidases. In the final step, the cystine residue in the conjugate is acetylated.

Conjugates and their metabolites can be excreted from cells in phase III of their metabolism, with the anionic groups acting as affinity tags for a variety of membrane transporters of the multidrug resistance protein (MRP) family. These proteins are members of the family of ATP-binding cassette transporters and can catalyse the ATP-dependent transport of a huge variety of hydrophobic anions, and thus act to remove phase II products to the extracellular medium, where they may be further metabolised or excreted.

Endogenous Toxins

The detoxification of endogenous reactive metabolites such as peroxides and reactive aldehydes often cannot be achieved by the system described above. This is the result of these species' being derived from normal cellular constituents and usually sharing their polar characteristics. However, since these compounds are few in number, it is possible for enzymatic systems to utilize specific molecular recognition to recognize and remove them. The similarity of these molecules to useful metabolites therefore means that different detoxification enzymes are usually required for the metabolism of each group of endogenous toxins. Examples of these specific detoxification systems are the glyoxalase system, which acts to dispose of the reactive aldehyde methylglyoxal, and the various antioxidant systems that remove reactive oxygen species.

Sites

Quantitatively, the smooth endoplasmic reticulum of the liver cell is the principal organ of drug metabolism, although every biological tissue has some ability to metabolize drugs. Factors responsible for the liver's contribution to drug metabolism include that it is a large organ, that it is the first organ perfused by chemicals absorbed in the gut, and that there are very high concentrations of most drug-metabolizing enzyme systems relative to other organs. If a drug is taken into the GI tract, where it enters hepatic circulation through the portal vein, it becomes well-metabolized and is said to show the *first pass effect*.

Other sites of drug metabolism include epithelial cells of the gastrointestinal tract, lungs, kidneys, and the skin. These sites are usually responsible for localized toxicity reactions.

Factors that Affect Drug Metabolism

The duration and intensity of pharmacological action of most lipophilic drugs are determined by the rate they are metabolized to inactive products. The Cytochrome P450 monooxygenase system is the most important pathway in this regard. In general, anything that *increases* the rate of metabolism (*e.g.*, enzyme induction) of a pharmacologically active metabolite will *decrease* the duration and intensity of the drug action. The opposite is also true (*e.g.*, enzyme inhibition). However, in cases where an enzyme is responsible for metabolizing a pro-drug into a drug, enzyme induction can speed up this conversion and increase drug levels, potentially causing toxicity.

Various *physiological* and *pathological* factors can also affect drug metabolism. Physiological factors that can influence drug metabolism include age, individual variation (*e.g.*, pharmacogenetics), enterohepatic circulation, nutrition, intestinal flora, or sex differences.

In general, drugs are metabolized more slowly in fetal, neonatal and elderly humans and animals than in adults.

Genetic variation (polymorphism) accounts for some of the variability in the effect of drugs. With N-acetyltransferases (involved in *Phase II* reactions), individual variation creates a group of people who acetylate slowly (*slow acetylators*) and those who acetylate quickly, split roughly 50:50 in the population of Canada. This variation may have dramatic consequences, as the slow acetylators are more prone to dose-dependent toxicity.

Cytochrome P450 monooxygenase system enzymes can also vary across individuals, with deficiencies occurring in 1 – 30% of people, depending on their ethnic background.

Pathological factors can also influence drug metabolism, including liver, kidney, or heart diseases.

In silico modelling and simulation methods allow drug metabolism to be predicted in virtual patient populations prior to performing clinical studies in human subjects. This can be used to identify individuals most at risk from adverse reaction.

History

Studies on how people transform the substances that they ingest began in the mid-nineteenth century, with chemists discovering that organic chemicals such as benzaldehyde could be oxidized and conjugated to amino acids in the human body. During the remainder of the nineteenth century, several other basic detoxification reactions were discovered, such as methylation, acetylation, and sulfonation.

In the early twentieth century, work moved on to the investigation of the enzymes and pathways that were responsible for the production of these metabolites. This field became defined as a separate area of study with the publication by Richard Williams of the book *Detoxication mechanisms* in 1947. This modern biochemical research resulted in the identification of glutathione *S*-transferases in 1961, followed by the discovery of cytochrome P450s in 1962, and the realization of their central role in xenobiotic metabolism in 1963.

Pharmacodynamics

Pharmacodynamics is the study of the biochemical and physiologic effects of drugs (especially pharmaceutical drugs). The effects can include those manifested within animals (including humans), microorganisms, or combinations of organisms (for example, infection). Pharmacodynamics is the study of how a drug affects an organism, whereas pharmacokinetics is the study of how the organism affects the drug. Both together influence dosing, benefit, and adverse effects. Pharmacodynamics is sometimes abbreviated as PD and pharmacokinetics as PK, especially in combined reference (for example, when speaking of PK/PD models).

Pharmacodynamics places particular emphasis on dose–response relationships, that is, the relationships between drug concentration and effect. One dominant example is drug-receptor interactions as modeled by

$$L + R \rightleftharpoons LR$$

where *L*, *R*, and *LR* represent ligand (drug), receptor, and ligand-receptor complex concentrations, respectively. This equation represents a simplified model of reaction dynamics that can be studied mathematically through tools such as free energy maps.

Effects on the Body

The majority of drugs either

(a) mimic or inhibit normal physiological/biochemical processes or inhibit pathological processes in animals or

(b) inhibit vital processes of endo- or ectoparasites and microbial organisms. There are 7 main drug actions:

- stimulating action through direct receptor agonism and downstream effects

- depressing action through direct receptor agonism and downstream effects (ex.: inverse agonist)

- blocking/antagonizing action (as with silent antagonists), the drug binds the receptor but does not activate it

- stabilizing action, the drug seems to act neither as a stimulant or as a depressant (ex.: some drugs possess receptor activity that allows them to stabilize general receptor activation, like buprenorphine in opioid dependent individuals or aripiprazole in schizophrenia, all depending on the dose and the recipient)

- exchanging/replacing substances or accumulating them to form a reserve (ex.: glycogen storage)

- direct beneficial chemical reaction as in free radical scavenging

- direct harmful chemical reaction which might result in damage or destruction of the cells, through induced toxic or lethal damage (cytotoxicity or irritation)

Desired Activity

The desired activity of a drug is mainly due to successful targeting of one of the following:

- Cellular membrane disruption

- Chemical reaction with downstream effects

- Interaction with enzyme proteins

- Interaction with structural proteins

- Interaction with carrier proteins

- Interaction with ion channels

- Ligand binding to receptors:

  o Hormone receptors

  o Neuromodulator receptors

  o Neurotransmitter receptors

General anesthetics were once thought to work by disordering the neural membranes, thereby altering the Na^+ influx. Antacids and chelating agents combine chemically in the body. Enzyme-substrate binding is a way to alter the production or metabolism of key endogenous chemicals, for example aspirin irreversibly inhibits the enzyme prostaglandin synthetase (cyclooxygenase) thereby preventing inflammatory response. Colchicine, a drug for gout, interferes with the function of the structural protein tubulin, while Digitalis, a drug still used in heart failure, inhibits the activity of the carrier molecule, Na-K-ATPase pump. The widest class of drugs act as ligands which bind to receptors which determine cellular effects. Upon drug binding, receptors can elicit their normal action (agonist), blocked action (antagonist), or even action opposite to normal (inverse agonist).

In principle, a pharmacologist would aim for a target plasma concentration of the drug for a desired level of response. In reality, there are many factors affecting this goal. Pharmacokinetic factors determine peak concentrations, and concentrations cannot be maintained with absolute consistency because of metabolic breakdown and excretory clearance. Genetic factors may exist which would alter metabolism or drug action itself, and a patient's immediate status may also affect indicated dosage.

Undesirable Effects

Undesirable effects of a drug include:

- Increased probability of cell mutation (carcinogenic activity)

- A multitude of simultaneous assorted actions which may be deleterious

- Interaction (additive, multiplicative, or metabolic)

- Induced physiological damage, or abnormal chronic conditions

Therapeutic Window

The therapeutic window is the amount of a medication between the amount that gives an effect (effective dose) and the amount that gives more adverse effects than desired effects. For instance, medication with a small pharmaceutical window must be administered with care and control, e.g. by frequently measuring blood concentration of the drug, since it easily loses effects or gives adverse effects.

Duration of Action

The *duration of action* of a drug is the length of time that particular drug is effective. Duration of action is a function of several parameters including plasma half-life, the time to equilibrate between plasma and target compartments, and the off rate of the drug from its biological target.

Receptor binding and effect

The binding of ligands (drug) to receptors is governed by the *law of mass action* which relates the large-scale status to the rate of numerous molecular processes. The rates of formation and un-formation can be used to determine the equilibrium concentration of bound receptors. The *equilibrium dissociation constant* is defined by:

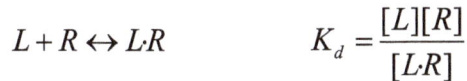

$$L + R \leftrightarrow L\cdot R \qquad\qquad K_d = \frac{[L][R]}{[L\cdot R]}$$

where L=ligand, R=receptor, square brackets [] denote concentration. The fraction of bound receptors is

$$Fraction\ Bound = \frac{[L\cdot R]}{[R]+[L\cdot R]} = \frac{1}{1+\dfrac{K_d}{[L]}}$$

This expression is one way to consider the effect of a drug, in which the response is related to the fraction of bound receptors. The fraction of bound receptors is known as occupancy. The relationship between occupancy and pharmacological response is usually non-linear. This explains the so-called *receptor reserve* phenomenon i.e. the concentration producing 50% occupancy is typically higher than the concentration producing 50% of maximum response. More precisely, receptor reserve refers to a phenomenon whereby stimulation of only a fraction of the whole receptor population apparently elicits the maximal effect achievable in a particular tissue.

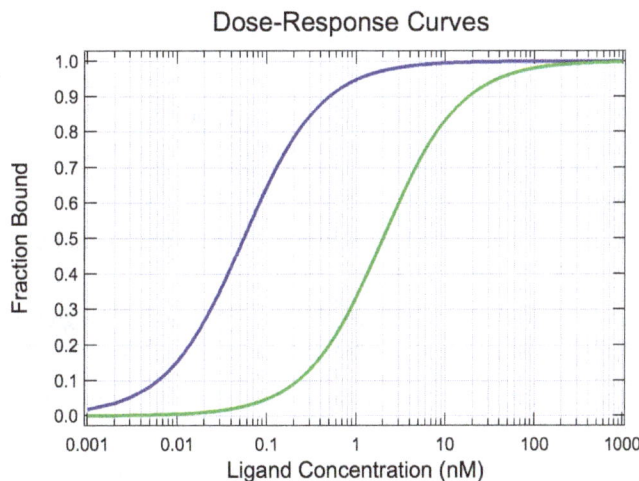

Semi-log plots of two agonists with different K_d. The blue curve represents the ligand with greater potency.

The simplest interpretation of receptor reserve is that it is a model that states there are excess receptors on the cell surface than what is necessary for full effect. Taking a more sophisticated approach, receptor reserve is an integrative measure of the response-inducing capacity of an agonist (in some receptor models it is termed intrinsic efficacy or intrinsic activity) and of the signal amplification capacity of the corresponding receptor (and its downstream signaling pathways). Thus, the existence (and magnitude) of receptor reserve depends on the agonist (efficacy), tissue (signal amplification ability) and measured effect (pathways activated to cause signal amplification). As receptor reserve is very sensitive to agonist's intrinsic efficacy, it is usually defined only for full (high-efficacy) agonists.

Often the response is determined as a function of $log[L]$ to consider many orders of magnitude of concentration. However, there is no biological or physical theory which relates effects to the log of concentration. It is just convenient for graphing purposes. It is useful to note that 50% of the receptors are bound when $[L]=K_d$.

The graph shown represents the conc-response for two hypothetical receptor agonists, plotted in a semi-log fashion. The curve toward the left represents a higher potency (potency arrow does not indicate direction of increase) since lower concentrations are needed for a given response. The effect increases as a function of concentration.

Multicellular Pharmacodynamics

The concept of pharmacodynamics has been expanded to include Multicellular Pharmacodynamics (MCPD). MCPD is the study of the static and dynamic properties and relationships between a set of drugs and a dynamic and diverse multicellular four-dimensional organization. It is the study of the workings of a drug on a minimal multicellular system (mMCS), both *in vivo* and *in silico*. Networked Multicellular Pharmacodynamics (Net-MCPD) further extends the concept of MCPD to model regulatory genomic networks together with signal transduction pathways, as part of a complex of interacting components in the cell.

Toxicodynamics

Pharmacokinetics and pharmacodynamics are termed toxicokinetics and toxicodynamics in the field of ecotoxicology. Here, the focus is on toxic effects on a wide range of organisms. The corresponding models are called toxicokinetic-toxicodynamic models.

References

- Koch HP, Ritschel WA (1986). "Liberation". Synopsis der Biopharmazie und Pharmakokinetik (in German). Landsberg, München: Ecomed. pp. 99–131. ISBN 3-609-64970-4.

- Michael E. Winter, Mary Anne Koda-Kimple, Lloyd Y. Young, Emilio Pol Yanguas Farmacocinética clínica básica Ediciones Díaz de Santos, 1994 pgs. 8-14 ISBN 84-7978-147-5, 9788479781477.

- Joaquín Herrera Carranza Manual de farmacia clínica y Atención Farmacéutica. Published by Elsevier España, 2003; page 159. ISBN 84-8174-658-4

- Simonetta Baroncini, Antonio Villani, Gianpaolo Serafini Anestesia neonatal y pediátrica. Published by Elsevier España, 2006; page 19. ISBN 84-458-1569-5

- Shargel, L.; Yu, A. B. (1999). Applied Biopharmaceutics & Pharmacokinetics (4th ed.). New York: McGraw-Hill. ISBN 0-8385-0278-4.

- Silk, Kenneth R.; Tyrer, Peter J. (2008). Cambridge textbook of effective treatments in psychiatry. Cambridge, UK: Cambridge University Press. p. 295. ISBN 0-521-84228-X.

Enzyme Inhibitor: An Overview

Enzyme inhibitor is a molecule that helps in binding enzymes. They are also used in decreasing the activities of enzymes; decreasing the activities of enzymes helps in correcting metabolic imbalances and is also used in pesticides. The features elucidated are dissociation constant, homeostasis, cytochrome P450, alcohol dehydrogenase and epoxide hydrolase. This section is an overview on enzyme inhibitors.

Enzyme Inhibitor

An enzyme inhibitor is a molecule that binds to an enzyme and decreases its activity. Since blocking an enzyme's activity can kill a pathogen or correct a metabolic imbalance, many drugs are enzyme inhibitors. They are also used in pesticides. Not all molecules that bind to enzymes are inhibitors; *enzyme activators* bind to enzymes and increase their enzymatic activity, while enzyme substrates bind and are converted to products in the normal catalytic cycle of the enzyme.

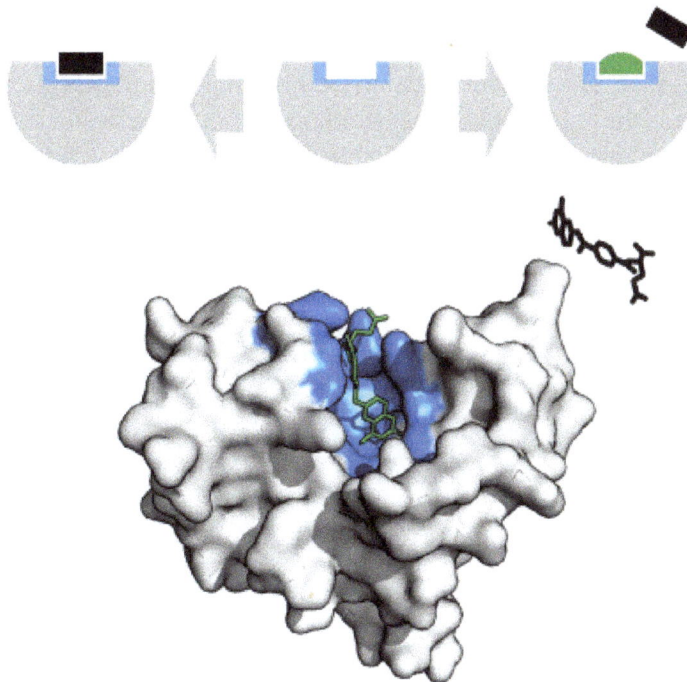

An enzyme binding site that would normally bind substrate can alternatively bind a competitive inhibitor, preventing substrate access. Dihydrofolate reductase is inhibited by methotrexate which prevents binding of its substrate, folic acid. Binding site in blue, inhibitor in green, and substrate in black. (PDB: 4QI9)

The binding of an inhibitor can stop a substrate from entering the enzyme's active site and/or hinder the enzyme from catalyzing its reaction. Inhibitor binding is either reversible or irreversible. Irreversible inhibitors usually react with the enzyme and change it chemically (e.g. via covalent bond formation). These inhibitors modify key amino acid residues needed for enzymatic activity. In contrast, reversible inhibitors bind non-covalently and different types of inhibition are produced depending on whether these inhibitors bind to the enzyme, the enzyme-substrate complex, or both.

Many drug molecules are enzyme inhibitors, so their discovery and improvement is an active area of research in biochemistry and pharmacology. A medicinal enzyme inhibitor is often judged by its specificity (its lack of binding to other proteins) and its potency (its dissociation constant, which indicates the concentration needed to inhibit the enzyme). A high specificity and potency ensure that a drug will have few side effects and thus low toxicity.

Enzyme inhibitors also occur naturally and are involved in the regulation of metabolism. For example, enzymes in a metabolic pathway can be inhibited by downstream products. This type of negative feedback slows the production line when products begin to build up and is an important way to maintain homeostasis in a cell. Other cellular enzyme inhibitors are proteins that specifically bind to and inhibit an enzyme target. This can help control enzymes that may be damaging to a cell, like proteases or nucleases. A well-characterised example of this is the ribonuclease inhibitor, which binds to ribonucleases in one of the tightest known protein–protein interactions. Natural enzyme inhibitors can also be poisons and are used as defences against predators or as ways of killing prey.

Reversible Inhibitors

Types of Reversible Inhibitors

Reversible inhibitors attach to enzymes with non-covalent interactions such as hydrogen bonds, hydrophobic interactions and ionic bonds. Multiple weak bonds between the inhibitor and the active site combine to produce strong and specific binding. In contrast to substrates and irreversible inhibitors, reversible inhibitors generally do not undergo chemical reactions when bound to the enzyme and can be easily removed by dilution or dialysis.

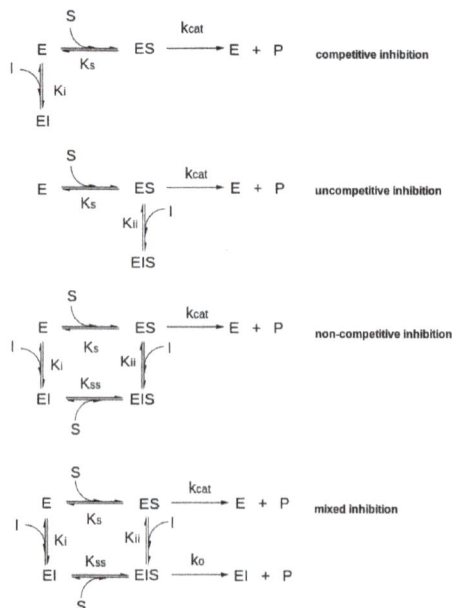

Types of inhibition. This classification was introduced by W.W. Cleland.

There are four kinds of reversible enzyme inhibitors. They are classified according to the effect of varying the concentration of the enzyme's substrate on the inhibitor.

- In competitive inhibition, the substrate and inhibitor cannot bind to the enzyme at the same time, as shown in the figure on the right. This usually results from the inhibitor having an affinity for the active site of an enzyme where the substrate also binds; the substrate and inhibitor *compete* for access to the enzyme's active site. This type of inhibition can be overcome by sufficiently high concentrations of substrate (V_{max} remains constant), i.e., by out-competing the inhibitor. However, the apparent K_m will increase as it takes a higher concentration of the substrate to reach the K_m point, or half the V_{max}. Competitive inhibitors are often similar in structure to the real substrate.

- In uncompetitive inhibition, the inhibitor binds only to the substrate-enzyme complex. This type of inhibition causes V_{max} to decrease (maximum velocity decreases as a result of removing activated complex) and K_m to decrease (due to better binding efficiency as a result of Le Chatelier's principle and the effective elimination of the ES complex thus decreasing the K_m which indicates a higher binding affinity).

- In non-competitive inhibition, the binding of the inhibitor to the enzyme reduces its activity but does not affect the binding of substrate. As a result, the extent of inhibition depends only on the concentration of the inhibitor. V_{max} will decrease due to the inability for the reaction to proceed as efficiently, but K_m will remain the same as the actual binding of the substrate, by definition, will still function properly.

- In mixed inhibition, the inhibitor can bind to the enzyme at the same time as the enzyme's substrate. However, the binding of the inhibitor affects the binding of the substrate, and vice versa. This type of inhibition can be reduced, but not overcome by increasing concentrations of substrate. Although it is possible for mixed-type inhibitors to bind in the active site, this type of inhibition generally results from an allosteric effect where the inhibitor binds to a different site on an enzyme. Inhibitor binding to this allosteric site changes the conformation (i.e., tertiary structure or three-dimensional shape) of the enzyme so that the affinity of the substrate for the active site is reduced.

Quantitative Description of Reversible Inhibition

Reversible inhibition can be described quantitatively in terms of the inhibitor's binding to the enzyme and to the enzyme-substrate complex, and its effects on the kinetic constants of the enzyme. In the classic Michaelis-Menten scheme below, an enzyme (E) binds to its substrate (S) to form the enzyme–substrate complex ES. Upon catalysis, this complex breaks down to release product P and free enzyme. The inhibitor (I) can bind to either E or ES with the dissociation constants K_i or K_i', respectively.

When an enzyme has multiple substrates, inhibitors can show different types of inhibition depending on which substrate is considered. This results from the active site containing two different binding sites within the active site, one for each substrate. For example, an inhibitor might compete with substrate A for the first binding site, but be a non-competitive inhibitor with respect to substrate B in the second binding site.

- Competitive inhibitors can bind to E, but not to ES. Competitive inhibition increases K_m (i.e., the inhibitor interferes with substrate binding), but does not affect V_{max} (the inhibitor does not hamper catalysis in ES because it cannot bind to ES).

- Uncompetitive inhibitors bind to ES. Uncompetitive inhibition decreases both K_m' and 'V_{max}. *The inhibitor affects substrate binding by increasing the enzyme's affinity for the substrate (decreasing K_m) as well as hampering catalysis (decreases V_{max}).*

- Non-competitive inhibitors have identical affinities for E and ES ($K_i = K_i$'). Non-competitive inhibition does not change K_m (i.e., it does not affect substrate binding) but decreases V_{max} (i.e., inhibitor binding hampers catalysis).

- Mixed-type inhibitors bind to both E and ES, but their affinities for these two forms of the enzyme are different ($K_i \neq K_i$'). Thus, mixed-type inhibitors interfere with substrate binding (increase K_m) and hamper catalysis in the ES complex (decrease V_{max}).

Kinetic scheme for reversible enzyme inhibitors

Measuring the Dissociation Constants of a Reversible Inhibitor

As noted above, an enzyme inhibitor is characterised by its two dissociation constants, K_i and K_i', to the enzyme and to the enzyme-substrate complex, respectively. The enzyme-inhibitor constant K_i can be measured directly by various methods; one extremely accurate method is isothermal titration calorimetry, in which the inhibitor is titrated into a solution of enzyme and the heat released or absorbed is measured. However, the other dissociation constant K_i' is difficult to measure directly, since the enzyme-substrate complex is short-lived and undergoing a chemical reaction to form the product. Hence, K_i' is usually measured indirectly, by observing the enzyme activity under various substrate and inhibitor concentrations, and fitting the data to a modified Michaelis–Menten equation

$$V = \frac{V_{max}[S]}{\alpha K_m + \alpha'[S]} = \frac{(1/\alpha')V_{max}[S]}{(\alpha/\alpha')K_m + [S]}$$

where the modifying factors α and α' are defined by the inhibitor concentration and its two dissociation constants

$$\alpha = 1 + \frac{[I]}{K_i}$$

$$\alpha' = 1 + \frac{[I]}{K_i'}.$$

Thus, in the presence of the inhibitor, the enzyme's effective K_m and V_{max} become $(\alpha/\alpha')K_m$ and $(1/\alpha')V_{max}$, respectively. However, the modified Michaelis-Menten equation assumes that binding of the inhibitor to the enzyme has reached equilibrium, which may be a very slow process for inhibitors with sub-nanomolar dissociation constants. In these cases, it is usually more practical to treat the tight-binding inhibitor as an irreversible inhibitor; however, it can still be possible to estimate K_i' kinetically if K_i is measured independently.

The effects of different types of reversible enzyme inhibitors on enzymatic activity can be visualized using graphical representations of the Michaelis–Menten equation, such as Lineweaver–Burk and Eadie-Hofstee plots. For example, in the Lineweaver–Burk plots at the right, the competitive inhibition lines intersect on the y-axis, illustrating that such inhibitors do not affect V_{max}. Similarly, the non-competitive inhibition lines intersect on the x-axis, showing these inhibitors do not affect K_m. However, it can be difficult to estimate K_i and K_i' accurately from such plots, so it is advisable to estimate these constants using more reliable nonlinear regression methods, as described above.

Reversible Inhibitors

Traditionally reversible enzyme inhibitors have been classified as competitive, uncompetitive, or non-competitive, according to their effects on K_m and V_{max}. These different effects result from the inhibitor binding to the enzyme E, to the enzyme–substrate complex ES, or to both, respectively. The division of these classes arises from a problem in their derivation and results in the need to use two different binding constants for one binding event. The binding of an inhibitor and its effect on the enzymatic activity are two distinctly different things, another problem the traditional equations fail to acknowledge. In noncompetitive inhibition the binding of the inhibitor results in 100% inhibition of the enzyme only, and fails to consider the possibility of anything in between. The common form of the inhibitory term also obscures the relationship between the inhibitor binding to the enzyme and its relationship to any other binding term be it the Michaelis–Menten equation or a dose response curve associated with ligand receptor binding. To demonstrate the relationship the following rearrangement can be made:

$$\frac{V_{max}}{1 + \frac{[I]}{K_i}} = \frac{V_{max}}{\frac{[I] + K_i}{K_i}}$$

Adding zero to the bottom ([I]-[I])

$$\frac{\frac{V_{max}}{[I] + K_i}}{[I] + K_i - [I]}$$

Dividing by $[I] + K_i$

$$\frac{V_{max}}{1 - \dfrac{[I]}{[I]+K_i}} = V_{max} - V_{max}\frac{[I]}{[I]+K_i}$$

This notation demonstrates that similar to the Michaelis–Menten equation, where the rate of reaction depends on the percent of the enzyme population interacting with substrate.

fraction of the enzyme population bound by substrate

$$\frac{[S]}{[S]+K_m}$$

fraction of the enzyme population bound by inhibitor

$$\frac{[I]}{[I]+K_i}$$

the effect of the inhibitor is a result of the percent of the enzyme population interacting with inhibitor. The only problem with this equation in its present form is that it assumes absolute inhibition of the enzyme with inhibitor binding, when in fact there can be a wide range of effects anywhere from 100% inhibition of substrate turn over to just >0%. To account for this the equation can be easily modified to allow for different degrees of inhibition by including a delta V_{max} term.

$$V_{max} - \Delta V_{max}\frac{[I]}{[I]+K_i}$$

or

$$V_{max1} - (V_{max1} - V_{max2})\frac{[I]}{[I]+K_i}$$

This term can then define the residual enzymatic activity present when the inhibitor is interacting with individual enzymes in the population. However the inclusion of this term has the added value of allowing for the possibility of activation if the secondary V_{max} term turns out to be higher than the initial term. To account for the possibly of activation as well the notation can then be rewritten replacing the inhibitor "I" with a modifier term denoted here as "X".

$$V_{max1} - (V_{max1} - V_{max2})\frac{[X]}{[X]+K_x}$$

While this terminology results in a simplified way of dealing with kinetic effects relating to the maximum velocity of the Michaelis–Menten equation, it highlights potential problems with the term used to describe effects relating to the K_m. The K_m relating to the affinity of the enzyme for the substrate should in most cases relate to potential changes in the binding site of the enzyme which would directly result from enzyme inhibitor interactions. As such a term similar to the one proposed above to modulate V_{max} should be appropriate in most situations:

$$K_{m1} - (K_{m1} - K_{m2})\frac{[X]}{[X]+K_x}$$

Special Cases

- The mechanism of partially competitive inhibition is similar to that of non-competitive, except that the EIS complex has catalytic activity, which may be lower or even higher (partially competitive activation) than that of the enzyme–substrate (ES) complex. This inhibition typically displays a lower V_{max}, but an unaffected K_m value.

- Uncompetitive inhibition occurs when the inhibitor binds only to the enzyme–substrate complex, not to the free enzyme; the EIS complex is catalytically inactive. This mode of inhibition is rare and causes a decrease in both V_{max} and the K_m value.

- Substrate and product inhibition is where either the substrate or product of an enzyme reaction inhibit the enzyme's activity. This inhibition may follow the competitive, uncompetitive or mixed patterns. In substrate inhibition there is a progressive decrease in activity at high substrate concentrations. This may indicate the existence of two substrate-binding sites in the enzyme. At low substrate, the high-affinity site is occupied and normal kinetics are followed. However, at higher concentrations, the second inhibitory site becomes occupied, inhibiting the enzyme. Product inhibition is often a regulatory feature in metabolism and can be a form of negative feedback.

- Slow-tight inhibition occurs when the initial enzyme–inhibitor complex EI undergoes isomerisation to a second more tightly held complex, EI*, but the overall inhibition process is reversible. This manifests itself as slowly increasing enzyme inhibition. Under these conditions, traditional Michaelis–Menten kinetics give a false value for K_i, which is time–dependent. The true value of K_i can be obtained through more complex analysis of the on (k_{on}) and off (k_{off}) rate constants for inhibitor association.

Examples of Reversible Inhibitors

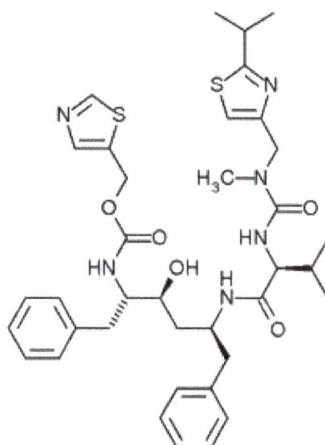

Peptide-based HIV-1 protease inhibitor ritonavir

As enzymes have evolved to bind their substrates tightly, and most reversible inhibitors bind in the active site of enzymes, it is unsurprising that some of these inhibitors are strikingly similar in structure to the substrates of their targets. An example of these substrate mimics are the protease inhibitors, a very successful class of antiretroviral drugs used to treat HIV. The structure of ritonavir, a protease inhibitor based on a peptide and containing three peptide bonds, is shown on the right. As this drug resembles the protein that is the substrate of the HIV protease, it competes with this substrate in the enzyme's active site.

Enzyme inhibitors are often designed to mimic the transition state or intermediate of an enzyme-catalyzed reaction. This ensures that the inhibitor exploits the transition state stabilising effect of the enzyme, resulting in a better binding affinity (lower K_i) than substrate-based designs. An example of such a transition state inhibitor is the antiviral drug oseltamivir; this drug mimics the planar nature of the ring oxonium ion in the reaction of the viral enzyme neuraminidase.

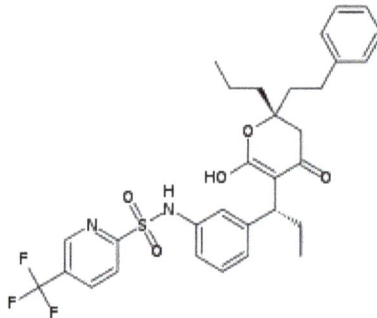

Nonpeptidic HIV-1 protease inhibitor tipranavir

However, not all inhibitors are based on the structures of substrates. For example, the structure of another HIV protease inhibitor tipranavir is shown on the left. This molecule is not based on a peptide and has no obvious structural similarity to a protein substrate. These non-peptide inhibitors can be more stable than inhibitors containing peptide bonds, because they will not be substrates for peptidases and are less likely to be degraded.

In drug design it is important to consider the concentrations of substrates to which the target enzymes are exposed. For example, some protein kinase inhibitors have chemical structures that are similar to adenosine triphosphate, one of the substrates of these enzymes. However, drugs that are simple competitive inhibitors will have to compete with the high concentrations of ATP in the cell. Protein kinases can also be inhibited by competition at the binding sites where the kinases interact with their substrate proteins, and most proteins are present inside cells at concentrations much lower than the concentration of ATP. As a consequence, if two protein kinase inhibitors both bind in the active site with similar affinity, but only one has to compete with ATP, then the competitive inhibitor at the protein-binding site will inhibit the enzyme more effectively.

Irreversible Inhibitors

Types of Irreversible Inhibition

Irreversible inhibitors usually covalently modify an enzyme, and inhibition can therefore not be reversed. Irreversible inhibitors often contain reactive functional groups such as nitrogen mustards, aldehydes, haloalkanes, alkenes, Michael acceptors, phenyl sulfonates, or fluorophosphonates.

These electrophilic groups react with amino acid side chains to form covalent adducts. The residues modified are those with side chains containing nucleophiles such as hydroxyl or sulfhydryl groups; these include the amino acids serine (as in DFP, right), cysteine, threonine, or tyrosine.

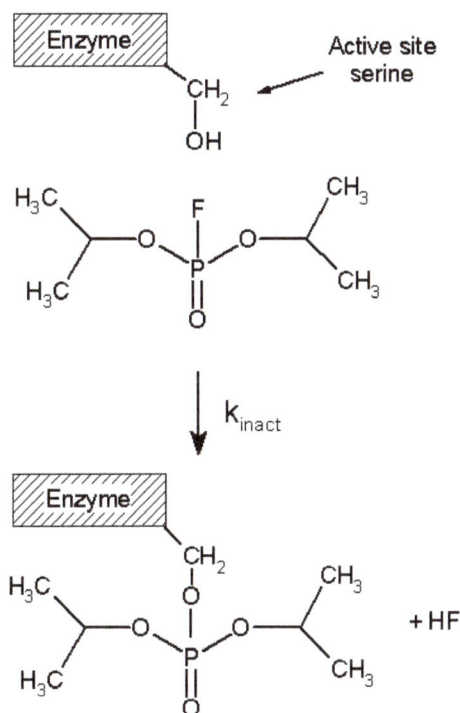

Reaction of the irreversible inhibitor diisopropylfluorophosphate (DFP) with a serine protease

Irreversible inhibition is different from irreversible enzyme inactivation. Irreversible inhibitors are generally specific for one class of enzyme and do not inactivate all proteins; they do not function by destroying protein structure but by specifically altering the active site of their target. For example, extremes of pH or temperature usually cause denaturation of all protein structure, but this is a non-specific effect. Similarly, some non-specific chemical treatments destroy protein structure: for example, heating in concentrated hydrochloric acid will hydrolyse the peptide bonds holding proteins together, releasing free amino acids.

Irreversible inhibitors display time-dependent inhibition and their potency therefore cannot be characterised by an IC_{50} value. This is because the amount of active enzyme at a given concentration of irreversible inhibitor will be different depending on how long the inhibitor is pre-incubated with the enzyme. Instead, $k_{obs}/[I]$ values are used, where k_{obs} is the observed pseudo-first order rate of inactivation (obtained by plotting the log of % activity vs. time) and $[I]$ is the concentration of inhibitor. The $k_{obs}/[I]$ parameter is valid as long as the inhibitor does not saturate binding with the enzyme (in which case $k_{obs} = k_{inact}$).

Analysis of Irreversible Inhibition

Irreversible inhibitors form a reversible non-covalent complex with the enzyme (EI or ESI) and this then reacts to produce the covalently modified "dead-end complex" EI*. The rate at which

EI* is formed is called the inactivation rate or k_{inact}. Since formation of EI may compete with ES, binding of irreversible inhibitors can be prevented by competition either with substrate or with a second, reversible inhibitor. This protection effect is good evidence of a specific reaction of the irreversible inhibitor with the active site.

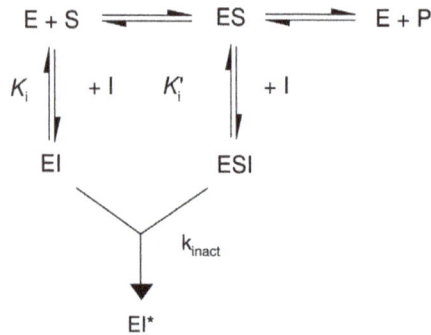

Kinetic scheme for irreversible inhibitors

The binding and inactivation steps of this reaction are investigated by incubating the enzyme with inhibitor and assaying the amount of activity remaining over time. The activity will be decreased in a time-dependent manner, usually following exponential decay. Fitting these data to a rate equation gives the rate of inactivation at this concentration of inhibitor. This is done at several different concentrations of inhibitor. If a reversible EI complex is involved the inactivation rate will be saturable and fitting this curve will give k_{inact} and K_i.

Another method that is widely used in these analyses is mass spectrometry. Here, accurate measurement of the mass of the unmodified native enzyme and the inactivated enzyme gives the increase in mass caused by reaction with the inhibitor and shows the stoichiometry of the reaction. This is usually done using a MALDI-TOF mass spectrometer. In a complementary technique, peptide mass fingerprinting involves digestion of the native and modified protein with a protease such as trypsin. This will produce a set of peptides that can be analysed using a mass spectrometer. The peptide that changes in mass after reaction with the inhibitor will be the one that contains the site of modification.

Special Cases

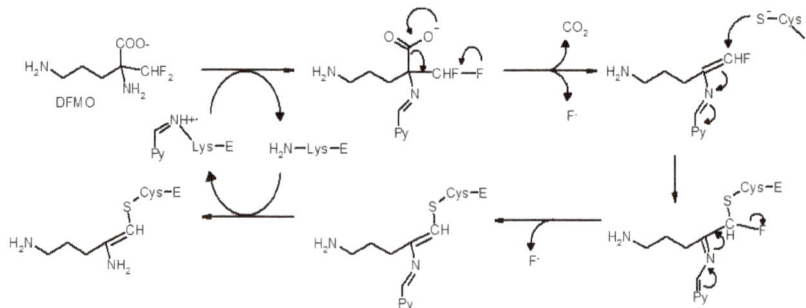

Chemical mechanism for irreversible inhibition of ornithine decarboxylase by DFMO. Pyridoxal 5'-phosphate (Py) and enzyme (E) are not shown. Adapted from

Not all irreversible inhibitors form covalent adducts with their enzyme targets. Some reversible inhibitors bind so tightly to their target enzyme that they are essentially irreversible. These tight-binding inhibitors may show kinetics similar to covalent irreversible inhibitors. In these cases, some of these inhibitors rapidly bind to the enzyme in a low-affinity EI complex and this then undergoes a slower rearrangement to a very tightly bound EI* complex (see figure above). This kinetic behaviour is called slow-binding. This slow rearrangement after binding often involves a conformational change as the enzyme "clamps down" around the inhibitor molecule. Examples of slow-binding inhibitors include some important drugs, such methotrexate, allopurinol, and the activated form of acyclovir.

Examples of Irreversible Inhibitors

Diisopropylfluorophosphate (DFP) is shown as an example of an irreversible protease inhibitor in the figure above right. The enzyme hydrolyses the phosphorus–fluorine bond, but the phosphate residue remains bound to the serine in the active site, deactivating it. Similarly, DFP also reacts with the active site of acetylcholine esterase in the synapses of neurons, and consequently is a potent neurotoxin, with a lethal dose of less than 100 mg.

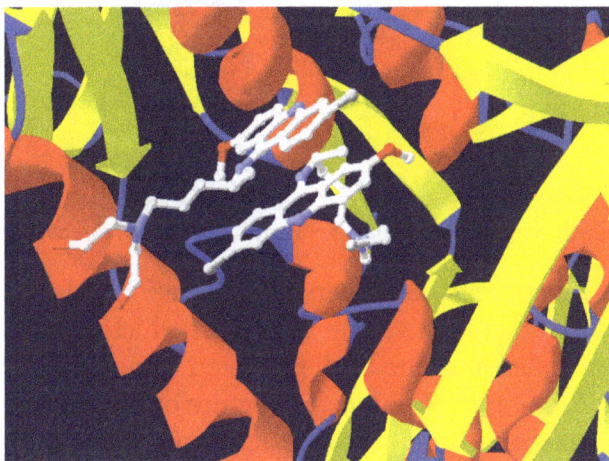

Trypanothione reductase with the lower molecule of an inhibitor bound irreversibly and the upper one reversibly. Created from PDB 1GXF.

Suicide inhibition is an unusual type of irreversible inhibition where the enzyme converts the inhibitor into a reactive form in its active site. An example is the inhibitor of polyamine biosynthesis, α-difluoromethylornithine or DFMO, which is an analogue of the amino acid ornithine, and is used to treat African trypanosomiasis (sleeping sickness). Ornithine decarboxylase can catalyse the decarboxylation of DFMO instead of ornithine, as shown above. However, this decarboxylation reaction is followed by the elimination of a fluorine atom, which converts this catalytic intermediate into a conjugated imine, a highly electrophilic species. This reactive form of DFMO then reacts with either a cysteine or lysine residue in the active site to irreversibly inactivate the enzyme.

Since irreversible inhibition often involves the initial formation of a non-covalent EI complex, it is sometimes possible for an inhibitor to bind to an enzyme in more than one way. For example, in the figure showing trypanothione reductase from the human protozoan parasite *Trypanosoma cruzi*, two molecules of an inhibitor called *quinacrine mustard* are bound in its active site. The top molecule is bound reversibly, but the lower one is bound covalently as it has reacted with an amino acid residue through its nitrogen mustard group.

Discovery and Design of Inhibitors

New drugs are the products of a long drug development process, the first step of which is often the discovery of a new enzyme inhibitor. In the past the only way to discover these new inhibitors was by trial and error: screening huge libraries of compounds against a target enzyme and hoping that some useful leads would emerge. This brute force approach is still successful and has even been extended by combinatorial chemistry approaches that quickly produce large numbers of novel compounds and high-throughput screening technology to rapidly screen these huge chemical libraries for useful inhibitors.

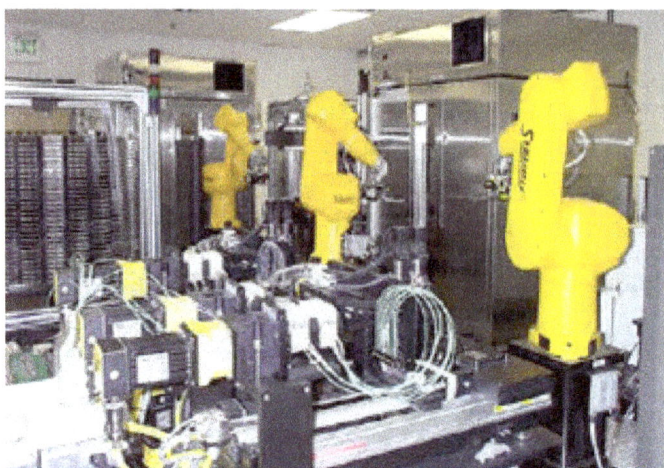

Robots used for the high-throughput screening of chemical libraries to discover new enzyme inhibitors

More recently, an alternative approach has been applied: rational drug design uses the three-dimensional structure of an enzyme's active site to predict which molecules might be inhibitors. These predictions are then tested and one of these tested compounds may be a novel inhibitor. This new inhibitor is then used to try to obtain a structure of the enzyme in an inhibitor/enzyme complex to show how the molecule is binding to the active site, allowing changes to be made to the inhibitor to try to optimise binding. This test and improve cycle is then repeated until a sufficiently potent inhibitor is produced. Computer-based methods of predicting the affinity of an inhibitor for an enzyme are also being developed, such as molecular docking and molecular mechanics.

Uses of Inhibitors

Enzyme inhibitors are found in nature and are also designed and produced as part of pharmacology and biochemistry. Natural poisons are often enzyme inhibitors that have evolved to defend a plant or animal against predators. These natural toxins include some of the most poisonous compounds known. Artificial inhibitors are often used as drugs, but can also be insecticides such as malathion, herbicides such as glyphosate, or disinfectants such as triclosan. Other artificial enzyme inhibitors block acetylcholinesterase, an enzyme which breaks down acetylcholine, and are used as nerve agents in chemical warfare.

Chemotherapy

The most common uses for enzyme inhibitors are as drugs to treat disease. Many of these inhibitors target a human enzyme and aim to correct a pathological condition. However, not all drugs are enzyme inhibitors. Some, such as anti-epileptic drugs, alter enzyme activity by causing more or less of the enzyme to be produced. These effects are called enzyme induction and inhibition and are alterations in gene expression, which is unrelated to the type of enzyme inhibition discussed here. Other drugs interact with cellular targets that are not enzymes, such as ion channels or membrane receptors.

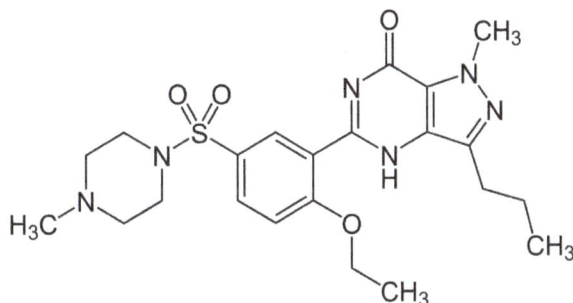

The structure of sildenafil (Viagra)

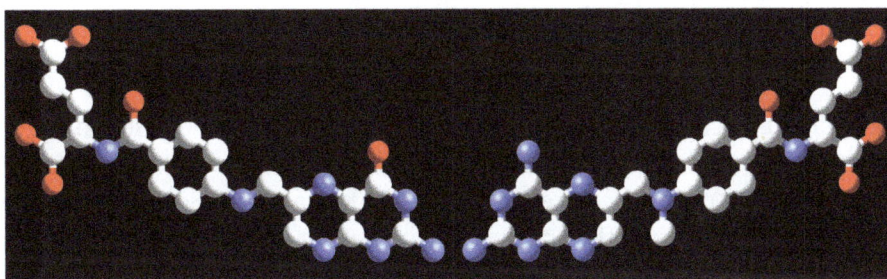

The coenzyme folic acid (left) compared to the anti-cancer drug methotrexate (right)

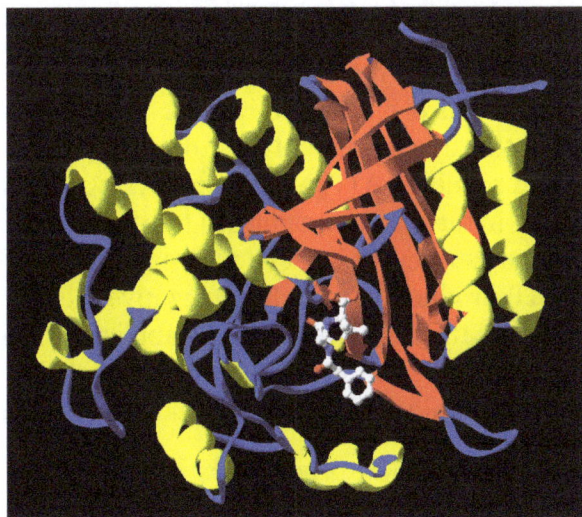

The structure of a complex between penicillin G and the *Streptomyces* transpeptidase. Generated from PDB 1PWC.

An example of a medicinal enzyme inhibitor is sildenafil (Viagra), a common treatment for male erectile dysfunction. This compound is a potent inhibitor of cGMP specific phosphodiesterase type 5, the enzyme that degrades the signalling molecule cyclic guanosine monophosphate. This signalling molecule triggers smooth muscle relaxation and allows blood flow into the corpus cavernosum, which causes an erection. Since the drug decreases the activity of the enzyme that halts the signal, it makes this signal last for a longer period of time.

Another example of the structural similarity of some inhibitors to the substrates of the enzymes they target is seen in the figure comparing the drug methotrexate to folic acid. Folic acid is a substrate of dihydrofolate reductase, an enzyme involved in making nucleotides that is potently inhibited by methotrexate. Methotrexate blocks the action of dihydrofolate reductase and thereby halts the production of nucleotides. This block of nucleotide biosynthesis is more toxic to rapidly growing cells than non-dividing cells, since a rapidly growing cell has to carry out DNA replication, therefore methotrexate is often used in cancer chemotherapy.

Antibiotics

Drugs also are used to inhibit enzymes needed for the survival of pathogens. For example, bacteria are surrounded by a thick cell wall made of a net-like polymer called peptidoglycan. Many antibiotics such as penicillin and vancomycin inhibit the enzymes that produce and then cross-link the strands of this polymer together. This causes the cell wall to lose strength and the bacteria to burst. In the figure, a molecule of penicillin (shown in a ball-and-stick form) is shown bound to its target, the transpeptidase from the bacteria *Streptomyces* R61 (the protein is shown as a ribbon-diagram).

Antibiotic drug design is facilitated when an enzyme that is essential to the pathogen's survival is absent or very different in humans. In the example above, humans do not make peptidoglycan, therefore inhibitors of this process are selectively toxic to bacteria. Selective toxicity is also produced in antibiotics by exploiting differences in the structure of the ribosomes in bacteria, or how they make fatty acids.

Metabolic Control

Enzyme inhibitors are also important in metabolic control. Many metabolic pathways in the cell are inhibited by metabolites that control enzyme activity through allosteric regulation or substrate inhibition. A good example is the allosteric regulation of the glycolytic pathway. This catabolic pathway consumes glucose and produces ATP, NADH and pyruvate. A key step for the regulation of glycolysis is an early reaction in the pathway catalysed by phosphofructokinase-1 (PFK1). When ATP levels rise, ATP binds an allosteric site in PFK1 to decrease the rate of the enzyme reaction; glycolysis is inhibited and ATP production falls. This negative feedback control helps maintain a steady concentration of ATP in the cell. However, metabolic pathways are not just regulated through inhibition since enzyme activation is equally important. With respect to PFK1, fructose 2,6-bisphosphate and ADP are examples of metabolites that are allosteric activators.

Physiological enzyme inhibition can also be produced by specific protein inhibitors. This mechanism occurs in the pancreas, which synthesises many digestive precursor enzymes known as zymogens. Many of these are activated by the trypsin protease, so it is important to inhibit the activity of trypsin in the pancreas to prevent the organ from digesting itself. One way in which the activity of trypsin is controlled is the production of a specific and potent trypsin inhibitor protein in the pancreas. This inhibitor binds tightly to trypsin, preventing the trypsin activity that would otherwise be detrimental to the organ. Although the trypsin inhibitor is a protein, it avoids being hydrolysed as a substrate by the protease by excluding water from trypsin's active site and destabilising the transition state. Other examples of physiological enzyme inhibitor proteins include the barstar inhibitor of the bacterial ribonuclease barnase and the inhibitors of protein phosphatases.

Pesticides

Many pesticides are enzyme inhibitors. Acetylcholinesterase (AChE) is an enzyme found in animals from insects to humans. It is essential to nerve cell function through its mechanism of breaking down the neurotransmitter acetylcholine into its constituents, acetate and choline. This is somewhat unique among neurotransmitters as most, including serotonin, dopamine, and norepinephrine, are absorbed from the synaptic cleft rather than cleaved. A large number of AChE inhibitors are used in both medicine and agriculture. Reversible competitive inhibitors, such as edrophonium, physostigmine, and neostigmine, are used in the treatment of myasthenia gravis and in anaesthesia. The carbamate pesticides are also examples of reversible AChE inhibitors. The organophosphate pesticides such as malathion, parathion, and chlorpyrifos irreversibly inhibit acetylcholinesterase.

The herbicide glyphosate is an inhibitor of 3-phosphoshikimate 1-carboxyvinyltransferase, other herbicides, such as the sulfonylureas inhibit the enzyme acetolactate synthase. Both these enzymes are needed for plants to make branched-chain amino acids. Many other enzymes are inhibited by herbicides, including enzymes needed for the biosynthesis of lipids and carotenoids and the processes of photosynthesis and oxidative phosphorylation.

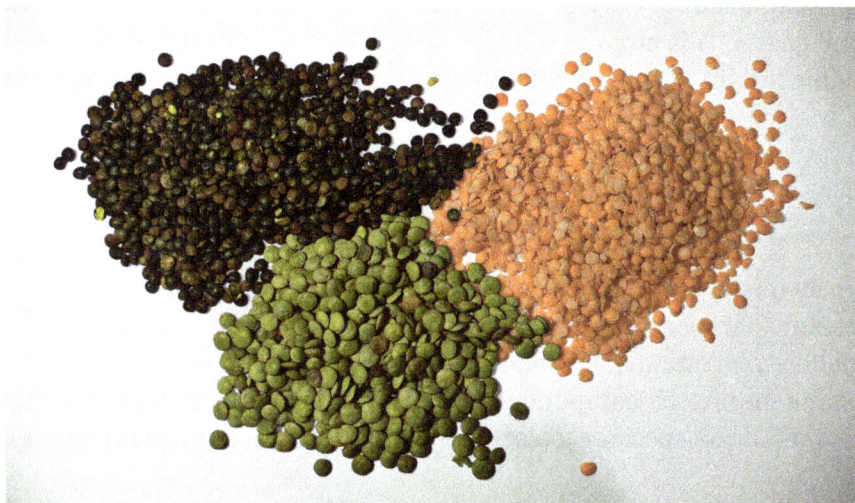

To discourage seed predators, pulses contain trypsin inhibitors that interfere with digestion.

Natural Poisons

Animals and plants have evolved to synthesise a vast array of poisonous products including secondary metabolites, peptides and proteins that can act as inhibitors. Natural toxins are usually small organic molecules and are so diverse that there are probably natural inhibitors for most metabolic processes. The metabolic processes targeted by natural poisons encompass more than enzymes in metabolic pathways and can also include the inhibition of receptor, channel and structural protein functions in a cell. For example, paclitaxel (taxol), an organic molecule found in the Pacific yew tree, binds tightly to tubulin dimers and inhibits their assembly into microtubules in the cytoskeleton.

Many natural poisons act as neurotoxins that can cause paralysis leading to death and have functions for defence against predators or in hunting and capturing prey. Some of these natural inhibitors, despite their toxic attributes, are valuable for therapeutic uses at lower doses. An example of a neurotoxin are the glycoalkaloids, from the plant species in the *Solanaceae* family (includes potato, tomato and eggplant), that are acetylcholinesterase inhibitors. Inhibition of this enzyme causes an uncontrolled increase in the acetylcholine neurotransmitter, muscular paralysis and then death. Neurotoxicity can also result from the inhibition of receptors; for example, atropine from deadly nightshade (*Atropa belladonna*) that functions as a competitive antagonist of the muscarinic acetylcholine receptors.

Although many natural toxins are secondary metabolites, these poisons also include peptides and proteins. An example of a toxic peptide is alpha-amanitin, which is found in relatives of the death cap mushroom. This is a potent enzyme inhibitor, in this case preventing the RNA polymerase II enzyme from transcribing DNA. The algal toxin microcystin is also a peptide and is an inhibitor of protein phosphatases. This toxin can contaminate water supplies after algal blooms and is a known carcinogen that can also cause acute liver hemorrhage and death at higher doses.

Proteins can also be natural poisons or antinutrients, such as the trypsin inhibitors (discussed above) that are found in some legumes, as shown in the figure above. A less common class of toxins are toxic enzymes: these act as irreversible inhibitors of their target enzymes and work by chemically modifying their substrate enzymes. An example is ricin, an extremely potent protein toxin found in castor oil beans. This enzyme is a glycosidase that inactivates ribosomes. Since ricin is a catalytic irreversible inhibitor, this allows just a single molecule of ricin to kill a cell.

Dissociation Constant

In chemistry, biochemistry, and pharmacology, a dissociation constant (K_d) is a specific type of equilibrium constant that measures the propensity of a larger object to separate (dissociate) reversibly into smaller components, as when a complex falls apart into its component molecules, or when a salt splits up into its component ions. The dissociation constant is the inverse of the association constant. In the special case of salts, the dissociation constant can also be called an ionization constant.

For a general reaction:

$$A_x B_y <=> xA + yB$$

in which a complex $A_x B_y$ breaks down into x A subunits and y B subunits, the dissociation constant is defined

$$K_d = \frac{[A]^x [B]^y}{[A_x B_y]}$$

where [A], [B], and [$A_x B_y$] are the concentrations of A, B, and the complex $A_x B_y$, respectively. One reason for the popularity of the dissociation constant in biochemistry and pharmacology is that in the frequently encountered case where x=y=1, K_d has a simple physical interpretation: when

$[A] = K_d$, $[B] = [AB]$ or equivalently $\frac{[AB]}{[B]+[AB]} = \frac{1}{2}$.. That is, K_d, which has the dimensions of concentration, equals the concentration of free A at which half of the total molecules of B are associated with A. This simple interpretation does not apply for higher values of x or y. It also presumes the absence of competing reactions, though the derivation can be extended to explicitly allow for and describe competitive binding. It is useful as a quick description of the binding of a substance, in the same way that EC50 and IC50 describe the biological activities of substances.

Concentration of Bound Molecules

Molecules with One Binding Site

Experimentally, the concentration of the molecule complex [AB] is obtained indirectly from the measurement of the concentration of a free molecules, either [A] or [B]. In principle, the total amounts of molecule $[A]_0$ and $[B]_0$ added to the reaction are known. They separate into free and bound components according to the mass conservation principle:

$$[A]_0 = [A] + [AB]$$
$$[B]_0 = [B] + [AB]$$

To track the concentration of the complex [AB], one substitutes the concentration of the free molecules ([A] or [B]), of the respective conservation equations, by the definition of the dissociation constant,

$$[A]_0 = K_d \frac{[AB]}{[B]} + [AB]$$

This yields the concentration of the complex related to the concentration of either one of the free molecules

$$[AB] = \frac{[A]_0[B]}{K_d + [B]} = \frac{[B]_0[A]}{K_d + [A]}$$

Macromolecules with Identical Independent Binding Sites

Many biological proteins and enzymes can possess more than one binding site. Usually, when a ligand L binds with a macromolecule M , it can influence binding kinetics of other ligands L binding to the macromolecule. A simplified mechanism can be formulated if the affinity of all binding sites can be considered independent of the number of ligands bound to the macromolecule. This is valid for macromolecules composed of more than one, mostly identical, subunits. It can be then assumed that each of these n subunits are identical, symmetric and that they possess only one single binding site. Then, the concentration of bound ligands $[L]_{bound}$ becomes

$$[L]_{bound} = \frac{n[M]_0[L]}{K_d + [L]}$$

In this case, $[L]_{bound} \neq [LM]$, but comprises all partially saturated forms of the macromolecule:

$$[L]_{bound} = [LM] + 2[L_2M] + 3[L_3M] + \ldots + n[L_nM]$$

where the saturation occurs stepwise

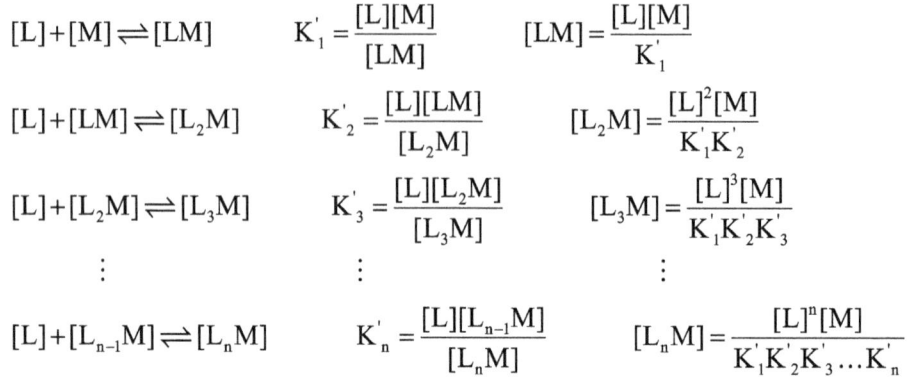

$$[L] + [M] \rightleftharpoons [LM] \qquad K_1' = \frac{[L][M]}{[LM]} \qquad [LM] = \frac{[L][M]}{K_1'}$$

$$[L] + [LM] \rightleftharpoons [L_2M] \qquad K_2' = \frac{[L][LM]}{[L_2M]} \qquad [L_2M] = \frac{[L]^2[M]}{K_1'K_2'}$$

$$[L] + [L_2M] \rightleftharpoons [L_3M] \qquad K_3' = \frac{[L][L_2M]}{[L_3M]} \qquad [L_3M] = \frac{[L]^3[M]}{K_1'K_2'K_3'}$$

$$\vdots \qquad\qquad \vdots \qquad\qquad \vdots$$

$$[L] + [L_{n-1}M] \rightleftharpoons [L_nM] \qquad K_n' = \frac{[L][L_{n-1}M]}{[L_nM]} \qquad [L_nM] = \frac{[L]^n[M]}{K_1'K_2'K_3'\ldots K_n'}$$

For the derivation of the general binding equation a saturation function r is defined as the quotient from the portion of bound ligand to the total amount of the macromolecule:

$$r = \frac{[L]_{bound}}{[M]_0} = \frac{[LM] + 2[L_2M] + 3[L_3M] + \ldots + n[L_nM]}{[M] + [LM] + [L_2M] + [L_3M] + \ldots + [L_nM]} = \frac{\sum\limits_{i=1}^{n}\left(\dfrac{i[L]^i}{\prod\limits_{j=1}^{i}K_{j'}}\right)}{1 + \sum\limits_{i=1}^{n}\left(\dfrac{[L]^i}{\prod\limits_{j=1}^{i}K_{j'}}\right)}$$

Even if all microscopic dissociation constants are identical, they differ from the macroscopic ones and there are differences between each binding step. The general relationship between both types of dissociation constants for n binding sites is

$$K_{i'} = K_d \frac{1}{n-i+1}$$

Hence, the ratio of bound ligand to macromolecules becomes

$$r = \frac{\sum\limits_{i=1}^{n} i\left(\prod\limits_{j=1}^{i}\dfrac{n-j+1}{j}\right)\left(\dfrac{[L]}{K_d}\right)^i}{1 + \sum\limits_{i=1}^{n}\left(\prod\limits_{j=1}^{i}\dfrac{n-j+1}{j}\right)\left(\dfrac{[L]}{K_d}\right)^i} = \frac{\sum\limits_{i=1}^{n} i\binom{n}{i}\left(\dfrac{[L]}{K_d}\right)^i}{1 + \sum\limits_{i=1}^{n}\binom{n}{i}\left(\dfrac{[L]}{K_d}\right)^i}$$

where $\binom{n}{i} = \dfrac{n!}{(n-i)!i!}$ is the binomial coefficient. Then, the first equation is proved by applying the binomial rule

$$r = \frac{n\left(\dfrac{[L]}{K_d}\right)\left(1+\dfrac{[L]}{K_d}\right)^{n-1}}{\left(1+\dfrac{[L]}{K_d}\right)^n} = \frac{n\left(\dfrac{[L]}{K_d}\right)}{\left(1+\dfrac{[L]}{K_d}\right)} = \frac{n[L]}{K_d+[L]} = \frac{[L]_{bound}}{[M]_0}$$

Protein-ligand Binding

The dissociation constant is commonly used to describe the affinity between a ligand L (such as a drug) and a protein P ; i.e., how tightly a ligand binds to a particular protein. Ligand-protein affinities are influenced by non-covalent intermolecular interactions between the two molecules such as hydrogen bonding, electrostatic interactions, hydrophobic and van der Waals forces. Affinities can also be affected by high concentrations of other macromolecules, which causes macromolecular crowding.

The formation of a ligand-protein complex LP can be described by a two-state process

$$L + P \rightleftharpoons LP$$

the corresponding dissociation constant is defined

$$K_d = \frac{[L][P]}{[LP]}$$

where [P], [L] and [LP] represent molar concentrations of the protein, ligand and complex, respectively.

The dissociation constant has molar units (M), which correspond to the concentration of ligand [L] at which the binding site on a particular protein is half occupied, i.e., the concentration of ligand at which the concentration of protein with ligand bound [LP] equals the concentration of protein with no ligand bound [P]. The smaller the dissociation constant, the more tightly bound the ligand is, or the higher the affinity between ligand and protein. For example, a ligand with a nanomolar (nM) dissociation constant binds more tightly to a particular protein than a ligand with a micromolar (μM) dissociation constant.

Sub-picomolar dissociation constants as a result of non-covalent binding interactions between two molecules are rare. Nevertheless, there are some important exceptions. Biotin and avidin bind with a dissociation constant of roughly 10^{-15} M = 1 fM = 0.000001 nM. Ribonuclease inhibitor proteins may also bind to ribonuclease with a similar 10^{-15} M affinity. The dissociation constant for a particular ligand-protein interaction can change significantly with solution conditions (e.g., temperature, pH and salt concentration). The effect of different solution conditions is to effectively modify the strength of any intermolecular interactions holding a particular ligand-protein complex together.

Drugs can produce harmful side effects through interactions with proteins for which they were not meant to or designed to interact. Therefore, much pharmaceutical research is aimed at designing drugs that bind to only their target proteins (Negative Design) with high affinity (typically 0.1-10 nM) or at improving the affinity between a particular drug and its *in-vivo* protein target (Positive Design).

Antibodies

In the specific case of antibodies (Ab) binding to antigen (Ag), usually the term affinity constant refers to the association constant.

$$Ab + Ag <=> AbAg$$

$$K_a = \frac{[AbAg]}{[Ab][Ag]} = \frac{1}{K_d}$$

This chemical equilibrium is also the ratio of the on-rate ($k_{forward}$) and off-rate (k_{back}) constants. Two antibodies can have the same affinity, but one may have both a high on- and off-rate constant, while the other may have both a low on- and off-rate constant.

$$K_a = \frac{k_{forward}}{k_{back}} = \frac{\text{on-rate}}{\text{off-rate}}$$

Acid–base Reactions

For the deprotonation of acids, K is known as K_a, the acid dissociation constant. Stronger acids, for example sulfuric or phosphoric acid, have larger dissociation constants; weaker acids, like acetic acid, have smaller dissociation constants.

(The symbol K_a, used for the acid dissociation constant, can lead to confusion with the association constant and it may be necessary to see the reaction or the equilibrium expression to know which is meant.)

Acid dissociation constants are sometimes expressed by pK_a, which is defined as:

$$pK_a = -\log_{10} K_a$$

This pK notation is seen in other contexts as well; it is mainly used for covalent dissociations (i.e., reactions in which chemical bonds are made or broken) since such dissociation constants can vary greatly.

A molecule can have several acid dissociation constants. In this regard, that is depending on the number of the protons they can give up, we define *monoprotic*, *diprotic* and *triprotic* acids. The first (e.g., acetic acid or ammonium) have only one dissociable group, the second (carbonic acid, bicarbonate, glycine) have two dissociable groups and the third (e.g., phosphoric acid) have three dissociable groups. In the case of multiple pK values they are designated by indices: pK_1, pK_2, pK_3 and so on. For amino acids, the pK_1 constant refers to its carboxyl (-COOH) group, pK_2 refers to its amino (-NH$_3$) group and the pK_3 is the pK value of its side chain.

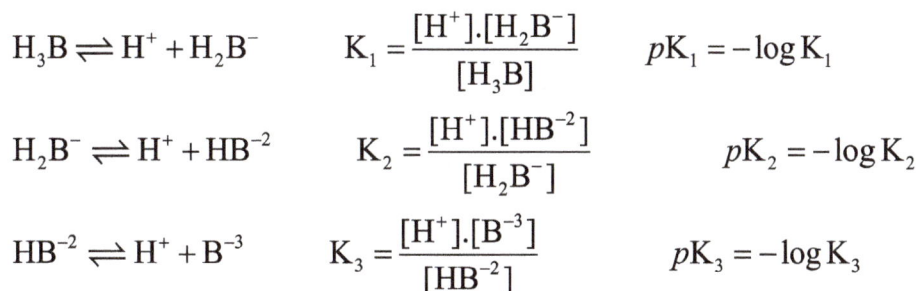

$$H_3B \rightleftharpoons H^+ + H_2B^- \qquad K_1 = \frac{[H^+].[H_2B^-]}{[H_3B]} \qquad pK_1 = -\log K_1$$

$$H_2B^- \rightleftharpoons H^+ + HB^{-2} \qquad K_2 = \frac{[H^+].[HB^{-2}]}{[H_2B^-]} \qquad pK_2 = -\log K_2$$

$$HB^{-2} \rightleftharpoons H^+ + B^{-3} \qquad K_3 = \frac{[H^+].[B^{-3}]}{[HB^{-2}]} \qquad pK_3 = -\log K_3$$

Dissociation Constant of Water

The dissociation constant of water is denoted K_w:

$$K_w = [H^+][OH^-]$$

The concentration of water H_2O is omitted by convention, which means that the value of K_w differs from the value of K_{eq} that would be computed using that concentration.

The value of K_w varies with temperature, as shown in the table below. This variation must be taken into account when making precise measurements of quantities such as pH.

Water temperature	K_w / 10^{-14}	pK_w
0 °C	0.112	14.95
25 °C	1.023	13.99
50 °C	5.495	13.26
75 °C	19.95	12.70
100 °C	56.23	12.25

Homeostasis

Homeostasis or homoeostasis is the property of a system in which a variable (for example, the concentration of a substance in solution, or its temperature) is actively regulated to remain very nearly constant. This regulation occurs inside a defined environment (mostly within a living organism's body). Examples of homeostasis include the regulation of the body temperature of an animal, the pH of its extracellular fluids, or the concentrations of sodium (Na$^+$) and calcium (Ca^{2+}) ions or of glucose in the blood plasma, despite changes in the animal's environment, or what it has eaten, or what it is doing (for example, resting or exercising). Each of these variables is controlled by a separate "homeostat" (or regulator), which, together, maintain life. Homeostats are energy-consuming physiological mechanisms.

The concept was described by French physiologist Claude Bernard in 1865 and the word was coined by Walter Bradford Cannon in 1926.

Although the term was originally used to refer to processes within living organisms, it is frequently applied to technological control systems such as thermostats. A homeostat has an absolute requirement for a sensor to detect changes in the controlled entity's value, as well as an effector mechanism that reverses any detected deviation from the desired value (or "setpoint") of the regulated entity. Since the correction of any error detected by the sensor is always in the opposite direction to the error, a homeostat relies on what is known as a negative feedback connection between the sensor and effector. The effector's corrective effects are monitored by the sensor, which turns the corrective measures off when setpoint conditions have been restored. Negative feedback systems are therefore referred to as "closed loop", or "negative feedback loops", to distinguish them from "open loop" systems where a stimulus (acting on a sensor) results in an, often, all-or-none response that is not subject to modification once it has been set in motion.

Biological

The metabolic processes of all living organisms can only take place in very specific physical and chemical environments. The conditions vary with each organism, and with whether the chemical processes take place inside the cell or in the fluids bathing the cells in multicellular creatures. The best known homeostats in human and other mammalian bodies are regulators that keep the composition of the extracellular fluids (or the "internal environment") constant, especially with regard to the temperature, pH, osmolality, and the concentrations of Na^+, K^+, Ca^{2+}, glucose and CO_2 and O_2. However, a great many other homeostats, encompassing many aspects of human physiology, control other entities in the body.

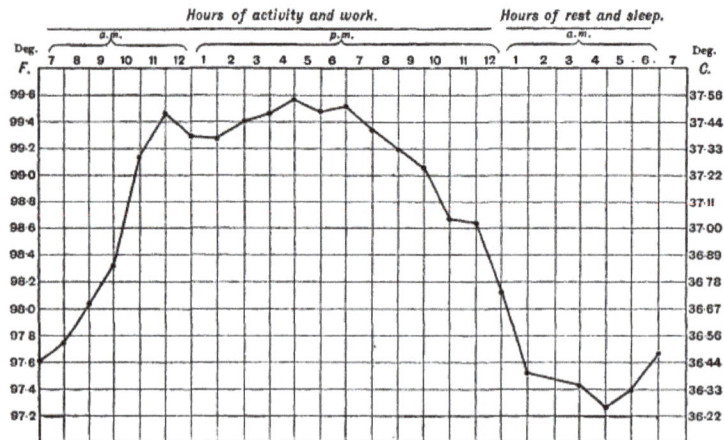

Circadian variation in body temperature, ranging from about 37.5 °C from 10 a.m. to 6 p.m., and falling to about 36.4 °C from 2 a.m. to 6 a.m.

If an entity is homeostatically controlled it does not imply that its value is necessarily absolutely steady in health. Core body temperature is, for instance, regulated by a homeostat with temperature sensors in, amongst others, the hypothalamus of the brain. However the set point of the regulator is regularly reset. For instance, core body temperature in humans varies during the course of the day (i.e. has a circadian rhythm), with the lowest temperatures occurring at night, and the highest in the afternoons (see diagram on the right). The temperature regulator's set point is also readjusted in adult women at the start of the luteal phase of the menstrual cycle (see the diagram on the right, below). The temperature regulator's set point is also reset during infections to produce a fever.

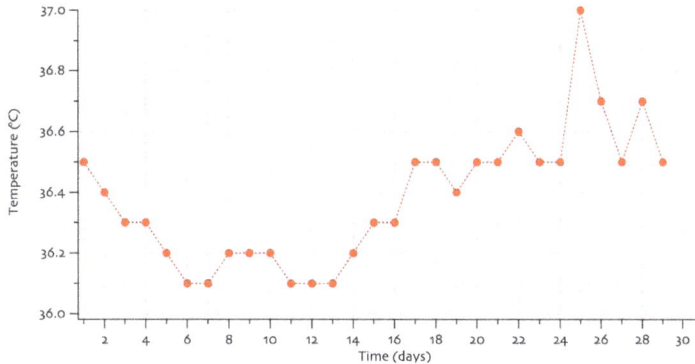

An example of a basal body temperature chart in an adult woman. Day 1 is the first day after the last menstrual period. The rise in temperature between days 14 and 18 is indicative of ovulation. Temperature was taken orally with a regular fever thermometer. Temperature reading is very sensitive to breaks in the regular sleep-rhythm (e.g. "sleeping in" on day 25).

Homeostasis doesn't govern every activity in the body. For instance the signal (be it via neurons or hormones) from the sensor to the effector is, of necessity, highly variable in order to convey information about the direction and magnitude of the error detected by the sensor. Similarly the effector's response needs to be highly adjustable to reverse the error – in fact it should be very nearly in proportion (but in the opposite direction) to the error that is threatening the internal environment. For instance, the arterial blood pressure in mammals is homeostatically controlled, and measured by sensors in the aorta and carotid arteries. The sensors send messages via sensory nerves to the medulla oblongata of the brain indicating whether the blood pressure has fallen or risen, and by how much. The medulla oblongata then distributes messages along motor or efferent nerves belonging to the autonomic nervous system to a wide variety of effector organs, whose activity is consequently changed to reverse the error in the blood pressure. One of the effector organs is the heart whose rate is stimulated to rise (tachycardia) when the arterial blood pressure falls, or to slow down (bradycardia) when the pressure rises above set point. Thus the heart rate (for which there is no sensor in the body) is not homeostatically controlled, but is one of effector responses to errors in the arterial blood pressure. Another example is the rate of sweating. This is one of the effectors in the homeostatic control of body temperature, and therefore highly variable in rough proportion to the heat load that threatens to destabilize the body's core temperature, for which there is a sensor in the hypothalamus of the brain.

Apart from the entities that are homeostatically controlled in the internal environment of the body, and the mechanisms that are responsible for this regulation, there are variables that are neither homeostatically controlled nor involved in the operation of homeostats. The blood urea concentration is an example. Mammals do not have "urea sensors". Instead the concentration of urea is determined by a dynamic equilibrium, in much the same way that the water level in a river at any particular point along its course is determined. The level of a river is simply dependent on the rate at which water flows into a particular section and how fast it flows away from there. It therefore varies with the rainfall in the catchment area and obstructions or otherwise to the flow down stream – there is no energy consuming "regulation". The blood urea concentration is comparable to the water level in a natural river. It is manufactured by the liver from the amino groups of the amino acids of proteins that are being degraded in this organ. It is then excreted by the kidneys which simply pass most of the urea in the glomerular filtrate on into the urine without active re-sorption or excretion by the renal tubules (a relatively small proportion of the urea in the tubules diffuses passively back into the blood as its concentration in the tubules rises when water, without urea, is removed from the tubular fluid). A high protein diet therefore produces high blood urea concentrations, and a protein-poor diet produced low blood plasma urea concentrations, without any physiological attempt to correct or mitigate these fluctuations in the level of urea in the extra-cellular fluids.

Examples of Some of the Better Understood Physiological Homeostats

The Core Body Temperature Homeostat

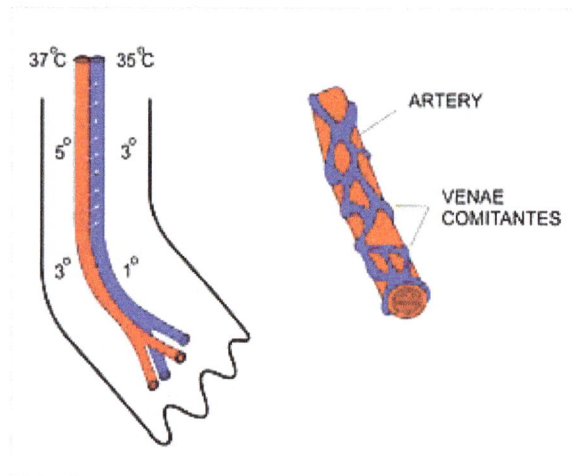

The counter-current flow of blood into a limb in a cold environment. On the left a cartoon of the blood flow into the flipper of a seal in icy water. The arterial blood blood is in close proximity to, indeed surrounded by, veins carrying cold blood back to the torso from the flipper which is almost at the same temperature as the icy water. The arterial blood is cooled by this counter-current flow of cold venous blood and arrives in the flipper at only a few degrees above the environmental temperature. As the blood returns in the veins it is warmed by the arterial blood, and arrives back in the torso at almost core temperature. Effectively the body heat has been short-circuited and does not enter the ice-cold flipper. The diagram on the right shows, in slightly more realistic form, the arrangement of the deep veins around the arteries in the limbs of mammals, all of whom can make use of the same mechanism as the seal to prevent heat loss from the body in cold weather.

Mammals regulate their core temperatures, using hypothalamic temperature sensors in their brains, but also elsewhere in their bodies. When core body temperature falls behavioral changes are set in motion, which, in humans, include the donning of warmer clothes, the seeking out of wind-free, warmer environments, and, eventually, the curling up in the "fetal position" to reduce the surface area (skin) exposed to the cold.

The blood flow to the limbs is reduced to a minimum via sympathetic nerves which constrict the limb arteries. The blood returns from the limb through the deep veins which surround the artery like a coarsely knitted stocking. These deep veins are called venae comitantes (see diagram on the right). This counter-current flow of blood into and out of a cold limb ensures that the arterial blood is cooled on its way into the limb, and is then re-warmed before it returns to the torso. The body heat is thus short-circuited before entering the inevitably cold limb, and relatively little heat is lost by the blood flow into that limb. The superficial subcutaneous veins of the limbs (which are very prominently visible in warm weather) are tightly constricted, as is the capillary blood flow to the skin in general, thus separating the blood as far as possible from the cold surroundings.

The metabolic rate is increased, initially by non-shivering thermogenesis, followed by shivering thermogenesis if the earlier reactions are insufficient to correct the hypothermia.

When body temperature rises, or skin heat sensors detect a threatening rise in body temperature, behavioral changes cause the animal to seek shade, and, in humans, the sweat glands in the skin are stimulated via cholinergic sympathetic nerves to secrete a dilute watery fluid called sweat onto the skin, which, when it evaporates, cools the skin and the blood flowing through it. Panting is an alternative effector in many vertebrates, which cools the body also by the evaporation of water, but this time from the mucous membranes of the throat and mouth.

The Blood Glucose Homeostat

All animals regulate the glucose concentration in their extracellular fluids. In mammals the primary sensor is situated in the beta cells of the pancreatic islets. The beta cells respond to a rise in the blood sugar level by secreting insulin into the blood, and simultaneously inhibiting their neighboring alpha cells from secreting glucagon into the blood. This combination (high blood insulin levels and low glucagon levels) act on effector tissues, chief of which are the liver, fat cells and muscle cells. The liver is inhibited from producing glucose, taking it up instead, and converting it to glycogen and triglycerides. The glycogen is stored in the liver, but the triglycerides are secreted into the blood as very low-density lipoprotein (VLDL) particles which are taken up by adipose tissue, there to be stored as fats. The fat cells take up glucose through special glucose transporters (GLUT4), whose numbers in the cell wall are increased as a direct effect of insulin acting on these cells. The glucose that enters the fat cells in this manner is converted into triglycerides (via the same metabolic pathways as are used by the liver) and then stored in those fat cells together with the VLDL-derived triglycerides that were made in the liver. Muscle cells also take glucose up through insulin-sensitive GLUT4 glucose channels, and convert it into muscle glycogen.

When the beta cells in the pancreatic islets detect lower than normal blood glucose levels, insulin secretion into the blood ceases and the alpha cells are stimulated to secrete glucagon into the blood. This inhibits the uptake of glucose from the blood by the liver, fats cells and muscle. Instead the liver is strongly stimulated to manufacture glucose from glycogen (through glycogenolysis) and from non-carbohydrate sources (such as lactate and de-aminated amino acids) using a process known as gluconeogenesis. The glucose thus produced is discharged into the blood correcting the detected error (hypoglycemia). The glycogen stored in muscles remains in the muscles, and is only broken down, during exercise, to glucose-6-phosphate and thence to pyruvate to be fed into the citric acid cycle or turned into lactate. It is only the lactate and the waste products of the citric acid cycle that are returned to the blood. The liver can take up only the lactate, and by the process of energy consuming gluconeogenesis convert it back to glucose.

The Plasma Ionized Calcium Homeostat

The plasma ionized calcium (Ca^{2+}) concentration is very tightly controlled by a pair of homeostats. The sensor for the one is situated in the parathyroid glands, where the chief cells sense the Ca^{2+}

level by means of specialized calcium receptors in their membranes. The sensors for the second homeostat are the parafollicular cells in the thyroid gland. The parathyroid chief cells secrete parathyroid hormone (PTH) in response to a fall in the plasma ionized calcium level; the parafollicular cells of the thyroid gland secrete calcitonin in response to a rise in the plasma ionized calcium level.

The effector organs of the first homeostat are the skeleton, the kidney, and, via a hormone released into the blood by the kidney in response to high PTH levels in the blood, the duodenum and jejunum. Parathyroid hormone (in high concentrations in the blood) causes bone resorption, releasing calcium into the plasma. This is a very rapid action which can correct a threatening hypocalcemia within minutes. High PTH concentrations cause the excretion of phosphate ions via the urine. Since phosphates combine with calcium ions to form insoluble salts, a decrease in the level of phosphates in the blood, releases free calcium ions into the plasma ionized calcium pool. PTH has a second action on the kidneys. It stimulates the manufacture and release, by the kidneys, of calcitriol (or 1,25 dihydroxycholecalciferol, or 1,25 dihydroxyvitamin D_3) into the blood. This steroid hormone acts on the epithelial cells of the upper small intestine, increasing their capacity to absorb calcium from the gut contents into the blood.

The second homeostat, with its sensors in the thyroid gland, releases calcitonin into the blood when the blood ionized calcium rises. This hormone acts primarily on bone, causing the rapid removal of calcium from the blood and depositing it, in insoluble form, in the skeleton.

The two homeostats working through PTH on the one hand, and calcitonin on the other, can very rapidly correct any impending error in the plasma ionized calcium level by either removing calcium from the blood and depositing it in the skeleton, or by removing calcium from it. The skeleton acts as an extremely large calcium store (about 1 kg) compared with the plasma calcium store (about 180 mg). Longer term regulation occurs through calcium absorption or loss from the gut.

The Blood Partial Pressure of Oxygen and Carbon Dioxide Homeostats

The partial pressure of oxygen (P_{O_2}) in the arterial blood is measured in the aortic and carotid bodies, near the splitting of the common carotid artery into the internal and external carotid arteries. The partial pressure of carbon dioxide (P_{CO_2}) is measured on the surface of medulla oblongata of the brain. Information from these sets of sensors is sent to the respiratory center in the medulla oblongata of the brain which activates the effector organs, which, in this case, are the skeletal muscles of respiration (particularly the diaphragm). An increase in the P_{CO_2} of the blood, or a decrease in the P_{O_2} , causes deeper and more rapid breathing (hyperventilation) thus increasing the ventilation rate of the lung alveoli, which blows CO_2 off, out of the blood, and into the outside air, while increasing the uptake of O_2 from the alveolar air into the blood.

Too little CO_2, and, to a lesser extent, too much O_2, in the blood can temporarily halt breathing, which breath-holding divers use to prolong the time they can stay underwater.

The P_{CO_2} homeostat is an important component of the pH of the extracellular fluid homeostat. At sea level it receives priority over the P_{O_2} homeostat. But above elevations of about 2500 m (or approximately 8000 ft) the rate of breathing is determined by the arterial P_{O_2} rather than the P_{CO_2} . (At 2500 m the atmospheric pressure and partial pressure of oxygen are 75% of what they are at sea level.) At higher elevations than this, the P_{CO_2} is allowed to fall, while hyperventilation now keeps the P_{O_2} constant. To keep the plasma pH at 7.4, despite the very low P_{CO_2} levels as climbers ascend to these high elevations, the kidneys are stimulated secrete hydrogen ions (H^+) into the blood while excreting of bicarbonate ions ($HCO-3$) into the urine. This is an important contribution to the acclimatization to high altitude.

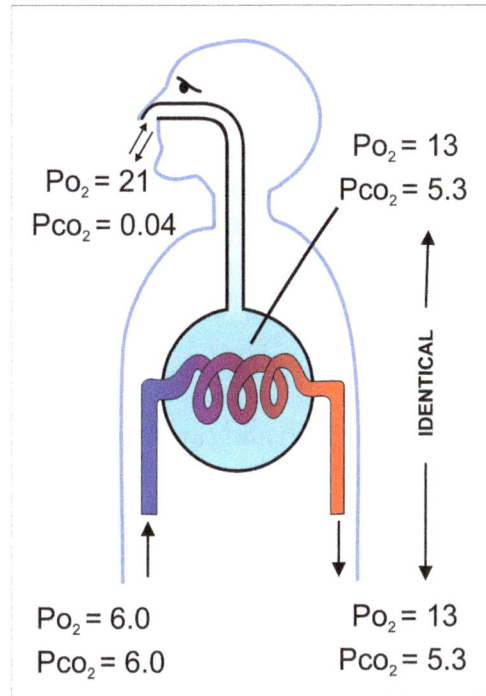

A cartoon of the effector mechanism employed by the blood gas homeostat. The partial pressures of the gases in the blood flowing through the mammalian lungs equilibrates with those in the approximately 3 liters of alveolar air that is always present in the lungs even after normal exhalation (indicated in the diagram by the light blue color in the sphere which represents the 3 liters of alveolar air). With each breath at rest, only about 350 ml of this alveolar air is replaced with ambient air (i.e. air from outside). This means that the composition of the alveolar air changes only minutely with each breath. Furthermore, the relatively long narrow tube separating the alveolar air from the ambient air allows the composition of the alveolar air to differ significantly from fresh atmospheric air: the oxygen concentration in the alveolar air is only about 60% of what it is in the atmosphere, while the carbon dioxide concentration, which is present only in trace quantities in the outside air, has a concentration of just over 5% in the alveoli. These alveolar concentrations of oxygen and carbon dioxide are kept constant by measuring the partial pressures of these gases in the blood that exits from the lungs (indicated in red on the right, in the diagram), in the aortic and carotid bodies, and adjusting the rate and depth of breathing accordingly. All the gas tensions are in kPa. To convert to mm Hg, multiply by 7.5.

The Blood Oxygen Content Homeostat

The kidneys measure the oxygen content (rather than the P_{O_2}) of the arterial blood. When the oxygen content of the blood is chronically low, these oxygen-sensitive cells secrete erythropoietin (EPO) into the blood. The effector tissue in this case is the red bone marrow which produces red blood cells (or erythrocytes). This tissue is stimulated by high levels of erythropoietin to increase the rate of red cell production, which leads to an increase in the hematocrit of the blood, and a consequent increase in its oxygen carrying capacity (due to the now high hemoglobin content of the blood). This is the mechanism whereby high altitude dwellers have higher hematocrits than sea-level residents, and also why persons with pulmonary insufficiency or right-to-left shunts in the heart (through which venous blood by-passes the lungs and goes directly into the systemic circulation) have similarly high hematocrits.

The distinction between the P_{O_2} of the arterial blood and its oxygen content (or oxygen concentration) is important. The P_{O_2} is the pressure with which the oxygen has been forced into the blood in the alveoli of the lungs. The amount of oxygen that is consequently carried in the blood (at a given P_{O_2}) depends on the hemoglobin concentration in the blood. The greater the hemoglobin concentration the greater the amount of oxygen that can be carried per liter of blood at that P_{O_2}. Thus, in anemia the P_{O_2} of the arterial blood is normal but the oxygen content is below normal. The oxygen content sensors in the kidneys detect this lower than normal oxygen concentration in the arterial blood, and increase their secretion of erythropoietin into the blood. This stimulates a greater rate of red blood cell production in the red bone marrow. This will correct the anemia, and therefore the oxygen concentration in the blood, if there are enough raw materials and co-factors (e.g. iron, vitamin B_{12} and folic acid) to manufacture the extra red cells.

The Arterial Blood Pressure Homeostat

Stretch receptors in the walls of the aortic arch and carotid sinus (at the beginning of the internal carotid artery) act as arterial blood pressure sensors. As the pressure rises the arteries balloon out, stretching their walls. This information is then conveyed, via sensory nerves, to the medulla oblongata of the brain stem. From here motor nerves belonging to the autonomic nervous system are stimulated to influence the activity of chiefly the heart and the smallest diameter arteries, called arterioles. The arterioles are the main resistance vessels in the arterial tree, and small changes in diameter cause large changes in the resistance to flow through them. When the arterial blood pressure rises the arterioles are stimulated to dilate making it easier for blood to leave the arteries, thus deflating them, and bringing the blood pressure down, back to normal. At the same time the heart is stimulated via cholinergic parasympathetic nerves to beat more slowly (called bradycardia), ensuring that the inflow of blood into the arteries is reduced, thus adding to the reduction in pressure, and correction of the original error.

If the pressure in the arteries falls, the opposite reflex is elicited: constriction of the arterioles, and a speeding up of the heart rate (called tachycardia). If the drop in blood pressure is very rapid or excessive, the medulla oblongata stimulates the adrenal medulla, via "preganglionic" sympathetic nerves, to secrete epinephrine (adrenaline) into the blood. This hormone enhances the tachycardia and causes severe vasoconstriction of the arterioles to all but the essential organ in the body (especially the heart, lungs and brain). These reactions usually correct the low arterial blood pressure (hypotension) very effectively.

The Extracellular Sodium Concentration Homeostat

The sodium concentration homeostat is rather more complex than most of the other homeostats described on this page.

The sensor is situated in the juxtaglomerular apparatus of kidneys, which senses the plasma sodium concentration in a surprisingly indirect manner. Instead of measuring it directly in the blood flowing past the juxtaglomerular cells, these cells respond to the sodium concentration in the renal tubular fluid after it has already undergone a certain amount of modification in the proximal convoluted tubule and loop of Henle. These cells also respond to rate of blood flow through the juxtaglomerular apparatus, which, under normal circumstances, is directly proportional to the arterial blood pressure, making this tissue an ancillary arterial blood pressure sensor.

In response to a lowering of the plasma sodium concentration, or to a fall in the arterial blood pressure, the juxtaglomerular cells release renin into the blood. Renin is an enzyme which cleaves a decapeptide (a short protein chain, 10 amino acids long) from a plasma α-2-globulin called angiotensinogen. This decapeptide is known as angiotensin I. It has no known biological activity. However, when the blood circulates through the lungs a pulmonary capillary endothelial enzyme called angiotensin-converting enzyme (ACE) cleaves a further two amino acids from angiotensin I to form an octapeptide known as angiotensin II. Angiotensin II is a hormone which acts on the adrenal cortex, causing the release into the blood of the steroid hormone, aldosterone. Angiotensin II also acts on the smooth muscle in the walls of the arterioles causing these small diameter vessels to constrict, thereby restricting the outflow of blood from the arterial tree, causing the arterial blood pressure to rise. This therefore reinforces the measures described above (under the heading of *The arterial blood pressure homeostat*), which defend the arterial blood pressure against changes, especially hypotension.

The angiotensin II-stimulated aldosterone released from the zona glomerulosa of the adrenal glands has an effect on particularly the epithelial cells of the distal convoluted tubules and collecting ducts of the kidneys. Here it causes the reabsorption of sodium ions from the renal tubular fluid, in exchange for potassium ions which are secreted from the blood plasma into the tubular fluid to exit the body via the urine. The reabsorption of sodium ions from the renal tubular fluid halts further sodium ion losses from the body, and therefore preventing the worsening of hyponatremia. The hyponatremia can only be *corrected* by the consumption of salt in the diet. However, it is not certain whether a "salt hunger" can be initiated by hyponatremia, or by what mechanism this might come about.

When the plasma sodium ion concentration is higher than normal (hypernatremia), the release of renin from the juxtaglomerular apparatus is halted, ceasing the production of angiotensin II, and its consequent aldosterone-release into the blood. The kidneys respond by excreting sodium ions into the urine, thereby normalizing the plasma sodium ion concentration. The low angiotensin II levels in the blood lower the arterial blood pressure as an inevitable concomitant response.

The reabsorption of sodium ions from the tubular fluid as a result of high aldosterone levels in the blood does not, of itself, cause renal tubular water to be returned to the blood from the distal convoluted tubules or collecting ducts. This is because sodium is reabsorbed in exchange for potassium and therefore causes only a modest change in the osmotic gradient between the blood and the tubular fluid. Furthermore, the epithelium of the distal convoluted tubules and collecting ducts is impermeable to water in the absence of antidiuretic hormone (ADH) in the blood. ADH is part of the body water homeostat. Its levels in the blood vary with the osmolality of the plasma, which is measured in the hypothalamus of the brain. Aldosterone's action on the kidney tubules does not *add* sodium to the extracellular fluids (ECF) - it simply prevents further loss. So there is no change in the osmolality of the ECF, and therefore no change in the ADH concentration of the plasma. However, low aldosterone levels cause a loss of sodium ions from the ECF, which could potentially cause a change in extracellular osmolality and therefore of ADH levels in the blood.

The Extracellular Potassium Concentration Homeostat

The extracellular potassium ion (K^+) concentration is sensed by the zona glomerulosa cells of the outer layer of the adrenal cortex, as well as, probably, by sensors in the carotid arteries. High potassium concentrations in the plasma cause depolarization of the zona glomerulosa cells' membranes. This causes the release of aldosterone into the blood.

Aldosterone acts primarily on the distal convoluted tubules and collecting ducts of the kidneys, stimulating them to excrete potassium ions into the tubular fluid, and thus into the urine. It does so, however, by activating the basolateral Na^+/K^+ pumps of the tubular epithelial cells. These sodium/potassium exchangers pump three sodium ions out of the cell, into the interstitial fluid and two potassium ions into the cell from the interstitial fluid. This creates concentration gradients which result in the reabsorption of sodium (Na^+) ions from the tubular fluid into the blood, and secreting potassium (K^+) ions from the blood into the urine (lumen of collecting duct).

This obviously implies that excess potassium in the plasma can only be excreted at the expense of sodium retention by the body. The fact that the sodium and potassium homeostats seem to rely entirely on the same effector, but in opposite directions, implies that the body can only excrete potassium while retaining sodium, or vice versa. It cannot simultaneously excrete sodium and potassium ions in higher than modest quantities (when aldosterone is at an intermediate concentration in the plasma), and has no way of retaining both of them if there is a shortage in the body of the two cations. How these two conflicting homeostats (using the same effector) are disentangled to allow the plasma sodium and potassium ion levels to be regulated independently is currently not clear.

The Volume of Body Water Homeostat

The volume of water in the body is measured by stretch receptors in the heart atria, and, somewhat indirectly, by the measurement of the osmolality of the plasma by the hypothalamus. Measurement of the plasma osmolality to give an indication of the water content of the body, relies on the fact that water losses from the body, through sweat, gut fluids (normal fecal water losses, and through vomiting and diarrhea), and the exhaled air, are all hypotonic, meaning that they are less salty than the body fluids (compare, for instance, the taste of saliva with that of tears. The latter have almost the same salt content as the extracellular fluids, whereas the former is hypotonic with respect to plasma. Saliva does not taste salty, whereas tears are decidedly salty). Nearly all normal and abnormal losses of body water therefore cause the extracellular fluids to become hyperosmolar. Conversely excessive water intake (in the form of most regular beverages) dilutes the extracellular fluids causing the hypothalamus to register hypo-osmolar conditions.

When the hypothalamus detects a hyperosmolar extracellular environment, it causes the secretion from the posterior pituitary gland of a peptide hormone called antidiuretic hormone (ADH), which acts on the effector organ, which in this case is the kidney. The effect of ADH on the kidney tubules is to reabsorb water from the distal convoluted tubules and collecting ducts, thus preventing aggravation of the water loss via the urine. The hypothalamus simultaneously stimulates the nearby thirst center causing an almost irresistible (if the hyperosmolarity is severe enough) urge to drink water. The cessation of urine flow prevents the hypovolemia and hypertonicity from getting worse; the drinking of water corrects the defect.

Hypo-osmolality results in very low plasma ADH levels. This results in the inhibition of water re-absorption from the kidney tubules, causing high volumes of very dilute urine to be excreted, thus getting rid of the excess water in the body.

Note that urinary water loss, when the body water homeostat is intact, is a *compensatory* water loss, *correcting* any water excess in the body. However, since the kidneys cannot generate water, the thirst reflex is the all important second effector mechanism of the body water homeostat, *correcting* any water deficit in the body.

Stretching of the right atrium of the heart, usually a sign of an excessive blood volume, causes stretch receptors to secrete a hormone known as atrial natriuretic peptide (ANP) into the blood. This also acts on the kidneys causing sodium, and accompanying water loss into the urine, thereby reducing the volume of circulating blood.

The Extracellular Fluid pH Homeostat

The pH of the extracellular fluids (which includes the blood plasma) is regulated by adjusting the ratio of the concentration of carbonic acid (H_2CO_3) to that of the bicarbonate ions (HCO–3) to equal 1:20. This ratio and its relationship to the pH is described by the Henderson–Hasselbalch equation, which, when applied to the bicarbonate buffering system in the extracellular fluids, states that:

$$pH = pK_{a\,H_2CO_3} + \log_{10}\left(\frac{[HCO_3^-]}{[H_2CO_3]}\right),$$

where:

- $pK_{a\,H2CO3}$ is the cologarithm of the acid dissociation constant of carbonic acid. It is equal to 6.1.

- [HCO–3] is the concentration of bicarbonate in the blood plasma

- [H_2CO_3] is the concentration of carbonic acid in the blood plasma

However, since the carbonic acid concentration is directly proportional to the P_{CO_2} in the extracellular fluid, the Henderson–Hasselbalch equation can be rewritten as follows:

$$pH = 6.1 + \log_{10}\left(\frac{[HCO_3^-]}{0.0307 \times P_{CO_2}}\right),$$

where:

- pH is the acidity in the plasma

- [HCO–3] is the concentration of bicarbonate in the plasma

- P_{CO2} is the partial pressure of carbon dioxide in the arterial blood plasma

There are therefore at least two homeostats responsible for the regulation of the plasma pH. The first is the P_{CO_2} homeostat described above which keeps the arterial blood P_{CO_2} at 5.3 kPa (or 40 mm Hg). The sensor is on the surface of the medulla oblongata of the brain stem, which is also sensitive to the pH of the cerebrospinal fluid. The effector organs are the muscles of respiration, which are stimulated via motor nerves to breathe faster and more deeply (hyperventilation) when the P_{CO_2} rises and the plasma pH falls, or more slowly and less deeply (hypoventilation) when the P_{CO_2} falls and the pH rises. Changes in the rate and depth of breathing can change the pH of the arterial plasma within a few seconds.

The sensor for the plasma HCO–3 concentration is not known for certain. It is very probable that the renal tubular cells of the distal convoluted tubules are themselves sensitive to the pH of the plasma. The metabolism of these cells produces CO_2, which is rapidly converted to H^+ and HCO–3 through the action of carbonic anhydrase. When the extracellular fluids tend towards acidity, the renal tubular cells secrete the H^+ ions into the tubular fluid from where they exit the body via the urine. The HCO–3 ions are simultaneously secreted into the blood plasma, thus raising the bicarbonate ion concentration in the plasma, increasing the $[HCO_3^-]:P_{CO_2}$ ratio, and consequently the pH of the plasma. The converse happens when the plasma pH rises above normal: bicarbonate ions are excreted into the urine, and hydrogen ions into the plasma.

Homeostatic Breakdown

Many diseases are the result of the failure of one or more homeostat(s). Almost any functional component of any homeostat can malfunction, either as a result of an inherited defect, or an acquired disease. Some of the homeostats have inbuilt redundancies, which insures that life is not immediately threatened if a component malfunctions; but in other cases malfunction of a homeostat causes severe disease, which can be fatal if not treated. Here only a few well known examples of homeostat dysfunction are described.

Type 1 diabetes mellitus is probably the best known example. Here the blood glucose homeostat ceases to function because the beta cells of the pancreatic islets are destroyed. This means that the glucose sensor is absent, and its effector pathway (the insulin level in the blood) remains unchanged at zero. The blood glucose concentration therefore rises to very high levels, while the body's proteins are degraded into amino acids which are turned at a very high rate into glucose, via gluconeogenesis, by the liver. The condition is fatal if not treated.

The plasma ionized calcium homeostat can be disrupted by the constant, unchanging, over-production of parathyroid hormone by a parathyroid adenoma resulting in the typically features of hyperparathyroidism, namely high plasma ionized Ca^{2+} levels and the resorption of bone, which can lead to spontaneous fractures. The abnormally high plasma ionized calcium concentrations cause conformational changes in many cell-surface proteins (especially ion channels and hormone or neurotransmitter receptors) giving rise to lethargy, muscle weakness, anorexia, constipation and labile emotions.

The body water homeostat can be compromised by the inability to secrete ADH in response to even the normal daily water losses via the exhaled air, the feces, and insensible sweating. On receiving a zero blood ADH signal, the kidneys produce huge unchanging volumes of very dilute urine, causing dehydration and death if not treated.

As organisms age, the efficiency of their control systems becomes reduced. The inefficiencies gradually result in an unstable internal environment that increases the risk of illness, and leads to the physical changes associated with aging.

Chronic Disease Compensation and Decompensation

Various chronic diseases are kept under control by homeostatic compensation, which masks a problem by compensating for it (making up for it) in another way. However, the compensating mechanisms eventually wear out or are disrupted by a new complicating factor (such as the advent of a concurrent acute viral infection), which sends the body reeling through a new cascade of events. Such decompensation unmasks the underlying disease, worsening its symptoms. Common examples include decompensated heart failure, kidney failure, and liver failure.

Examples from Technology

The following are all examples of familiar technological homeostatic mechanisms:

- A thermostat operates by switching heaters or air-conditioners on and off in response to the output of a temperature sensor.

- Cruise control adjusts a car's throttle in response to changes in speed.

- An autopilot operates the steering controls of an aircraft or ship in response to deviation from a pre-set compass bearing or route.

- Process control systems in a chemical plant or oil refinery maintain fluid levels, pressures, temperature, chemical composition, etc. by controlling heaters, pumps and valves.

- The centrifugal governor of a steam engine, as designed by James Watt in 1788, reduces the throttle valve in response to increases in the engine speed, or opens the valve if the speed falls below the pre-set rate.

Biosphere

In the Gaia hypothesis, James Lovelock stated that the entire mass of living matter on Earth (or any planet with life) functions as a vast homeostatic superorganism that actively modifies its planetary environment to produce the environmental conditions necessary for its own survival. In this view, the entire planet maintains several homeostats (the primary one being temperature homeostasis). Whether this sort of system is present on Earth is open to debate. However, some relatively simple homeostatic mechanisms are generally accepted. For example, it is sometimes claimed that when atmospheric carbon dioxide levels rise, certain plants may be able to grow better and thus act to remove more carbon dioxide from the atmosphere. However, warming has exacerbated droughts, making water the actual limiting factor on land. When sunlight is plentiful and atmospheric temperature climbs, it has been claimed that the phytoplankton of the ocean surface waters, acting as global sunshine, and therefore heat sensors, may thrive and produce more dimethyl sulfide (DMS). The DMS molecules act as cloud condensation nuclei, which produce more clouds, and thus increase the atmospheric albedo, and this feeds back to lower the temperature of the atmosphere. However, rising sea temperature has stratified the oceans, separating warm, sunlit waters from cool, nutrient-rich waters. Thus, nutrients have become the limiting factor, and plankton levels have actually fallen over the past 50 years, not risen. As scientists discover more about Earth, vast numbers of positive and negative feedback loops are being discovered, that, together, maintain a metastable condition, sometimes within very broad range of environmental conditions.

Predictive

Predictive homeostasis is an anticipatory response to an expected challenge in the future, such as the stimulation of insulin secretion by gut hormones which enter the blood in response to a meal. This insulin secretion occurs before the blood sugar level rises, lowering the blood sugar level in anticipation of a large influx into the blood of glucose resulting from the digestion of carbohydrates in the gut. Such anticipatory reactions are open loop systems which are based, essentially, on "guess work", and are not self-correcting. Anticipatory responses always require a closed loop negative feedback system to correct the over- and undershoots to which the anticipatory systems are prone.

Other Fields

The term has come to be used in other fields, for example:

Risk

An actuary may refer to *risk homeostasis*, where (for example) people ***who*** have anti-lock brakes have no better safety record than those without anti-lock brakes, because the former unconsciously compensate for the safer vehicle via less-safe driving habits. Previous to the innovation of anti-lock brakes, certain maneuvers involved minor skids, evoking fear and avoidance: Now the anti-lock system moves the boundary for such feedback, and behavior patterns expand into the no-longer punitive area. It has also been suggested that ecological crises are an instance of risk homeostasis in which a particular behavior continues until proven dangerous or dramatic consequences actually occur.

Stress

Sociologists and psychologists may refer to *stress homeostasis*, the tendency of a population or an individual to stay at a certain level of stress, often generating artificial stresses if the "natural" level of stress is not enough.

Jean-François Lyotard, a postmodern theorist, has applied this term to societal 'power centers' that he describes as being 'governed by a principle of homeostasis,' for example, the scientific hierarchy, which will sometimes ignore a radical new discovery for years because it destabilises previously accepted norms.

History of Discovery

The conceptual origins of homeostasis reach back to Greek concepts such as balance, harmony, equilibrium, and steady-state; all believed to be fundamental attributes of life and health. Thus, the philosopher Empedocles (495-435 BC) postulated that all matter consisted of elements and qualities that were in dynamic opposition or alliance to one another, and that balance or harmony was a necessary condition for the survival of living organisms. Following these hypotheses, Hippocrates (460-375 BC) compared health to the harmonious balance of the elements, and illness and disease to the systematic disharmony of these elements.

Nearly 150 years ago, Claude Bernard published his seminal work, stating that the maintenance of the internal environment, or milieu intérieur, surrounding the body's cells, was essential for the life of the organism. In 1929, Walter B. Cannon published an extrapolation from Bernard's 1865 work naming his theory "homeostasis". Cannon postulated that homeostasis was a process of synchronized adjustments in the internal environment resulting in the maintenance of specific physiological variables within defined parameters; and that these precise parameters included blood pressure, temperature, pH, and others; all with clearly defined "normal" ranges. Cannon further posited that threats to homeostasis might originate from the external environment (e.g., temperature extremes, traumatic injury) or the internal environment (e.g., pain, infection), and could be physical or psychological, as in emotional distress. Cannon's work outlined that maintenance of this internal physical and psychological balance, homeostasis, demands an internal network of communication, with sensors capable of identifying deviations from the acceptable ranges and effectors to return those deviations back within acceptable limits. Cannon identified these negative feedback systems and emphasized that, regardless of the nature of the threat to homeostasis, the response he mapped within the body would be the same.

Ribonuclease Inhibitor

Ribonuclease inhibitor (RI) is a large (~450 residues, ~49 kDa), acidic (pI ~4.7), leucine-rich repeat protein that forms extremely tight complexes with certain ribonucleases. It is a major cellular protein, comprising ~0.1% of all cellular protein by weight, and appears to play an important role in regulating the lifetime of RNA.

RI has a surprisingly high cysteine content (~6.5%, cf. 1.7% in typical proteins) and is sensitive to oxidation. RI is also rich in leucine (21.5%, compared to 9% in typical proteins) and commensurately lower in other hydrophobic residues, esp. valine, isoleucine, methionine, tyrosine, and phenylalanine.

Structure

RI is the classic leucine-rich repeat protein, consisting of alternating α-helices and β-strands along its backbone. These secondary structure elements wrap around in a curved, right-handed solenoid that resembles a horseshoe. The parallel β-strands and α-helices form the inner and outer wall of the horseshoe, respectively. The structure appears to be stabilized by buried asparagines at the base of each turn, as it passes from α-helix to β-strand. The αβ repeats alternate between 28 and 29 residues in length, effectively forming a 57-residue unit that corresponds to its genetic structure (each exon codes for a 57-residue unit).

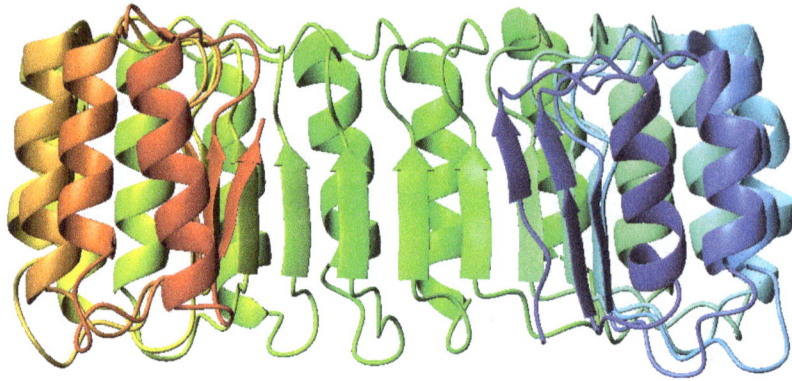

Side view of porcine ribonuclease inhibitor; ribbon is colored from blue (N-terminus) to red (C-terminus).

Binding to Ribonucleases

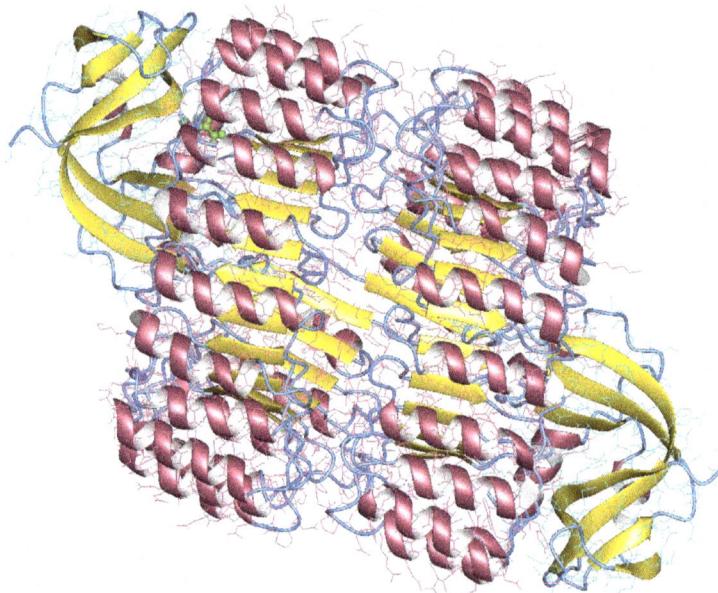

Ribonuclease I (yellow) and inhibitor (pink helixes) complex heterotetramer, Human.

The affinity of RI for ribonucleases is among the highest for any protein-protein interaction; the dissociation constant of the RI-RNase A complex is in the femtomolar (fM) range under physiological conditions while that for the RI-angiogenin complex is less than 1 fM. Despite this high affinity, RI is able to bind a wide variety of RNases A despite their relatively low sequence identity. Both biochemical studies and crystallographic structures of RI-RNase A complexes suggest that the interaction is governed largely by electrostatic interactions, but also involves substantial buried surface area. RI's affinity for ribonucleases is important, since many ribonucleases have cytotoxic and cytostatic effects that correlate well with ability to bind RI.

Mammalian RIs are unable to bind certain pancreatic ribonuclease family members from other species. In particular, amphibian RNases, such ranpirnase and amphinase from the Northern leopard frog, escape mammalian RI and have been noted to have differential cytotoxicity against cancer cells.

Cytochrome P450

Cytochromes P450 (CYPs) are proteins of the superfamily containing heme as a cofactor and, therefore, are hemoproteins. CYPs use a variety of small and large molecules as substrates in enzymatic reactions. They are, in general, the terminal oxidase enzymes in electron transfer chains, broadly categorized as P450-containing systems. The term *P450* is derived from the spectrophotometric peak at the wavelength of the absorption maximum of the enzyme (450 nm) when it is in the reduced state and complexed with carbon monoxide.

CYP enzymes have been identified in all kingdoms of life: animals, plants, fungi, protists, bacteria, archaea, and even in viruses. However, they are not omnipresent; for example, they have not been found in *Escherichia coli*. More than 200,000 distinct CYP proteins are known.

Most CYPs require a protein partner to deliver one or more electrons to reduce the iron (and eventually molecular oxygen). Based on the nature of the electron transfer proteins, CYPs can be classified into several groups:

- Microsomal P450 systems, in which electrons are transferred from NADPH via cytochrome P450 reductase (variously CPR, POR, or CYPOR). Cytochrome b5 (cyb5) can also contribute reducing power to this system after being reduced by cytochrome b5 reductase (CYB5R).

- Mitochondrial P450 systems, which employ adrenodoxin reductase and adrenodoxin to transfer electrons from NADPH to P450.

- Bacterial P450 systems, which employ a ferredoxin reductase and a ferredoxin to transfer electrons to P450.

- CYB5R/cyb5/P450 systems, in which both electrons required by the CYP come from cytochrome b5.

- FMN/Fd/P450 systems, originally found in *Rhodococcus* species, in which a FMN-domain-containing reductase is fused to the CYP.

- P450 only systems, which do not require external reducing power. Notable ones include thromboxane synthase (CYP5), prostacyclin synthase (CYP8), and CYP74A (allene oxide synthase).

The most common reaction catalyzed by cytochromes P450 is a monooxygenase reaction, e.g., insertion of one atom of oxygen into the aliphatic position of an organic substrate (RH) while the other oxygen atom is reduced to water:

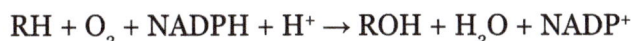

$$RH + O_2 + NADPH + H^+ \rightarrow ROH + H_2O + NADP^+$$

Many hydroxylation reactions (insertion of hydroxyl groups) use CYP enzymes.

Nomenclature

Genes encoding CYP enzymes, and the enzymes themselves, are designated with the root symbol CYP for the superfamily, followed by a number indicating the gene family, a capital letter indicating the subfamily, and another numeral for the individual gene. The convention is to *italicise* the name when referring to the gene. For example, *CYP2E1* is the gene that encodes the enzyme CYP2E1—one of the enzymes involved in paracetamol (acetaminophen) metabolism. The CYP nomenclature is the official naming convention, although occasionally CYP450 or CYP_{450} is used synonymously. However, some gene or enzyme names for CYPs may differ from this nomenclature, denoting the catalytic activity and the name of the compound used as substrate. Examples include CYP5A1, thromboxane A_2 synthase, abbreviated to TBXAS1 (ThromBoXane A_2 Synthase 1), and CYP51A1, lanosterol 14-α-demethylase, sometimes unofficially abbreviated to LDM according to its substrate (Lanosterol) and activity (DeMethylation).

The current nomenclature guidelines suggest that members of new CYP families share at least 40% amino acid identity, while members of subfamilies must share at least 55% amino acid identity. There are nomenclature committees that assign and track both base gene names (Cytochrome P450 Homepage) and allele names (CYP Allele Nomenclature Committee).

Mechanism

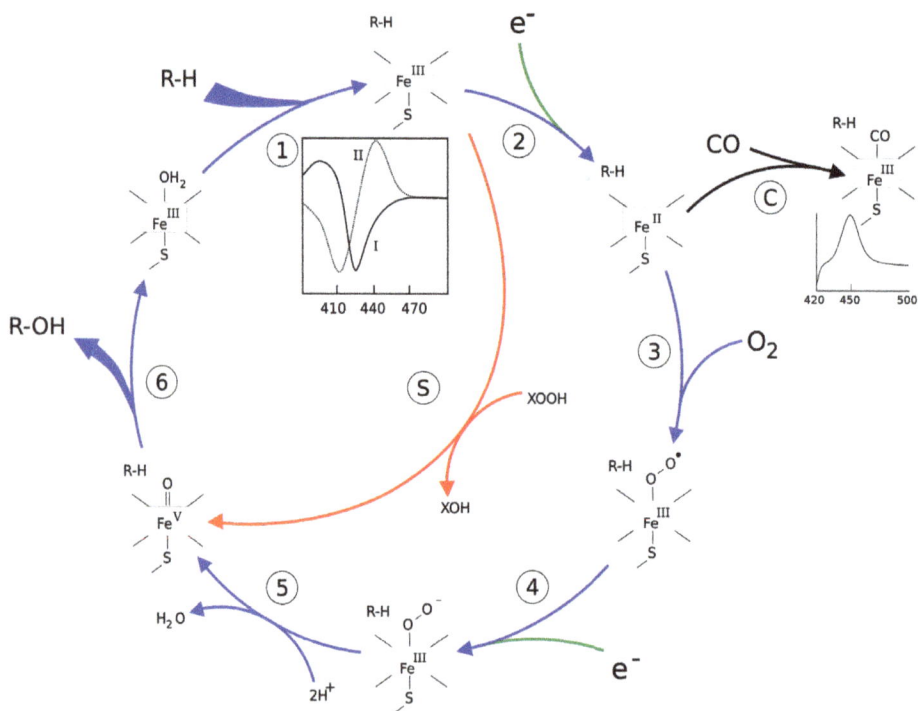

The "Fe(V) intermediate" at the bottom left is a simplification: it is an Fe(IV) with a radical heme ligand.

Structure

The active site of cytochrome P450 contains a heme-iron center. The iron is tethered to the protein via a cysteine thiolate ligand. This cysteine and several flanking residues are highly conserved in known CYPs and have the formal PROSITE signature consensus pattern [FW] - [SGNH] - x - [GD] - {F} - [RKHPT] - {P} - C - [LIVMFAP] - [GAD]. Because of the vast variety of reactions catalyzed by CYPs, the activities and properties of the many CYPs differ in many aspects. In general, the P450 catalytic cycle proceeds as follows:

Catalytic Cycle

1. Substrate binds in proximity to the heme group, on the side opposite to the axial thiolate. Substrate binding induces a change in the conformation of the active site, often displacing a water molecule from the distal axial coordination position of the heme iron, and changing the state of the heme iron from low-spin to high-spin.

2. Substrate binding induces electron transfer from NAD(P)H via cytochrome P450 reductase or another associated reductase.

3. Molecular oxygen binds to the resulting ferrous heme center at the distal axial coordination position, initially giving a dioxygen adduct not unlike oxy-myoglobin.

4. A second electron is transferred, from either cytochrome P450 reductase, ferredoxins, or cytochrome b5, reducing the Fe-O$_2$ adduct to give a short-lived peroxo state.

5. The peroxo group formed in step 4 is rapidly protonated twice, releasing one molecule of water and forming the highly reactive species referred to as P450 Compound 1 (or just Compound I). This highly reactive intermediate was isolated in 2010, P450 Compound 1 is an iron(IV) oxo (or ferryl) species with an additional oxidizing equivalent delocalized over the porphyrin and thiolate ligands. Evidence for the alternative perferryl iron(V)-oxo is lacking.

6. Depending on the substrate and enzyme involved, P450 enzymes can catalyze any of a wide variety of reactions. A hypothetical hydroxylation is shown in this illustration. After the product has been released from the active site, the enzyme returns to its original state, with a water molecule returning to occupy the distal coordination position of the iron nucleus.

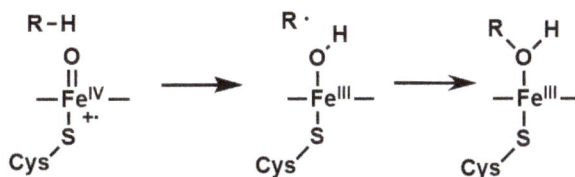

Oxygen rebound mechanism utilized by cytochrome P450 for conversion of hydrocarbons to alcohols via the action of "compound I", an iron(IV) oxide bound to a radical heme.

1. An alternative route for mono-oxygenation is via the "peroxide shunt" (path "S" in figure). This pathway entails oxidation of the ferric-substrate complex with oxygen-atom donors such as peroxides and hypochlorites. A hypothetical peroxide "XOOH" is shown in the diagram.

Spectroscopy

Binding of substrate is reflected in the spectral properties of the enzyme, with an increase in absorbance at 390 nm and a decrease at 420 nm. This can be measured by difference spectrometry and is referred to as the "type I" difference spectrum. Some substrates cause an opposite change in spectral properties, a "reverse type I" spectrum, by processes that are as yet unclear. Inhibitors and certain substrates that bind directly to the heme iron give rise to the type II difference spectrum, with a maximum at 430 nm and a minimum at 390 nm

If no reducing equivalents are available, this complex may remain stable, allowing the degree of binding to be determined from absorbance measurements *in vitro* C: If carbon monoxide (CO) binds to reduced P450, the catalytic cycle is interrupted. This reaction yields the classic CO difference spectrum with a maximum at 450 nm.

P450s in Humans

Human CYPs are primarily membrane-associated proteins located either in the inner membrane of mitochondria or in the endoplasmic reticulum of cells. CYPs metabolize thousands of endogenous and exogenous chemicals. Some CYPs metabolize only one (or a very few) substrates, such as *CYP19* (aromatase), while others may metabolize multiple substrates. Both of these characteristics account for their central importance in medicine. Cytochrome P450 enzymes are present in most tissues of the body, and play important roles in hormone synthesis and breakdown (including estrogen and testosterone synthesis and metabolism), cholesterol synthesis, and vitamin D metabolism. Cytochrome P450 enzymes also function to metabolize potentially toxic compounds, including drugs and products of endogenous metabolism such as bilirubin, principally in the liver.

The Human Genome Project has identified 57 human genes coding for the various cytochrome P450 enzymes.

Drug Metabolism

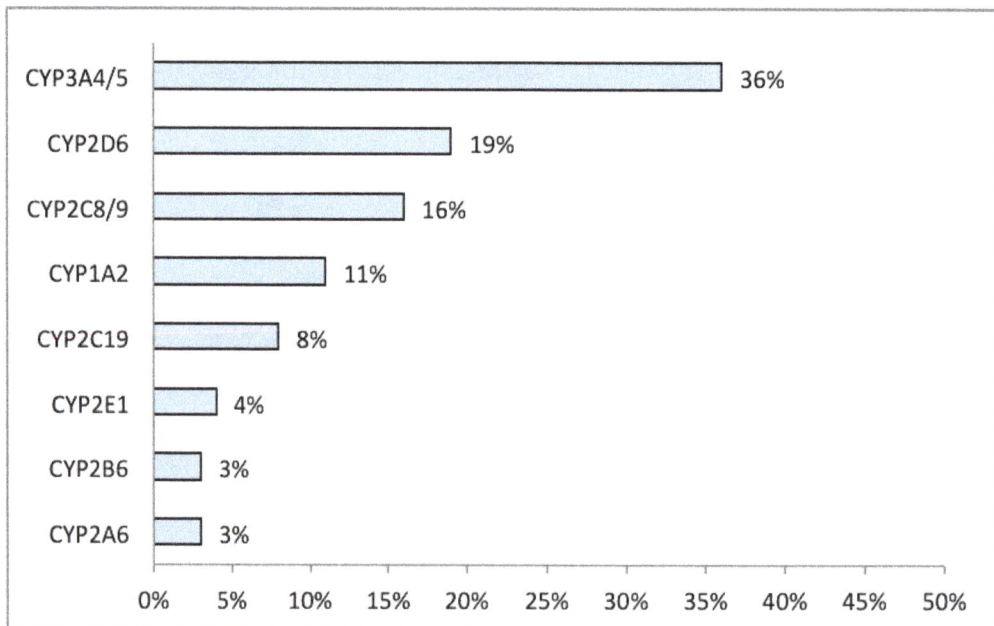

Proportion of antifungal drugs metabolized by different families of CYPs.

CYPs are the major enzymes involved in drug metabolism, accounting for about 75% of the total metabolism. Most drugs undergo deactivation by CYPs, either directly or by facilitated excretion from the body. Also, many substances are bioactivated by CYPs to form their active compounds.

Drug Interaction

Many drugs may increase or decrease the activity of various CYP isozymes either by inducing the biosynthesis of an isozyme (enzyme induction) or by directly inhibiting the activity of the CYP (enzyme inhibition). This is a major source of adverse drug interactions, since changes in CYP enzyme activity may affect the metabolism and clearance of various drugs. For example, if one drug inhibits the CYP-mediated metabolism of another drug, the second drug may accumulate within the body to toxic levels. Hence, these drug interactions may necessitate dosage adjustments or choosing drugs that do not interact with the CYP system. Such drug interactions are especially important to take into account when using drugs of vital importance to the patient, drugs with important side-effects and drugs with small therapeutic windows, but any drug may be subject to an altered plasma concentration due to altered drug metabolism.

A classical example includes anti-epileptic drugs. Phenytoin, for example, induces CYP1A2, CYP2C9, CYP2C19, and CYP3A4. Substrates for the latter may be drugs with critical dosage, like amiodarone or carbamazepine, whose blood plasma concentration may either increase because of enzyme inhibition in the former, or decrease because of enzyme induction in the latter.

Interaction of Other Substances

Naturally occurring compounds may also induce or inhibit CYP activity. For example, bioactive compounds found in grapefruit juice and some other fruit juices, including bergamottin, dihydroxybergamottin, and paradicin-A, have been found to inhibit CYP3A4-mediated metabolism of certain medications, leading to increased bioavailability and, thus, the strong possibility of overdosing. Because of this risk, avoiding grapefruit juice and fresh grapefruits entirely while on drugs is usually advised.

Other examples:

- Saint-John's wort, a common herbal remedy induces CYP3A4, but also inhibits CYP1A1, CYP1B1, and CYP2D6.

- Tobacco smoking induces CYP1A2 (example CYP1A2 substrates are clozapine, olanzapine, and fluvoxamine)

- At relatively high concentrations, starfruit juice has also been shown to inhibit CYP2A6 and other CYPs. Watercress is also a known inhibitor of the cytochrome P450 CYP2E1, which may result in altered drug metabolism for individuals on certain medications (e.g., chlorzoxazone).

- Tributyltin has been found to inhibit the function of Cytochrome P450, leading to masculinization of mollusks.

- Goldenseal, with its two notable alkaloids berberine and hydrastine, has been shown to alter P450-marker enzymatic activities (involving CYP2C9, CYP2D6, and CYP3A4).

Other Specific CYP Functions

Steroid Hormones

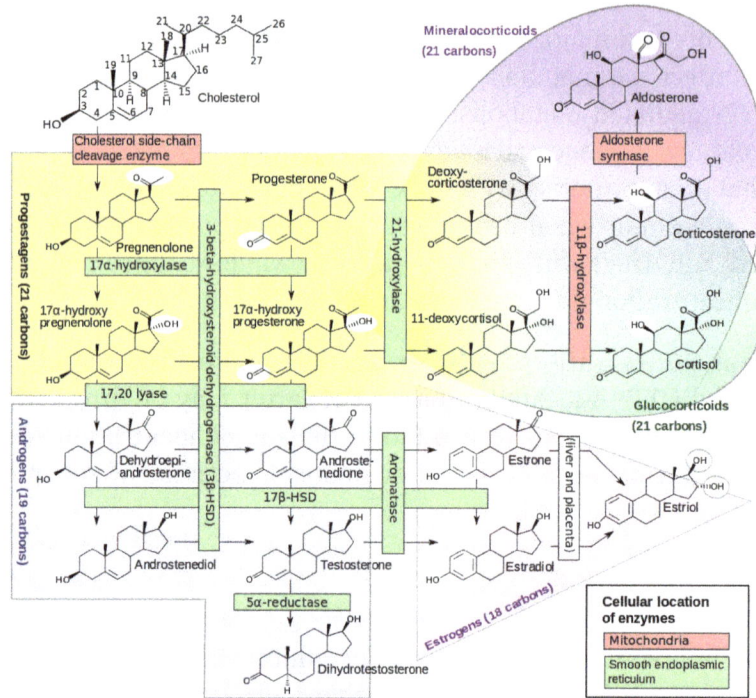

Steroidogenesis, showing many of the enzyme activities that are performed by cytochrome P450 enzymes. HSD: Hydroxysteroid dehydrogenase.

A subset of cytochrome P450 enzymes play important roles in the synthesis of steroid hormones (steroidogenesis) by the adrenals, gonads, and peripheral tissue:

- CYP11A1 (also known as P450scc or P450c11a1) in adrenal mitochondria affects "the activity formerly known as 20,22-desmolase" (steroid 20α-hydroxylase, steroid 22-hydroxylase, cholesterol side-chain scission).

- CYP11B1 (encoding the protein P450c11β) found in the inner mitochondrial membrane of adrenal cortex has steroid 11β-hydroxylase, steroid 18-hydroxylase, and steroid 18-methyloxidase activities.

- CYP11B2 (encoding the protein P450c11AS), found only in the mitochondria of the adrenal zona glomerulosa, has steroid 11β-hydroxylase, steroid 18-hydroxylase, and steroid 18-methyloxidase activities.

- CYP17A1, in endoplasmic reticulum of adrenal cortex has steroid 17α-hydroxylase and 17,20-lyase activities.

- CYP21A1 (P450c21) in adrenal cortex conducts 21-hydroxylase activity.

- CYP19A (P450arom, aromatase) in endoplasmic reticulum of gonads, brain, adipose tissue, and elsewhere catalyzes aromatization of androgens to estrogens.

Polyunsaturated Fatty Acids and Eicosanoids

Certain cytochrome P450 enzymes are critical in metabolizing polyunstaturated fatty acids (PU-FAs) to biologically active, intercellular cell signaling molecules (eicosanoids) and/or metabolize biologically active metabolites of the PUFA to less active or inactive products. These CYPs possess Cytochrome P450 omega hydroxylase and/or epoxygenase enzyme activity.

- CYP1A1, CYP1A2, and CYP2E1 metabolize endogenous PUFAs to signaling molecules: they metabolize arachidonic acid (i.e. AA) to 19-hydroxyeicosatetraenoic acid (i.e. 19-HETE; see 20-Hydroxyeicosatetraenoic acid); eicosapentaenoic acid (i.e. EPA) to epoxyeicosatetraenoic acids (i.e. EEQs); and docosahexaenoic acid (i.e. DHA) to epoxydocosapentaenoic acids (i.e. EDPs).

- CYP2C8, CYP2C9, CYP2C18, CYP2C19, and CYP2J2 metabolize endogenous PUFAs to signaling molecules: they metabolize AA to epoxyeicosatetraenoic acids (i.e. EETs); EPA to EEQs; and DHA to EDPs.

- CYP2S1 metabolizes PUFA to signaling molecules: it metabolizes AA to EETs ad EPA to EEQs.

- CYP3A4 metabolizes AA to EET signaling molecules.

- CYP4A11 metabolizes endogenous PUFAs to signaling molecules: it metabolizes AA to 20-HETE and EETs; it also hydroxylates DHA to 22-hydroxy-DHA (i.e. 12-HDHA).

- CYP4F2, CYP4F3A, and CYP4F3B metabolize PU-FAs to signaling molecules: they metabolizes AA to 20-HETE. They also metabolize EPA to 19-hydroxyeicosapentaenoic acid (19-HEPE) and 20-hydroxyeicosapentaenoic acid (20-HEPE) as well as metabolize DHA to 22-HDA. They also inactivate or reduce the activity of signaling molecules: they metabolize leukotriene B4 (LTB4) to 20-hy-droxy-LTB4, 5-hydroxyeicosatetraenoic acid (5-HETE) to 5,20-diHETE, 5-oxo-eico-satetraenoic acid (5-oxo-ETE) to 5-oxo,20-hydroxy-ETE, 12-hydroxyeicosatetraenoic acid (12-HETE) to 12,20-diHETE, EETs to 20-hydroxy-EETs, and lipoxins to 20-hydroxy products.

- CYP4F8 and CYP4F12 metabolize PUFAs to signaling molecules: they metabolizes EPA to EEQs and DHA to EDPs. They also metabolize AA to 18-hydroxyeicosatetraenoic acid (18-HETE) and 19-HETE.

- CYP4F11 inactivates or reduces the activity of signaling molecules: it metabolizes LTB4 to 20-hydroxy-LTB4, (5-HETE) to 5,20-diHETE, (5-oxo-ETE) to 5-oxo,20-hydroxy-ETE, (12-HETE) to 12,20-diHETE, EETs to 20-hydroxy-EETs, and lipoxins to 20-hydroxy products.

- CYP4F22 ω-hydroxylates extremely long "very long chain fatty acids", i.e. fatty acids that are 28 or more carbons long. The ω-hydroxylation of these special fatty acids is critical to creating and maintaining the skins water barrier function; autosomal recessive inactivating mutations of CYP4F22 are associated with the Lamellar ichthyosis subtype of Congenital ichthyosiform erythrodema in humans.

CYP Families in Humans

Humans have 57 genes and more than 59 pseudogenes divided among 18 families of cytochrome P450 genes and 43 subfamilies. This is a summary of the genes and of the proteins they encode.

Family	Function	Members	Names
CYP1	drug and steroid (especially estrogen) metabolism, benzo[*a*]pyrene toxification (forming (+)-benzo[*a*]pyrene-7,8-dihydrodiol-9,10-epoxide)	3 subfamilies, 3 genes, 1 pseudogene	CYP1A1, CYP1A2, CYP1B1
CYP2	drug and steroid metabolism	13 subfamilies, 16 genes, 16 pseudogenes	CYP2A6, CYP2A7, CYP2A13, CYP2B6, CYP2C8, CYP2C9, CYP2C18, CYP2C19, CYP2D6, CYP2E1, CYP2F1, CYP2J2, CYP2R1, CYP2S1, CYP2U1, CYP2W1
CYP3	drug and steroid (including testosterone) metabolism	1 subfamily, 4 genes, 2 pseudogenes	CYP3A4, CYP3A5, CYP3A7, CYP3A43
CYP4	arachidonic acid or fatty acid metabolism	6 subfamilies, 12 genes, 10 pseudogenes	CYP4A11, CYP4A22, CYP4B1, CYP4F2, CYP4F3, CYP4F8, CYP4F11, CYP4F12, CYP4F22, CYP4V2, CYP4X1, CYP4Z1
CYP5	thromboxane A_2 synthase	1 subfamily, 1 gene	CYP5A1
CYP7	bile acid biosynthesis 7-alpha hydroxylase of steroid nucleus	2 subfamilies, 2 genes	CYP7A1, CYP7B1
CYP8	*varied*	2 subfamilies, 2 genes	CYP8A1 (prostacyclin synthase), CYP8B1 (bile acid biosynthesis)
CYP11	steroid biosynthesis	2 subfamilies, 3 genes	CYP11A1, CYP11B1, CYP11B2
CYP17	steroid biosynthesis, 17-alpha hydroxylase	1 subfamily, 1 gene	CYP17A1
CYP19	steroid biosynthesis: aromatase synthesizes estrogen	1 subfamily, 1 gene	CYP19A1
CYP20	unknown function	1 subfamily, 1 gene	CYP20A1
CYP21	steroid biosynthesis	2 subfamilies, 1 gene, 1 pseudogene	CYP21A2
CYP24	vitamin D degradation	1 subfamily, 1 gene	CYP24A1
CYP26	retinoic acid hydroxylase	3 subfamilies, 3 genes	CYP26A1, CYP26B1, CYP26C1
CYP27	*varied*	3 subfamilies, 3 genes	CYP27A1 (bile acid biosynthesis), CYP27B1 (vitamin D_3 1-alpha hydroxylase, activates vitamin D_3), CYP27C1 (unknown function)
CYP39	7-alpha hydroxylation of 24-hydroxycholesterol	1 subfamily, 1 gene	CYP39A1
CYP46	cholesterol 24-hydroxylase	1 subfamily, 1 gene	CYP46A1
CYP51	cholesterol biosynthesis	1 subfamily, 1 gene, 3 pseudogenes	CYP51A1 (lanosterol 14-alpha demethylase)

P450s in Other Species

Animals

Many animals have as many or more CYP genes than humans do. Reported numbers range from 35 genes in the sponge *Amphimedon queenslandica* to 235 genes in the cephalochordate *Branchiostoma floridae*. Mice have genes for 101 CYPs, and sea urchins have even more (perhaps as many as 120 genes). Most CYP enzymes are presumed to have monooxygenase activity, as is the case for most mammalian CYPs that have been investigated (except for, e.g., CYP19 and CYP5). Gene and genome sequencing is far outpacing biochemical characterization of enzymatic function, though many genes with close homology to CYPs with known function have been found, giving clues to their functionality.

The classes of CYPs most often investigated in non-human animals are those either involved in development (e.g., retinoic acid or hormone metabolism) or involved in the metabolism of toxic compounds (such as heterocyclic amines or polyaromatic hydrocarbons). Often there are differences in gene regulation or enzyme function of CYPs in related animals that explain observed differences in susceptibility to toxic compounds (ex. canines inability to metabolize xanthines such as caffeine). Some drugs undergo metabolism in both species via different enzymes, resulting in different metabolites, while other drugs are metabolized in one species but excreted unchanged in another species. For this reason, one species's reaction to a substance is not a reliable indication of the substance's effects in humans.

CYPs have been extensively examined in mice, rats, dogs, and less so in zebrafish, in order to facilitate use of these model organisms in drug discovery and toxicology. Recently CYPs have also been discovered in avian species, in particular turkeys, that may turn out to be a great model for cancer research in humans. CYP1A5 and CYP3A37 in turkeys were found to be very similar to the human CYP1A2 and CYP3A4 respectively, in terms of their kinetic properties as well as in the metabolism of aflatoxin B1.

CYPs have also been heavily studied in insects, often to understand pesticide resistance. For example, CYP6G1 is linked to insecticide resistance in DDT-resistant Drosophila melanogaster and CYP6Z1 in the mosquito malaria vector Anopheles gambiae is capable of directly metabolizing DDT.

Microbial

Microbial cytochromes P450 are often soluble enzymes and are involved in diverse metabolic processes. In bacteria the distribution of P450s is very variable with many bacteria having no identified P450s (e.g. E.coli). Some bacteria, predominantly actinomycetes, have numerous P450s (e.g.,). Those so far identified are generally involved in either biotransformation of xenobiotic compounds (e.g. CYP105A1 from Streptomyces griseolus metabolizes sulfonylurea herbicides to less toxic derivatives,) or are part of specialised metabolite biosynthetic pathways (e.g. CYP170B1 catalyses production of the sesquiterpenoid albaflavenone in Streptomyces albus,). Although no P450 has yet been shown to be essential in a microbe, the CYP105 family is highly conserved with a representative in every streptomycete genome sequenced so far (). Due to the solubility of bacterial P450 enzymes, they are generally regarded as easier to work with than the predominantly membrane bound eukaryotic P450s. This, combined with the remarkable chemistry they catalyse, has led to many studies using the heterologously expressed proteins in vitro. Few studies have investigated what P450s do in vivo, what the natural substrate(s) are and how P450s contribute to survival of the bacteria in the natural environment.Three examples that have contributed significantly to structural and mechanistic studies are listed here, but many different families exist.

- Cytochrome P450cam (CYP101) originally from *Pseudomonas putida* has been used as a model for many cytochromes P450 and was the first cytochrome P450 three-dimensional protein structure solved by X-ray crystallography. This enzyme is part of a camphor-hydroxylating catalytic cycle consisting of two electron transfer steps from putidaredoxin, a 2Fe-2S cluster-containing protein cofactor.

- Cytochrome P450 eryF (CYP107A1) originally from the actinomycete bacterium *Saccharopolyspora erythraea* is responsible for the biosynthesis of the antibiotic erythromycin by C6-hydroxylation of the macrolide 6-deoxyerythronolide B.

- Cytochrome P450 BM3 (CYP102A1) from the soil bacterium *Bacillus megaterium* catalyzes the NADPH-dependent hydroxylation of several long-chain fatty acids at the $\omega-1$ through $\omega-3$ positions. Unlike almost every other known CYP (except CYP505A1, cytochrome P450 foxy), it constitutes a natural fusion protein between the CYP domain and an electron donating cofactor. Thus, BM3 is potentially very useful in biotechnological applications.

- Cytochrome P450 119 (CYP119) isolated from the thermophillic archea *Sulfolobus acidocaldarius* has been used in a variety of mechanistic studies. Because thermophillic enzymes evolved to function at high temperatures, they tend to function more slowly at room temperature (if at all) and are therefore excellent mechanistic models.

Fungi

The commonly used azole class antifungal drugs work by inhibition of the fungal cytochrome P450 14α-demethylase. This interrupts the conversion of lanosterol to ergosterol, a component of the fungal cell membrane. (This is useful only because humans' P450 have a different sensitivity; this is how this class of antifungals work.)

Significant research is ongoing into fungal P450s, as a number of fungi are pathogenic to humans (such as Candida yeast and Aspergillus) and to plants.

Cunninghamella elegans is a candidate for use as a model for mammalian drug metabolism.

Plants

Plant cytochrome P450s are involved in a wide range of biosynthetic reactions and target a diverse range of biomolecules. These reactions lead to various fatty acid conjugates, plant hormones, secondary metabolites, lignins, and a variety of defensive compounds. Plant genome annotations suggest that Cytochrome P450 genes make up as much as 1% of the plant genes. The number and diversity of P450 genes is responsible, in part, for the multitude of bioactive compounds.

P450s in Biotechnology

The remarkable reactivity and substrate promiscuity of P450s have long attracted the attention of chemists. Recent progress towards realizing the potential of using P450s towards difficult oxidations have included: (i) eliminating the need for natural co-factors by replacing them with inexpensive peroxide containing molecules, (ii) exploring the compatibility of p450s with organic solvents, and (iii) the use of small, non-chiral auxiliaries to predictably direct P450 oxidation.

InterPro Subfamilies

InterPro subfamilies:

- Cytochrome P450, B-class InterPro: *IPR002397*

- Cytochrome P450, mitochondrial InterPro: *IPR002399*

- Cytochrome P450, E-class, group I InterPro: *IPR002401*

- Cytochrome P450, E-class, group II InterPro: *IPR002402*

- Cytochrome P450, E-class, group IV InterPro: *IPR002403*

- Aromatase

Clozapine, imipramine, paracetamol, phenacetin Heterocyclic aryl amines Inducible and CYP1A2 5-10% deficient oxidize uroporphyrinogen to uroporphyrin (CYP1A2) in heme metabolism, but they may have additional undiscovered endogenous substrates. are inducible by some polycyclic hydrocarbons, some of which are found in cigarette smoke and charred food.

These enzymes are of interest, because in assays, they can activate compounds to carcinogens. High levels of CYP1A2 have been linked to an increased risk of colon cancer. Since the 1A2 enzyme can be induced by cigarette smoking, this links smoking with colon cancer.

Flavin-containing Monooxygenase

The flavin-containing monooxygenase (FMO) protein family specializes in the oxidation of xeno-substrates in order to facilitate the excretion of these compounds from living organisms. These enzymes can oxidize a wide array of heteroatoms, particularly soft nucleophiles, such as amines, sulfides, and phosphites. This reaction requires an oxygen, an NADPH cofactor, and an FAD prosthetic group. FMOs share several structural features, such as a NADPH binding domain, FAD binding domain, and a conserved arginine residue present in the active site. Recently, FMO enzymes have received a great deal of attention from the pharmaceutical industry both as a drug target for various diseases and as a means to metabolize pro-drug compounds into active pharmaceuticals. These monooxygenases are often misclassified because they share activity profiles similar to those of cytochrome P450 (CYP450), which is the major contributor to oxidative xenobiotic metabolism. However, a key difference between the two enzymes lies in how they proceed to oxidize their respective substrates; CYP enzymes make use of an oxygenated heme prosthetic group, while the FMO family utilizes FAD to oxidize its substrates.

History

Prior to the 1960s, the oxidation of xenotoxic materials was thought to be completely accomplished by CYP450. However, in the early 1970s, Dr. Daniel Ziegler from the University of Texas at Austin discovered a hepatic flavoprotein isolated from pig liver that was found to oxidize a vast array of various amines to their corresponding nitro state. This flavoprotein named "Ziegler's enzyme" exhibited unusual chemical and spectrometric properties. Upon further spectroscopic characterization and investigation of the substrate pool of this enzyme, Dr. Ziegler discovered that this enzyme solely bound FAD molecule that could form a C4a-hydroxyperoxyflavin intermediate, and that this enzyme could oxidize a wide variety of substrates with no common structural features, including phosphines, sulfides, selenium compounds, amongst others. Once this was noticed, Dr. Ziegler's enzyme was reclassified as a broadband flavin monooxygenase.

In 1984, the first evidence for multiple forms of FMOs was elucidated by two different laboratories when two distinct FMOs were isolated from rabbit lungs. Since then, over 150 different FMO enzymes have been successfully isolated from a wide variety of organisms. Up until 2002, only 5 FMO enzymes were successfully isolated from mammals. However, a group of researchers found a sixth FMO gene located on human chromosome 1. In addition to the sixth FMO discovered as of 2002, the laboratories of Dr. Ian Philips and Elizabeth Sheppard discovered a second gene cluster in humans that consists of 5 additional pseudogenes for FMO on human chromosome 1.

Evolution of FMO Gene Family

The FMO family of genes is conserved across all phyla that have been studied so far, therefore some form of the FMO gene family can be found in all studied eukaryotes. FMO genes are characterized by specific structural and functional constraints, which led to the evolution of different types of FMO's in order to perform a variety of functions. Divergence between the functional types of FMO's (FMO 1–5) occurred before the amphibians and mammals diverged into separate classes. FMO5 found in vertebrates appears to be evolutionarily older than other types of FMO's, making FMO5 the first functionally distinct member of the FMO family. Phylogenetic studies suggest that FMO1 and FMO3 are the most recent FMO's to evolve into enzymes with distinct functions. Although FMO5 was the first distinct FMO, it is not clear what function it serves since it does not oxygenate the typical FMO substrates involved in first-pass metabolism.

Analyses of FMO genes across several species have shown extensive silent DNA mutations, which indicate that the current FMO gene family exists because of selective pressure at the protein level rather than the nucleotide level. FMO's found in invertebrates are found to have originated polyphyletically; meaning that a phenotypically similar gene evolved in invertebrates which was not inherited from a common ancestor.

Classification and Characterization

FMOs are one subfamily of class B external flavoprotein monooxygenases (EC 1.14.13), which belong to the family of monooxygenase oxidoreductases, along with the other subfamilies Baeyer-Villiger monooxygenases and microbial N-hydroxylating monooxygenases. FMO's are found in fungi, yeast, plants, mammals, and bacteria.

Mammals

Developmental and tissue specific expression has been studied in several mammalian species, including humans, mice, rats, and rabbits. However, because FMO expression is unique to each animal species, it is difficult to make conclusions about human FMO regulation and activity based on other mammalian studies. It is likely that species-specific expression of FMO's contributes to differences in susceptibility to toxins and xenobiotics as well as the efficiency with excreting among different mammals.

Six functional forms of human FMO genes have been reported. However, FMO6 is considered to be a pseudogene. FMOs 1–5 share between 50–58% amino acid identity across the different species. Recently, five more human FMO genes were discovered, although they fall in the category of pseudogenes.

- FMO1, FMO2, FMO3, FMO4, FMO5, FMO6

Yeast

Unlike mammals, yeast (*Saccharomyces cerevisiae*) do not have several isoforms of FMO, but instead only have one called yFMO. This enzyme does not accept xenobiotic compounds. Instead, yFMO helps to fold proteins that contain disulfide bonds by catalyzing O_2 and NADPH-dependent oxidations of biological thiols, just like mammalian FMO's. An example is the oxidation of glutathione to glutathione disulfide, both of which form a redox buffering system in the cell between the endoplasmic reticulum and the cytoplasm. yFMO is localized in the cytoplasm in order to maintain the optimum redox buffer ratio necessary for proteins containing disulfide bonds to fold properly. This non-xenobiotic role of yFMO may represent the original role of the FMO's before the rise of the modern FMO family of enzymes found in mammals.

Plants

Plant FMO's play a role in defending against pathogens and catalyze specific steps in the biosynthesis of auxin, a plant hormone. Plant FMO's also play a role in the metabolism of glucosinolates. These non-xenobiotic roles of plant FMO's suggest that other FMO functions could be identified in non-plant organisms.

Structure

Crystal structures have been determined for yeast (*Schizosaccharomyces pombe*) FMO (PDB: 1VQW) and bacterial (*Methylophaga aminisulfidivorans*) FMO (PDB: 2XVH). The crystal structures are similar to each other and they share 27% sequence identity. These enzymes share 22% and 31% sequence identity with human FMOs, respectively.

FMOs have a tightly bound FAD prosthetic group and a binding NADPH cofactor. Both dinucleotide binding motifs form Rossmann folds. The yeast FMO and bacterial FMO are dimers, with each monomer consisting of two structural domains: the smaller NADPH binding domain and the larger FAD-binding domain. The two domains are connected by a double linker. A channel between the two domains leads to the active site where NADPH binds both domains and occupies a cleft that blocks access to the flavin group of FAD, which is bound to the large domain along the channel together with a water molecule. The nicotinamide group of NADPH interacts with the flavin group of FAD, and the NADPH binding site overlaps with the substrate binding site on the flavin group.

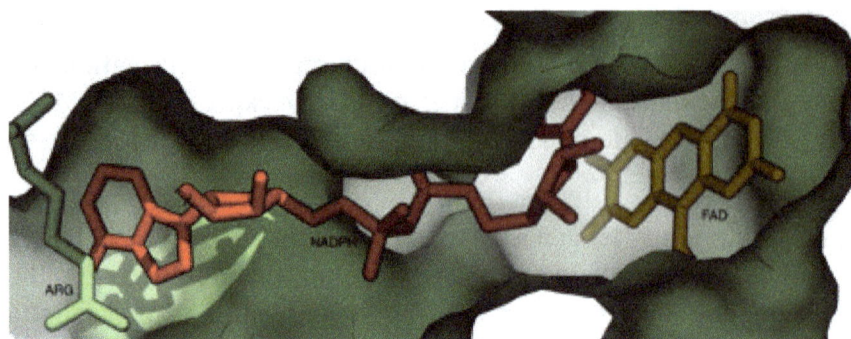

Channel and active site of bacterial FMO with bound NADPH and FAD (PDB: 2XVH).

FMOs contain several sequence motifs that are conserved across all domains:

- FAD-binding motif (GXGXXG)

- FMO identifying motif (FXGXXXHXXXF/Y)

- NADPH-binding motif (GXSXXA)

- F/LATGY motif

- arginine residue in the active site

The FMO identifying motif interacts with the flavin of FAD. The F/LATGY motif is a sequence motif common in *N*-hydroxylating enzymes. The arginine residue interacts with the phosphate group of NADPH.

Function

The general function of these enzymes is to metabolise xenobiotics. Hence, they are considered to be xenobiotic detoxication catalysts. These proteins catalyze the oxygenation of multiple heteroatom-containing compounds that are present in our diet, such as amine-, sulfide-, phosphorus-, and other nucleophilic heteroatom-containing compounds. FMOs have been implicated in the metabolism of a number of pharmaceuticals, pesticides and toxicants, by converting the lipophilic xenobiotics into polar, oxygenated, and readily excreted metabolites.

N-Oxidation

tertiary amines to amine oxides

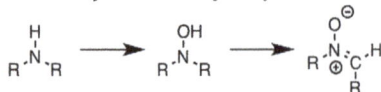

secondary amines to hydroxylamines to nitrones

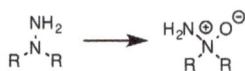

hydrazines

S-Oxidation

thiols to disulfides

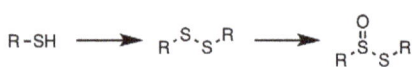

sulfides to sulfoxides to sulfones

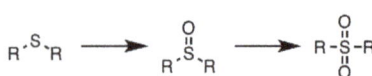

thiones

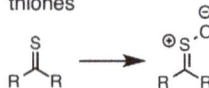

Reactions catalyzed by FMOs.

Substrate Diversity

FMO substrates are structurally diverse compounds. However, they all share similar characteristics:

- Soft nucleophiles (basic amines, sulfides, Se- or P-containing compounds)

- Neutral or single-positively charged

Zwitterions, anions and dications are considered to be unfavorable substrates. There are several drugs reported to be typical substrates for FMOs.

Typical Drug Substrates		
Albendazole	Clindamycin	Pargyline
Benzydamine	Fenbendazole	Ranitidine
Chlorpheniramine	Itopride	Thioridazine
Cimetidine	Olopatadine	Sulindac sulfide
Xanomeline	Zimeldine	

The majority of drugs function as alternate substrate competitive inhibitors to FMOs (i.e. good nucleophiles that compete with the drug for FMO oxygenation), since they are not likely to serve as FMO substrates. Only a few true FMO competitive inhibitors have been reported. Those include indole-3-carbinol and N,N-dimethylamino stilbene carboxylates. A well-known FMO inhibitor is methimazole (MMI).

Mechanism

Catalytic cycle of FMOs together with the redox state of the FAD prosthetic group.

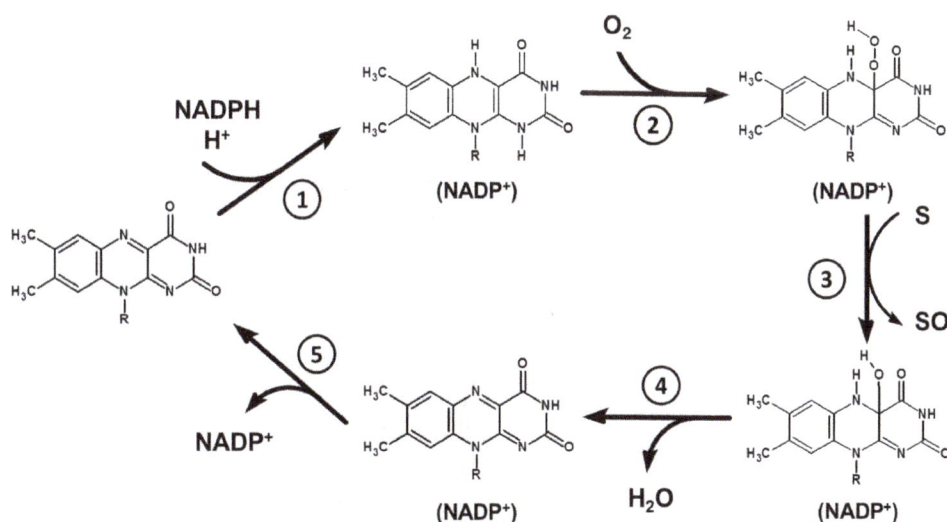

The FMO catalytic cycle proceeds as follows:

1. The cofactor NADPH binds to the oxidized state of the FAD prosthetic group, reducing it to $FADH_2$.

2. Molecular oxygen binds to the formed NADP⁺-FADH₂-enzyme complex and is reduced, resulting in 4a-hydroperoxyflavin (4a-HPF or FADH-OOH). This specie is stabilized by $NADP^+$ in the catalytic site of the enzyme. These first two steps in the cycle are fast.

3. In the presence of a substrate (S), a nucleophilic attack occurs on the distal O-atom of the prosthetic group. The substrate is oxygenated to SO, forming the 4a-hydroxyflavin (FADH-OH). Only when the flavin is in the hydroperoxy form is when the xenobiotic substrate will react.

4. The flavin product then breaks down with release of water to reform FAD.

5. Due to the low dissociation constant of the $NADP^+$-enzyme complex, $NADP^+$ is released by the end of the cycle and the enzyme returns to its original state. The rate-limiting step involves either the breakdown of FADH-OH to water or the release of $NADP^+$.

6. Quantum mechanics simulations showed the N-hydroxylation catalyzed by flavin-containing monooxygenases initiated by homolysis of the O-O bond in the C4a-hydroperoxyflavin intermediate resulting in the formation of an internal hydrogen bonded hydroxyl radical.

Cellular Expression in Humans

Expression of each type of FMO relies on several factors including, cofactor supply, physiological & environmental factors, as well as diet. Because of these factors, each type of FMO is expressed differently depending on the species and tissue. In humans, expression of FMO's is mainly concentrated to the human liver, lungs, and kidneys, where most of the metabolism of xenobiotics occur. However, FMO's can also be found in the human brain and small intestine. While FMO1-5 can be found in the brain, liver, kidneys, lungs, and small intestine, the distribution of each type of FMO differs depending on the tissue and the developmental stage of the person.

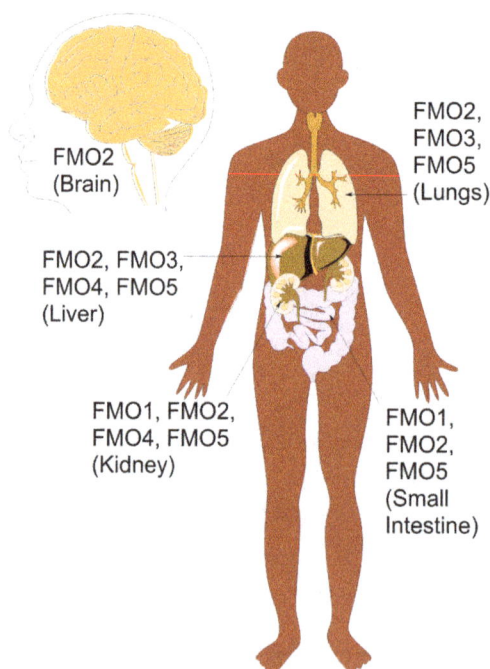

FMO2
(Brain)

FMO2,
FMO3,
FMO5
(Lungs)

FMO2, FMO3,
FMO4, FMO5
(Liver)

FMO1, FMO2,
FMO4, FMO5
(Kidney)

FMO1,
FMO2,
FMO5
(Small
Intestine)

Main distributions of different types of Flavin-containing Monooxygenases (FMO) in adult human tissues.

Expression in Adult Tissues

In an adult, FMO1 is predominately expressed in the kidneys and to a lesser extent in the lungs and small intestine. FMO2 is the most abundant of the FMO's and is mostly expressed in the lungs and kidneys, with lower expression in the liver and small intestine. FMO3 is highly concentrated in the liver, but is also expressed in the lungs. FMO4 is expressed mostly in the liver and kidneys. FMO5 is highly expressed in the liver, but also has substantial expression in the lungs and small intestine. Though FMO2 is the most expressed FMO in the brain, it only constitutes about 1% of that found in the lungs, making FMO expression in the brain fairly low.

Expression in Fetal Tissues

The distribution of FMO's in various types of tissues changes as a person continues to develop, making the fetal distribution of FMO's quite different than adult distribution of FMO's. While the adult liver is dominated by the expression of FMO3 and FMO5, the fetal liver is dominated by the expression of FMO1 and FMO5. Another difference is in the brain, where adults mostly express FMO2 and fetuses mostly express FMO1.

Clinical Significance

Drug Development

Drug metabolism is one of the most important factors to consider when developing new drugs for therapeutic applications. The degradation rate of these new drugs in an organism's system determines the duration and intensity of their pharmacological action. During the past few years, FMOs have gained a lot of attention in drug development since these enzymes are not readily induced or inhibited by the chemicals or drugs surrounding their environment. CYPs are the primary enzymes involved in drug metabolism. However, recent efforts have been directed towards the development of drug candidates that incorporate functional groups that can be metabolized by FMOs. By doing this, the number of potential adverse drug-drug interactions is minimized and the reliance on CYP450 metabolism is decreased. Several approaches have been made to screen potential drug interactions. One of them includes human FMO3 (hFMO3), which is described as the most vital FMO regarding drug interactions. In order to successfully screen hFMO3 in a high throughput fashion hFMO3 was successfully fixed to graphene oxide chips in order to measure the change in electrical potential generated as a result of the drug being oxidized when it interacts with the enzyme.

Hypertension

There is evidence that FMOs are associated to the regulation of blood pressure. FMO3 is involved in the formation of TMA N-oxides (TMAO). Some studies indicate that hypertension can develop when there are no organic osmolytes (i.e. TMAO) that can counteract an increase in osmotic pressure and peripheral resistance. Individuals with deficient FMO3 activity have a higher prevalence of hypertension and other cardiovascular diseases, since there is a decrease in formation of TMA N-oxides to counterbalance the effects of a higher osmotic pressure and peripheral resistance.

Fish Odor Syndrome

The trimethylaminuria disorder, also known as fish odor syndrome, causes abnormal FMO3-mediated metabolism or a deficiency of this enzyme in an individual. A person with this disorder has a low capacity to oxidize the trimethylamine (TMA) that comes from their diet to its odourless metabolite TMAO. When this happens, large amounts of TMA are excreted through the individual's urine, sweat, and breath, with a strong fish-like odor. As of today, there is no known cure or treatment for this disorder. However, doctors recommend patients to avoid foods containing choline, carnitine, nitrogen, sulfur and lecithin.

Other Diseases

FMOs have also been associated with other diseases, such as cancer and diabetes. Yet, additional studies are imperative to elucidate what is the relationship between FMO function and these diseases, as well as to define these enzymes' clinical relevance.

Alcohol Dehydrogenase

Alcohol dehydrogenases (ADH) (EC 1.1.1.1) are a group of dehydrogenase enzymes that occur in many organisms and facilitate the interconversion between alcohols and aldehydes or ketones with the reduction of nicotinamide adenine dinucleotide (NAD^+ to NADH). In humans and many other animals, they serve to break down alcohols that otherwise are toxic, and they also participate in generation of useful aldehyde, ketone, or alcohol groups during biosynthesis of various metabolites. In yeast, plants, and many bacteria, some alcohol dehydrogenases catalyze the opposite reaction as part of fermentation to ensure a constant supply of NAD^+.

Evolution

Genetic evidence from comparisons of multiple organisms showed that a glutathione-dependent formaldehyde dehydrogenase, identical to a class III alcohol dehydrogenase (ADH-3/ADH5), is presumed to be the ancestral enzyme for the entire ADH family. Early on in evolution, an effective method for eliminating both endogenous and exogenous formaldehyde was important and this capacity has conserved the ancestral ADH-3 through time. Gene duplication of ADH-3, followed by series of mutations, the other ADHs evolved.

The ability to produce ethanol from sugar (which is the basis of how alcoholic beverages are made) is believed to have initially evolved in yeast. Though this feature is not adaptive from an energy point of view, by making alcohol in such high concentrations so that they would be toxic to other organisms, yeast cells could effectively eliminate their competition. Since rotting fruit can contain more than 4% of ethanol, animals eating the fruit needed a system to metabolize exogenous ethanol. This was thought to explain the conservation of ethanol active ADH in other species than yeast, though ADH-3 is now known to also have a major role in nitric oxide signaling.

In humans, sequencing of the ADH1B gene (responsible for production of an alcohol dehydrogenase polypeptide) shows two variants, in which there is an SNP (single nucleotide polymorphism) that leads to either a Histidine or an Arginine residue in the enzyme catalyzing the conversion of ethanol into acetaldehyde. In the Histidine variant, the enzyme is much more effective at the aforementioned conversion. The enzyme responsible for the conversion of acetaldehyde to acetate, however, remains unaffected, which leads to differential rates of substrate catalysis and causes a buildup of toxic acetaldehyde, causing cell damage. In humans, various haplotypes arising from this mutation are more concentrated in regions near Eastern China, a region also known for its low alcohol tolerance and dependence.

A study was conducted in order to find a correlation between allelic distribution and alcoholism, and the results suggest that the allelic distribution arose along with rice cultivation in the region between 12,000 and 6,000 years ago. In regions where rice was cultivated, rice was also fermented into ethanol. The results of increased alcohol availability led to alcoholism and abuse by those able to acquire it, resulting in lower reproductive fitness. Those with the variant allele have little tolerance for alcohol, thus lowering chance of dependence and abuse. The hypothesis posits that those individuals with the His variant enzyme were sensitive enough to the effects of alcohol that differential reproductive success arose and the corresponding alleles were passed through the generations.

Classical Darwinian evolution would act to select against the detrimental form of the enzyme (Arg variant) because of the lowered reproductive success of individuals carrying the allele. The result would be a higher frequency of the allele responsible for the His-variant enzyme in regions that had been under selective pressure the longest. The distribution and frequency of the His variant follows the spread of rice cultivation to inland regions of Asia, with higher frequencies of the His variant in regions that have cultivated rice the longest. The geographic distribution of the alleles seems to therefore be a result of natural selection against individuals with lower reproductive success, namely, those who carried the Arg variant allele and were more susceptible to alcoholism.

Discovery

The first-ever isolated alcohol dehydrogenase (ADH) was purified in 1937 from *Saccharomyces cerevisiae* (brewer's yeast). Many aspects of the catalytic mechanism for the horse liver ADH enzyme were investigated by Hugo Theorell and coworkers. ADH was also one of the first oligomeric enzymes that had its amino acid sequence and three-dimensional structure determined.

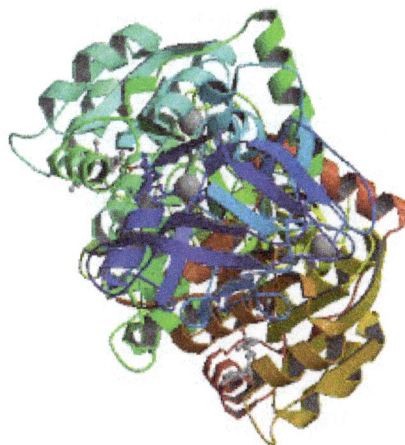

Horse LADH (Liver Alcohol Dehydrogenase)

In early 1960, it was discovered in fruit flies of the genus *Drosophila*.

Properties

The alcohol dehydrogenases comprise a group of several isozymes that catalyse the oxidation of primary and secondary alcohols to aldehydes and ketones, respectively, and also can catalyse the reverse reaction. In mammals this is a redox (reduction/oxidation) reaction involving the coenzyme nicotinamide adenine dinucleotide (NAD^+).

Alcohol dehydrogenase is a dimer with a mass of 80 kDa.

Oxidation of Alcohol

Steps

1. Binding of the coenzyme NAD^+

2. Binding of the alcohol substrate by coordination to zinc

3. Deprotonation of His-51

4. Deprotonation of nicotinamide ribose

5. Deprotonation of Thr-48

6. Deprotonation of the alcohol

7. Hydride transfer from the alkoxide ion to NAD^+, leading to NADH and a zinc bound aldehyde or ketone

8. Release of the product aldehyde.

The mechanism in yeast and bacteria is the reverse of this reaction. These steps are supported through kinetic studies.

Involved Subunits

The substrate is coordinated to the zinc and this enzyme has two zinc atoms per subunit. One is the active site, which is involved in catalysis. In the active site, the ligands are Cys-46, Cys-174, His-67, and one water molecule. The other subunit is involved with structure. In this mechanism, the hydride from the alcohol goes to NAD^+. Crystal structures indicate that the His-51 deprotonates the nicotinamide ribose, which deprotonates Ser-48. Finally, Ser-48 deprotonates the alcohol, making it an aldehyde. From a mechanistic perspective, if the enzyme adds hydride to the re face of NAD^+, the resulting hydrogen is incorporated into the pro-R position. Enzymes that add hydride to the re face are deemed Class A dehydrogenases.

Active Site

The active site of human ADH1 (PDB:1HSO) consists of a zinc atom, His-67, Cys-174, Cys-46, Thr-48, His-51, Ile-269, Val-292, Ala-317, and Leu-319. In the commonly studied horse liver isoform,

Thr-48 is a Ser, and Leu-319 is a Phe. The zinc coordinates the substrate (alcohol). The zinc is co-ordinated by Cys-46, Cys-174, and His-67. Leu-319, Ala-317, His-51, Ile-269 and Val-292 stabilize NAD$^+$ by forming hydrogen bonds. His-51 and Ile-269 form hydrogen bonds with the alcohols on nicotinamide ribose. Phe-319, Ala-317 and Val-292 form hydrogen bonds with the amide on NAD$^+$.

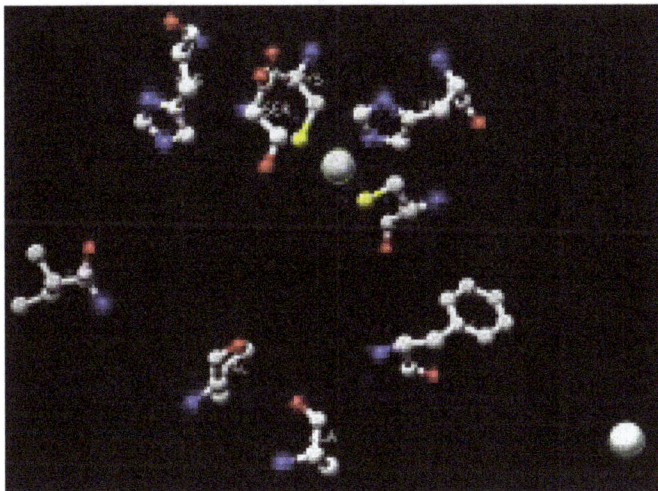

The active site of alcohol dehydrogenase

Structural Zinc Site

Mammalian alcohol dehydrogenases also have a structural zinc site. This Zn ion plays a structural role and is crucial for protein stability. The structures of the catalytic and structural zinc sites in horse liver alcohol dehydrogenase (HLADH) as revealed in crystallographic structures, which has been studied computationally with quantum chemical as well as with classical molecular dynamics methods. The structural zinc site is composed of four closely spaced cysteine ligands (Cys97, Cys100, Cys103, and Cys111 in the amino acid sequence) positioned in an almost symmetric tetra-hedron around the Zn ion. A recent study showed that the interaction between zinc and cysteine is governed by primarily an electrostatic contribution with an additional covalent contribution to the binding.

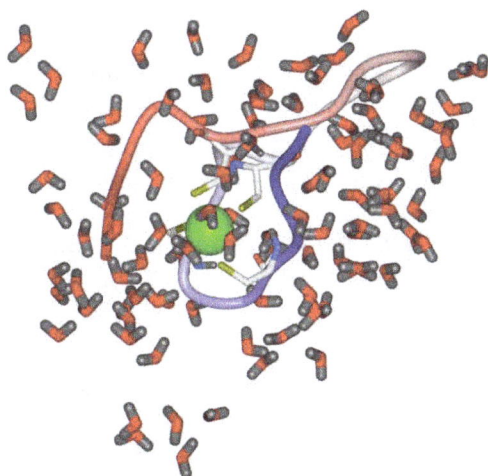

The structural zinc binding motif in alcohol dehydrogenase from a MD simulation

Types

Human

In humans, ADH exists in multiple forms as a dimer and is encoded by at least seven different genes. There are five classes (I-V) of alcohol dehydrogenase, but the hepatic form that is used primarily in humans is class 1. Class 1 consists of α, β, and γ subunits that are encoded by the genes ADH1A, ADH1B, and ADH1C. The enzyme is present at high levels in the liver and the lining of the stomach. It catalyzes the oxidation of ethanol to acetaldehyde (ethanal):

$$CH_3CH_2OH + NAD^+ \rightarrow CH_3CHO + NADH + H^+$$

This allows the consumption of alcoholic beverages, but its evolutionary purpose is probably the breakdown of alcohols naturally contained in foods or produced by bacteria in the digestive tract.

Another evolutionary purpose may be metabolism of the endogenous alcohol vitamin A (retinol), which generates the hormone retinoic acid, although the function here may be primarily the elimination of toxic levels of retinol.

alcohol dehydrogenase 1A, α polypeptide	
Identifiers	
Symbol	ADH1A
Alt. symbols	ADH1
Entrez	124
HUGO	249
OMIM	103700
RefSeq	NM_000667
UniProt	P07327
Other data	
EC number	1.1.1.1
Locus	Chr. 4 *q23*

alcohol dehydrogenase 1B, β polypeptide	
Identifiers	
Symbol	ADH1B
Alt. symbols	ADH2
Entrez	125
HUGO	250
OMIM	103720
RefSeq	NM_000668
UniProt	P00325
Other data	
EC number	1.1.1.1
Locus	Chr. 4 *q23*

alcohol dehydrogenase 1C, γ polypeptide	
Identifiers	
Symbol	ADH1C
Alt. symbols	ADH3
Entrez	126
HUGO	251
OMIM	103730
RefSeq	NM_000669
UniProt	P00326
Other data	
EC number	1.1.1.1
Locus	Chr. 4 *q23*

Alcohol dehydrogenase is also involved in the toxicity of other types of alcohol: For instance, it oxidizes methanol to produce formaldehyde and ethylene glycol to ultimately yield glycolic and oxalic acids. Humans have at least six slightly different alcohol dehydrogenases. Each is a dimer (i.e., consists of two polypeptides), with each dimer containing two zinc ions Zn^{2+}. One of those ions is crucial for the operation of the enzyme: It is located at the catalytic site and holds the hydroxyl group of the alcohol in place.

Alcohol dehydrogenase activity varies between men and women, between young and old, and among populations from different areas of the world. For example, young women are unable to process alcohol at the same rate as young men because they do not express the alcohol dehydrogenase as highly, although the inverse is true among the middle-aged. The level of activity may not be dependent only on level of expression but also on allelic diversity among the population.

The human genes that encode class II, III, IV, and V alcohol dehydrogenases are ADH4, ADH5, ADH7, and ADH6, respectively.

alcohol dehydrogenase 4 (class II), π polypeptide	
Identifiers	
Symbol	ADH4
Entrez	127
HUGO	252
OMIM	103740
RefSeq	NM_000670
UniProt	P08319
Other data	
EC number	1.1.1.1
Locus	Chr. 4 *q22*

alcohol dehydrogenase 5 (class III), χ polypeptide	
Identifiers	
Symbol	ADH5
Entrez	128
HUGO	253
OMIM	103710
RefSeq	NM_000671
UniProt	P11766
Other data	
EC number	1.1.1.1
Locus	Chr. 4 *q23*

alcohol dehydrogenase 6 (class V)	
Identifiers	
Symbol	ADH6
Entrez	130
HUGO	255
OMIM	103735
RefSeq	NM_000672
UniProt	P28332
Other data	
EC number	1.1.1.1
Locus	Chr. 4 *q23*

alcohol dehydrogenase 7 (class IV), μ or σ polypeptide	
Identifiers	
Symbol	ADH7
Entrez	131
HUGO	256
OMIM	600086
RefSeq	NM_000673
UniProt	P40394
Other data	
EC number	1.1.1.1
Locus	Chr. 4 *q23-q24*

Yeast and Bacteria

Unlike humans, yeast and bacteria (except lactic acid bacteria, and *E. coli* in certain conditions) do not ferment glucose to lactate. Instead, they ferment it to ethanol and CO_2. The overall reaction can be seen below:

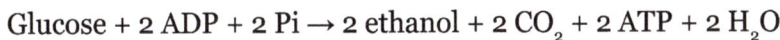

Glucose + 2 ADP + 2 Pi → 2 ethanol + 2 CO_2 + 2 ATP + 2 H_2O

In yeast and many bacteria, alcohol dehydrogenase plays an important part in fermentation: Pyruvate resulting from glycolysis is converted to acetaldehyde and carbon dioxide, and the acetaldehyde is then reduced to ethanol by an alcohol dehydrogenase called ADH1. The purpose of this latter step is the regeneration of NAD^+, so that the energy-generating glycolysis can continue. Humans exploit this process to produce alcoholic beverages, by letting yeast ferment various fruits or grains. It is interesting to note that yeast can produce and consume their own alcohol.

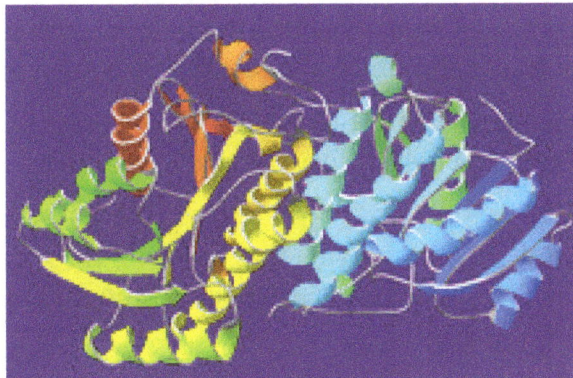

Alcohol Dehydrogenase

The main alcohol dehydrogenase in yeast is larger than the human one, consisting of four rather than just two subunits. It also contains zinc at its catalytic site. Together with the zinc-containing alcohol dehydrogenases of animals and humans, these enzymes from yeasts and many bacteria form the family of "long-chain"-alcohol dehydrogenases.

Brewer's yeast also has another alcohol dehydrogenase, ADH2, which evolved out of a duplicate version of the chromosome containing the ADH1 gene. ADH2 is used by the yeast to convert ethanol back into acetaldehyde, and it is expressed only when sugar concentration is low. Having these two enzymes allows yeast to produce alcohol when sugar is plentiful (and this alcohol then kills off competing microbes), and then continue with the oxidation of the alcohol once the sugar, and competition, is gone.

Plants

In plants, ADH catalyses the same reaction as in yeast and bacteria to ensure that there is a constant supply of NAD^+. Maize has two versions of ADH - ADH1 and ADH2, *Arabidopsis thaliana* contains only one ADH gene. The structure of *Arabidopsis* ADH is 47%-conserved, relative to ADH from horse liver. Structurally and functionally important residues, such as the seven residues that provide ligands for the catalytic and noncatalytic zinc atoms, however, are conserved, suggesting that the enzymes have a similar structure. ADH is constitutively expressed at low levels in the roots of young plants grown on agar. If the roots lack oxygen, the expression of *ADH* increases significantly. Its expression is also increased in response to dehydration, to low temperatures, and to abscisic acid, and it plays an important role in fruit ripening, seedlings development, and pollen development. Differences in the sequences of *ADH* in different species have been used to create phylogenies showing how closely related different species of plants are. It is an ideal gene to use due to its convenient size (2–3 kb in length with a ~1000 nucleotide coding sequence) and low copy number.

Iron-containing

A third family of alcohol dehydrogenases, unrelated to the above two, are iron-containing ones. They occur in bacteria and fungi. In comparison to enzymes the above families, these enzymes are oxygen-sensitive. Members of the iron-containing alcohol dehydrogenase family include:

- *Saccharomyces cerevisiae* alcohol dehydrogenase 4 (gene ADH4)

- *Zymomonas mobilis* alcohol dehydrogenase 2 (gene adhB)

- *Escherichia coli* propanediol oxidoreductase EC 1.1.1.77 (gene fucO), an enzyme involved in the metabolism of fucose and which also seems to contain ferrous ion(s).

- *Clostridium acetobutylicum* NADPH- and NADH-dependent butanol dehydrogenases EC 1.1.1.- (genes adh1, bdhA and bdhB), enzymes that have activity using butanol and ethanol as substrates.

- *E. coli* adhE, an iron-dependent enzyme that harbours three different activities: alcohol dehydrogenase, acetaldehyde dehydrogenase (acetylating) EC 1.2.1.10 and pyruvate-formate-lyase deactivase.

- Bacterial glycerol dehydrogenase EC 1.1.1.6 (gene gldA or dhaD).

- *Clostridium kluyveri* NAD-dependent 4-hydroxybutyrate dehydrogenase (4hbd) EC 1.1.1.61

- *Citrobacter freundii* and *Klebsiella pneumoniae* 1,3-propanediol dehydrogenase EC 1.1.1.202 (gene dhaT)

- *Bacillus methanolicus* NAD-dependent methanol dehydrogenase EC 1.1.1.244

- *E. coli* and *Salmonella typhimurium* ethanolamine utilization protein eutG.

- *E. coli* hypothetical protein yiaY.

Other Types

A further class of alcohol dehydrogenases belongs to quinoenzymes and requires quinoid cofactors (e.g., pyrroloquinoline quinone, PQQ) as enzyme-bound electron acceptors. A typical example for this type of enzyme is methanol dehydrogenase of methylotrophic bacteria.

Applications

In biotransformation, alcohol dehydrogenases are often used for the synthesis of enantiomerically pure stereoisomers of chiral alcohols. Often, high chemo- and enantioselectivity can be achieved. One example is the alcohol dehydrogenase from *Lactobacillus brevis* (*Lb*ADH), which is described to be a versatile biocatalyst. The high chemospecificity has been confirmed also in the case of substrates presenting two potential redox sites. For instance cinnamaldehyde presents both aliphatic double bond and aldehyde function. Unlike conventional catalysts, alcohol dehydrogenases are able to selectively act only on the latter, yielding exclusively cinnamyl alcohol.

In fuel cells, alcohol dehydrogenases can be used to catalyze the breakdown of fuel for an ethanol fuel cell. Scientists at Saint Louis University have used carbon-supported alcohol dehydrogenase with poly(methylene green) as an anode, with a nafion membrane, to achieve about 50 $\mu A/cm^2$.

In 1949, E. Racker defined one unit of alcohol dehydrogenase activity as the amount that causes a change in optical density of 0.001 per minute under the standard conditions of assay. Recently, the international definition of enzymatic unit (E.U.) has been more common: one unit of Alcohol Dehydrogenase will convert 1.0 μmole of ethanol to acetaldehyde per minute at pH 8.8 at 25 °C.

Clinical Significance

Alcoholism

There have been studies showing that ADH may have an influence on the dependence on ethanol metabolism in alcoholics. Researchers have tentatively detected a few genes to be associated with alcoholism. If the variants of these genes encode slower metabolizing forms of ADH2 and ADH3, there is increased risk of alcoholism. The studies have found that mutations of ADH2 and ADH3 are related to alcoholism in Northeast Asian populations. However, research continues in order to identify the genes and their influence on alcoholism.

Drug Dependence

Drug dependence is another problem associated with ADH, which researchers think might be linked to alcoholism. One particular study suggests that drug dependence has seven ADH genes associated with it. These results may lead to treatments that target these specific genes. However, more research is necessary.

Poisoning

Fomepizole, a drug that inhibits alcohol dehydrogenase, can be used in the setting of acute methanol or ethylene glycol toxicity. This prevents the conversion of methanol to its toxic metabolites, formic acid and formaldehyde.

Cytochrome P450 Reductase

Cytochrome P450 reductase (EC 1.6.2.4; also known as NADPH:ferrihemoprotein oxidoreductase, NADPH:hemoprotein oxidoreductase, NADPH:P450 oxidoreductase, P450 reductase, POR, CPR, CYPOR) is a membrane-bound enzyme required for electron transfer from NADPH to cytochrome P450 in the endoplasmic reticulum of the eukaryotic cell.

Function

In *Bacillus megaterium* and *Bacillus subtilis*, POR is a C-terminal domain of CYP102, a single-polypeptide self-sufficient soluble P450 system (P450 is an N-terminal domain). The general scheme of electron flow in the POR/P450 system is:

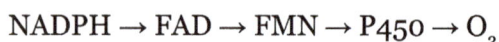

$$NADPH \rightarrow FAD \rightarrow FMN \rightarrow P450 \rightarrow O_2$$

The definitive evidence for the requirement of POR in cytochrome-P450-mediated reactions came from the work of Lu, Junk and Coon, who dissected the P450-containing mixed function oxidase system into three constituent components: POR, cytochrome P450, and lipids.

Since all microsomal P450 enzymes require POR for catalysis, it is expected that disruption of POR would have devastating consequences. POR knockout mice are embryonic lethal, probably due to lack of electron transport to extrahepatic P450 enzymes since liver-specific knockout of POR yields phenotypically and reproductively normal mice that accumulate hepatic lipids and have remarkably diminished capacity of hepatic drug metabolism.

The reduction of cytochrome P450 is not the only physiological function of POR. The final step of heme oxidation by mammalian heme oxygenase requires POR and O_2. In yeast, POR affects the ferrireductase activity, probably transferring electrons to the flavocytochrome ferric reductase.

Gene Organization

Human POR gene has 16 exons and the exons 2-16 code for a 677-amino acid POR protein (NCBI NP_000932.2). There is a single copy of 50 kb POR gene (NCBI NM_000941.2) in humans on chromosome 7 (7q11.23).

Mutations and Polymorphisms

Five missense mutations (A287P, R457H, V492E, C569Y, and V608F) and a splicing mutation in the POR genes have been found in patients who had hormonal evidence for combined deficiencies of two steroidogenic cytochrome P450 enzymes - P450c17 CYP17A1, which catalyzes steroid

17α-hydroxylation and 17,20 lyase reaction, and P450c21 21-Hydroxylase, which catalyzes steroid 21-hydroxylation. Another POR missense mutation Y181D has also been identified. Fifteen of nineteen patients having abnormal genitalia and disordered steroidogenesis were homozygous or apparent compound heterozygous for POR mutations that destroyed or dramatically inhibited POR activity.

More than 200 variations in POR gene have been identified.

POR Deficiency – Mixed Oxidase Disease

POR deficiency is the newest form of congenital adrenal hyperplasia first described in 2004. The index patient was a newborn 46,XX Japanese girl with craniosynostosis, hypertelorism, mid-face hypoplasia, radiohumeral synostosis, arachnodactyly and disordered steroidogenesis. However, the clinical and biochemical characteristics of patients with POR deficiency are long known in the literature as so-called mixed oxidase disease, as POR deficiency typically shows a steroid profile that suggests combined deficiencies of steroid 21-hydroxylase and 17α-hydroxylase/17,20 lyase activities. The clinical spectrum of POR deficiency ranges from severely affected children with ambiguous genitalia, adrenal insufficiency, and the Antley-Bixler skeletal malformation syndrome (ABS) to mildly affected individuals with polycystic ovary syndrome-like features. Some of the POR patients were born to mothers who became virilized during pregnancy, suggesting deficient placental aromatization of fetal androgens due to a lesion in microsomal aromatase resulting in low estrogen production, which was later confirmed by lower aromatase activities caused by POR mutations. However, it has also been suggested that fetal and maternal virilization in POR deficiency might be caused by increased dihydrotestosterone synthesis by the fetal gonad through an alternative "backdoor" pathway first described in the marsupials and later confirmed in humans . Gas chromatography/mass spectrometry analysis of urinary steroids from pregnant women carrying a POR-deficient fetus described in an earlier report also supports the existence of this pathway, and the relevance of the "backdoor" pathway along with POR dependent steroidogenesis have become clearer from recent studies. The role of POR mutations beyond CAH are being investigated; and questions such as how POR mutations cause bony abnormalities and what role POR variants play in drug metabolism by hepatic P450s are being addressed in recent publications. However, reports of ABS in some offsprings of mothers who were treated with fluconazole, an antifungal agent which interferes with cholesterol biosynthesis at the level of CYP51 activity - indicate that disordered drug metabolism may result from deficient POR activity.

Williams Syndrome

Williams syndrome is a genetic disorder characterized by the deletion of genetic material approximately 1.2 Mb from the POR gene (POR). Cells with this genetic deletion show reduced transcription of POR, it seems, due to the loss of a cis-regulatory element that alters expression of this gene. Some persons with Williams syndrome show characteristics of POR deficiency, including radio-ulnar synostosis and other skeletal abnormalities. Cases of mild impairment of cortisol and androgen synthesis have been noted, however, despite the fact that deficient POR impairs androgen synthesis, patients with Williams syndrome often show increased androgen levels. A similar increase in testosterone has been observed in a mouse model that has globally decreased POR expression.

Structure

The 3D crystal structure of human POR has been determined. The molecule is composed of four structural domains: the FMN-binding domain, the connecting domain, the FAD-binding domain, and NADPH-binding domain. The FMN-binding domain is similar to the structure of FMN-containing protein flavodoxin, whereas the FAD-binding domain and NADPH-binding domains are similar to those of flavoprotein ferredoxin-NADP$^+$ reductase (FNR). The connecting domain is situated between the flavodoxin-like and FNR-like domains.

POR Homologs

The other enzymes containing homologs of POR are nitric oxide synthase (EC 1.14.13.39), NADPH:sulfite reductase (EC 1.8.1.2), and methionine synthase reductase (EC 1.16.1.8).

Epoxide Hydrolase

Epoxide hydrolases (EH's), also known as epoxide hydratases, are enzymes that metabolize compounds that contain an epoxide residue; they convert this residue to two hydroxyl residues through a dihydroxylation reaction to form diol products. Several enzymes possess EH activity. Microsomal epoxide hydrolase (epoxide hydrolase 1, EH1, or mEH), soluble epoxide hydrolase (sEH, epoxide hydrolase 2, EH2, or cytoplasmic epoxide hydrolase), and the more recently discovered but not as yet well defined functionally, epoxide hydrolase 3 (EH3) and epoxide hydrolase 4 (EH4) are structurally closely related isozymes. Other enzymes with epoxide hydrolase activity include leukotriene A4 hydrolase, Cholesterol-5,6-oxide hydrolase, MEST (gene) (Peg1/MEST), and Hepoxilin-epoxide hydrolase. The hydrolases are distinguished from each other by their substrate preferences and, directly related to this, their functions.

Epoxide Hydrolase Types

mEH (EH1), sEH (EH2), EH3, and EH4 isozymes

Humans express four epoxide hydrolase isozymes: mEH, sEH, EH3, and EH4. These isozymes are known (mEH and sEH) or presumed (EH3 and EH4) to share a common structure that includes containing an Alpha/beta hydrolase fold and a common reaction mechanism wherein they add water to epoxides to form vicinal cis (see (cis-trans isomerism); see (epoxide#Olefin oxidation using organic peroxides and metal catalysts)) diol products. They differ, however, in subcellular location, substrate preferences, tissue expression, and/or function.

mEH

mEH is widely expressed in virtually all mammalian cells as an endoplasmic reticulum-bound (i.e. microsomal-bound) enzyme with its C terminal catalytic domain facing the cytoplasm; in some tissues, however, mEH has been found bound to the cell surface plasma membrane with its catalytic domain facing the extracellular space. The primary function of mEH is to convert potentially toxic xenobiotics and other compounds that possess epoxide residues (which is often due to their initial metabolism by cytochrome P450 enzymes to epoxides) to diols. Epoxides are highly reactive electrophilic compounds that form adducts with DNA and proteins and also cause strand breaks in DHA; in consequence, epoxides can cause gene mutations, cancer, and the inactivation of critical proteins. The diols thereby formed are usually not toxic or far less toxic than their epoxide predecessors, are readily further metabolized, and ultimately excreted in the urine. mEH also metabolizes certain epoxides of polyunsaturated fatty acids such as the epoxyeicosatrienoic acids (EETs) but its activity in doing this is far less than that of sEH; mEH therefore may play a minor role, compared to sEH, in limiting the bioactivity of these cell signaling compounds (see microsomal epoxide hydrolase).

sEH

sEH is widely expressed in mammalian cells as a cytosolic enzyme where it primarily serves the function of converting epoxyeicosatrienoic acids (EETs), epoxyeicosatetraenoic acids (EPAs), and epoxydocosapentaenoic acids (DPAs) to there corresponding diols, thereby limiting or ending their cell signaling actions; in this capacity, sEH appears to play a critical in vivo role in limiting the effects of these epoxides in animal models and possibly humans. However, sEH also metabolizes the epoxides of linoleic acid viz., Vernolic acid (leukotoxins) and Coronaric acids (isoleukotoxins) to there corresponding diols which are highly toxic in animal models and possibly humans (see Vernolic acid#toxicity, Coronaric acid#toxicity, and soluble epoxide hydrolase). sEH also possesses hepoxilin-epoxide hydrolase activity, converting bioactive hepoxilins to their inactive trioxilin products (see below section "Hepoxilin-epoxide hydrolase").

EH3

Human EH3 is a recently characterized protein with epoxy hydrolase activity for metabolizing epoxyeicosatrienoic acids (EETs) and vernolic acids (leukotoxins) to their corresponding diols; in these capacities they may thereby limit the cell signaling activity of the EETs and contribute to the toxicity of the leukotoxins. mRNA for EH3 is most strongly expressed in the lung, skin, and upper gastrointestinal tract tissues of mice. The function of EH3 in humans, mice, or other mammals has not yet been determined although the gene for EH3 has been validated as being hypermethylated on CpG sites in its promoter region in human prostate cancer tissue, particularly in the tissues of more advanced or morphologically-based (i.e. Gleason score) more aggressive cancers; this suggests that the gene silencing of EH3 due to this hypermethylation may contribute to the onset and/or progression of prostate cancer. Similar CpG site hypermethylations in the promoter of for the EH3 gene have been validated for other cancers. This promoter methylation pattern, although not yet validated, was also found in human malignant melanoma.

EH4

The gene for EH4, EPHX4, is projected to encode an epoxide hydrolase closely related in amino acid sequence and structure to mEH, sEH, and EH3. The activity and function of EH4 has not yet been defined.

Other Epoxy Hydrolases

Leukotriene A4 Hydrolase

Leukotriene A4 hydrolase (LTA4H) acts primarily, if not exclusively, to hydrolyze leukotriene A4 (LTA4, i.e. 5S,6S-oxido-7E,9E,11Z,14Z-eicosatetraenoic acid; IUPAC name 4-{(2S,3S)-3-[(1E,3E,5Z,8Z)-1,3,5,8-Tetradecatetraen-1-yl]-2-oxiranyl}butanoic acid) to its diol metabolite, leukotriene B4 (LTB4, i.e. 5S,12R-dihydroxy-6Z,8E,10E,14Z-icosatetraenoic acid; IUPA name 5S,6Z,8E,10E,12R,14Z)-5,12-Dihydroxy-6,8,10,14-icosatetraenoic acid). LTB4 is an important recruiter and activator of leukocytes involved in mediation in inflammatory responses and diseases. The enzyme also possess aminopeptidase activity, degrading, for example, the leukocyte chemotactic factor tripeptide, Pro-Gly-Pro (PGP); the function of the aminopeptidase activity of LTA4AH is unknown but has been proposed to be involved in limiting inflammatory reactions caused by this or other aminopeptidase-susceptible peptides.

Cholesterol-5,6-oxide Hydrolase

(Cholesterol epoxide hydrolase or ChEH), is located in the endoplasmic reticulum and to a lesser extent plasma membrane of various cell types but most highly express in liver. The enzyme catalyzes the conversion of certain 3-hydoxyl-5,6-epoxides of cholesterol to their 3,5,6-trihydroxy products (see Cholesterol-5,6-oxide hydrolase). The function of ChEH is unknown.

Peg1/MEST

The substrate(s) and physiological function of Peg1/MEST are not known; however, the protein may play a role in mammalian development and abnormalities in its expression by its gene (PEG1/MEST)by, for example, loss of Genomic imprinting, overexpression, or promoter switching, has been linked to certain types of cancer and tumors in humans such as invasive cervical cancer, uterine leiomyomas, and cancers of the breast, lung, and colon.

Hepoxilin-epoxide Hydrolase

Hepoxilin-epoxide hydrolase or hepoxilin hydrolase is currently best defined as an enzyme activity that converts the biologically active monohydroxy-epoxide metabolites of arachidonic acid hepoxilin A3s and hepoxilin B3s to essentially inactive trihydroxy products, the trioxilins. That is, hepoxilin A3s (8-hydroxy-11,12-oxido-5Z,9E,14Z-eicosatrienoic acid) are metabolized to trioxilin A3s (8,11,12-trihydroxy-5Z,9E,14Z-eicosatrienoic acids) and hepoxilins B3s (10-hydroxy-11,12-oxido-5Z,8Z,14Z-eicosatrienoic acids) are metabolized to trioxilin B3s (10,11,12-trihydroxy-5Z,8Z,14Z-eicosatrienoic acids). However, this activity has not been characterized at the purified protein or gene level and recent work indicate that sEH readily metabolizes an hepoxilin A3 to a trioxilin A3 and that hepoxilin-epoxide hydrolase activity is due to sEH, at least as it is detected in mouse liver.

Mycobacterium Tuberculosis

This causative agent of tuberculosis expresses at least six different forms of epoxide hydrolase (forms A-F). The structure of epoxide hydrolase B reveals that the enzyme is a monomer and contains an alpha/beta hydrolase fold. In addition to providing insights into the enzyme mechanism, this hydrolase currently serves as a platform for rational drug design of potent inhibitors. In particular, urea based inhibitors have been developed. These inhibitors directly target the catalytic cavity. It is hypothesized that the structure of epoxide hydrolase B may allow for drug design to inhibit all other Mycobacterium tuberculosis hydrolases as long as they contain similar alpha/beta folds. The structure of hydrolase B contains a cap domain, which is hypothesized to regulate the active site of the hydrolase. Furthermore, Asp104, His333, and Asp302 form the catalytic triad of the protein and is critical to function of the protein. At present, other structures of Mycobacterium tuberculosis hydrolase have not been solved. Model studies on pharmacological susceptibility of these epoxide hydrolases continue.

References

- *Irwin H. Segel, Enzyme Kinetics : Behavior and Analysis of Rapid Equilibrium and Steady-State Enzyme Systems. Wiley–Interscience; New edition (1993), ISBN 0-471-30309-7

- Walsh, Ryan (2012). "Ch. 17. Alternative Perspectives of Enzyme Kinetic Modeling". In Ekinci, Deniz. Medicinal Chemistry and Drug Design (PDF). InTech. pp. 357–371. ISBN 978-953-51-0513-8.

- Segel, Irwin H. (1993) Enzyme Kinetics : Behavior and Analysis of Rapid Equilibrium and Steady-State Enzyme Systems. Wiley-Interscience; New edition , ISBN 0-471-30309-7.

- Cohen, J.A.; Oosterbaan, R.A.; Berends, F. (1967). "[81] Organophosphorus compounds". Enzyme Structure. Methods in Enzymology. 11. p. 686. doi:10.1016/S0076-6879(67)11085-9. ISBN 978-0-12-181860-9.

- Price, Nicholas and Stevens, Lewis (1999) Fundamentals of Enzymology, Oxford University Press, ISBN 0-19-850229-X.

- Bisswanger, Hans (2008). Enzyme Kinetics: Principles and Methods (PDF). Weinheim: Wiley-VCH. p. 302. ISBN 978-3-527-31957-2.

- Zorea, Aharon (2014). Steroids (Health and Medical Issues Today). Westport, CT: Greenwood Press. p. 10. ISBN 978-1440802997.

- Marieb, Elaine N., Hoehn, Katja N. (2009). Essentials of Human Anatomy & Physiology (9th ed.). San Francisco, CA: Pearson/Benjamin Cummings. ISBN 0321513428.

- Tortora, Gerard J.; Anagnostakos, Nicholas P. (1987). Principles of Anatomy and Physiology (Fifth ed.). New York: Harper & Row, Publishers. pp. 657–658. ISBN 0-06-350729-3.

- Swedan, Nadya Gabriele (2001). Women's Sports Medicine and Rehabilitation. Lippincott Williams & Wilkins. p. 149. ISBN 0-8342-1731-7.

- Weschler, Toni (2002). Taking Charge of Your Fertility. New York: HarperCollins. pp. 52, 316, 361–362. ISBN 0-06-093764-5.

- Kluge, Matthew J. (2015). Fever: Its Biology, Evolution, and Function. Princeton University Press. p. 57. ISBN 9781400869831.

- Garmel, Gus M. (2012). "Fever in adults". In Mahadevan, S.V.; Garmel, Gus M. An introduction to clinical emergency medicine (2nd ed.). Cambridge: Cambridge University Press. p. 375. ISBN 0521747767.

Permissions

Index

www.ingramcontent.com/pod-product-compliance
Lightning Source LLC
Chambersburg PA
CBHW061318190326
41458CB00011B/3832